Stereotactic and Functional Neurosurgery

Advances in Stereoencephalotomy

Vol. 10

Editor:
Philip L. Gildenberg, Houston, Tex.

KARGER

Basel · München · Paris · London · New York · New Delhi · Singapore · Tokyo · Sydney

Proceedings of the
Ninth Meeting of the World Society for

Stereotactic and Functional Neurosurgery

Toronto, Ont., July 4–7, 1985

Editors:
R.R. Tasker, Toronto, Ont.;
I.M. Turnbull, Vancouver, B.C.;
Ph.L. Gildenberg, Houston, Tex.;
P.O. Franklin, Houston, Tex.

133 figures, 68 tables, 1986

KARGER

Basel · München · Paris · London · New York · New Delhi · Singapore · Tokyo · Sydney

Reprint from Applied Neurophysiology, Vol. 48, No. 1–6 (1985)

Advances in Stereoencephalotomy

Vol. 1–6: Please ask for details.
Vol. 7: Sixth Symposium of the International Society for Research in Stereoencephalotomy, Tokyo, October 12–13, 1973 (Reprint from Confinia Neurologica, Vol. 36, No. 4–6 and Vol. 37, No. 1–3).
Vol. 8: Seventh Symposium of the International Society for Research in Stereoencephalotomy, São Paulo, June 24, 1977 (Reprint from Applied Neurophysiology, Vol. 41, No. 1–4).
Vol. 9: Eighth Symposium of the World Society and the Fifth Symposium of the European Society for Stereotactic and Functional Neurosurgery, Zurich, July 9–11, 1981 (Reprint from Applied Neurophysiology, Vol. 45, No. 1–2, No. 3, No. 4–5).

Drug Dosage
The authors and the publisher have exerted every effort to ensure that drug selection and dosage set forth in this text are in accord with current recommendations and practice at the time of publication. However, in view of ongoing research, changes in government regulations, and the constant flow of information relating to drug therapy and drug reactions, the reader is urged to check the package insert for each drug for any change in indications and dosage and for added warnings and precautions. This is particularly important when the recommended agent is a new and/or infrequently employed drug.

Printed in Switzerland by Basler Zeitung, Basel
ISBN 3-8055-4401-4

Contents

Session IX: CT-Stereotaxis for Tumors

Remarks

Session I: Technical Advances

Proc. 9th Meeting World Soc. Stereotactic and Functional
Neurosurgery, Toronto 1985
Appl. Neurophysiol. *48:* 1-6 (1985)

Present and Future Developments of Stereotactic Technology

Patrick J. Kelly, Bruce A. Kall, Stephan Goerss, Franklin Earnest
Mayo Clinic, Rochester, Minn., USA

Key Words. Stereotactic techniques · Biopsy · Laser · Brain

Abstract. Incorporation of a surgical computer system into stereotactic methodology provides the facility for efficient utilization of the multiple data bases at the disposal of the modern stereotactician. Computed tomography, magnetic resonance imaging, and digital fluoroscopy data gathered in stereotactic conditions are digitized into a stereotactic surgical matrix for surgical planning and interactive surgical procedures. The advantages of this system are illustrated in stereotactic biopsy, interstitial irradiation, and laser resections of intracranial tumors.

Introduction

Stereotactic surgery has experienced a renaissance, primarily due to the incorporation of new imaging technologies into stereotactic techniques. Old procedures have been modified and others developed to exploit the new possibilities provided by computed tomography (CT), magnetic resonance imaging (MRI), and digital fluoroscopy (DF). New instrumentation has been developed to utilize new data bases in a more efficient manner and allow a performance of new procedures with greater efficiency and accuracy than ever before possible [3]. However, it is the operating room computer system which will provide the necessary substrate for technological advancement in stereotactic methodology. At present, the surgical computer system is used for data acquisition, surgical planning, and interactive data manipulation and calculations during the surgical procedure as described below.

Data Base Acquisition

Information from preoperatively gathered CT, MRI, and DF examinations performed under stereotactic conditions may be effectively stored in an operating room computer system and reformatted and displayed to the surgeon in a useful manner. In our system, patients undergo CT, MRI, and DF examinations with their heads fixed in a CT/MRI compatible stereotactic headframe which is fixed to the skull by carbon fiber pins inserted into the diploe [1, 7]. Detachable micrometers provide reference numbers which allow replacement of the stereotactic headholder if the data base acquisition and definitive surgical procedure are to be performed on separate days.

Fiducial localization systems which attach to the headholder create reference artifacts on each CT, MRI, and DF image which allows the translation of imaging data into the stereotactic coordinate system [1, 2, 5, 9].

The archived data tapes from CT, MRI, and DF examinations are input into the operating room computer system (Independent Physicians Diagnostic Console [IPDC] for General Electric 8800 CT Scanning Unit).

Utilization and Surgical Planning

CT, MRI, and DF images are displayed on a display console in the operating room or treatment planning area. Utilizing the system cursor and trackball, the surgeon inputs a point displayed from CT and/or MRI slices or DF images into a three-dimensional computer matrix. In addition, a volume may be interpolated from a series of digitized outlines on CT or MRI images [6, 8, 9]. Points selected from CT or MRI images may be displayed on lateral or AP arterial or venous phase images from digital angiography [5]. Lastly, functional procedures can be aided by a computer resident stereotactic atlas which may be overlayed on reformatted CT slices. Substructures of interest may then be digitized and the stereotactic coordinates easily calculated.

Applications

Intracranial Tumors

There are now more options than ever before for patients harboring deep-seated, intracranial, or intra-axial neoplasms. These include stereotactic biopsy, interstitial irradiation, and computer-assisted stereotactic laser resection.

Stereotactic Biopsy

A computer can easily calculate target points from stereotactic CT or MRI images and translate these to mechanical adjustments on stereotactic instruments. In our system, the surgeon simply positions a cursor over a point within the lesion on a displayed CT slice, and the point is then suspended within a three-dimensional computer matrix corresponding to the stereotactic coordinate system. In addition, entry and target points can be displayed on stereotactic DF images so that a safe avascular trajectory may be selected and viewed on sequential CT or MRI slices [5, 7].

Therapeutic Interventions

Although biopsy procedures require the calculation of single points in stereotactic space, accurate surgical planning for therapeutic procedures requires volumetric interpolation. In addition, volumes for both CT and MRI defined limits are interpolated with the three-dimensional computer image matrix [8]. The spatial histology defined by stereotactic serial biopsies performed at a separate reference procedure is used to define whether the CT or MRI defined limits of the tumor are to be used.

Interstitial Irradiation

Ideally, the isodose envelope generated by stereotactically implanted interstitial radionuclide sources should conform to the three-dimensional shape of the tumor. Placement of these sources may be simulated on the operating room computer for ideal source placements within the neoplasm such that a maximum amount of radiation is delivered to the tumor while minimal radiation exposure is delivered to the surrounding brain. In the simulation program, the computer slices the three-dimensional tumor volume along the implantation angles (stereotactic frame settings) and displays these slices on a video monitor display system. Using the cursor and trackball subsystems and deposit key, the surgeon simulates radionuclide source placements within sequential slices of the tumor. The computer then calculates and displays the aggregate isodoses for each slice. Superficial and deep slices may be displayed with the sources arranged to best fit the slice. Following simulation, the computer calculates the length of each source and the stereotactic frame settings for their placements. At our institution, we utilize temporary sources of iridium-192 employing a double catheter afterloading technique. The custom arc-quadrant, computer interactive and servomotor-controlled stereotactic frame, which is described in the next section, facilitates the placement of the afterloading system.

Computer-Assisted Stereotactic Laser Surgery

CT or MRI defined tumor volumes represented in stereotactic space can be resected with precision utilizing a computer-controlled, computer-monitored stereotactic CO_2 laser system as described below.

Instrumentation

A new stereotactic frame utilizing a three-dimensional servomotor-controlled slide system positions the patient's head in a fixed arc-quadrant [2]. A digital readout provided by optical encoders displays the stereotactic positions. A control panel is utilized for convenient activation of the servomotors and for the rapid productions of stereotactic coordinates. A 400-mm double gimballed arc system is attached to the stereotactic frame. An operating microscope and CO_2 laser manipulator system are directed toward the focal point of the stereotactic arc-quadrant. The CO_2 laser beam is directed from the stereotactic arc-quadrant by mirrors whose pitch is regulated by X and Y galvanometers. The axes rotation of the galvanometers are controlled by the digital to analog (D–A) output of the computer. The computer controls the laser beam by a preset computer program or by manual input from the surgeon manipulating a joystick which relays the intended position of the laser to the computer by means of optical encoders.

In either case, the computer displays the position of the laser as a cursor against slices of the tumor which are sliced perpendicular to the surgical viewline at the level at which the microscope and laser are focused [2, 6].

Deep-seated tumors are approached through the linear scalp incision, a 1½- to 2-inch trephine and incision through the subcortial white matter directed through nonessential brain tissue in a direction parallel to major white matter fibers. A stereotactically directed retractor maintains exposure. Tumors are vaporized slice by slice from the most superficial layer to the deepest. The position of the CO_2 laser and stereotactic retractor are displayed on an operating-room computer in relationship to slices of the tumor cut from MRI or CT defined tumor volumes. The computer also displays the position of the stereotactic retractor with respect to the tumor slice. These computer reconstructions of the surgical anatomy may be displayed in the microscope and upon the operative field by a recently developed 'heads up' display unit.

With this method, it is possible to resect all of a subcortical intracranial lesion defined by preoperative CT and/or MRI data bases. Significant reductions of the tumor burden in primary or metastatic lesions are possible in all subcortical and some brainstem locations. One hundred and twelve of these procedures have now been performed with acceptable postoperative results. In addition, this method has also been successfully employed for the selective stereotactic resection of abnormal CT or MRI defined cortical areas in the treatment of focal epilepsy and for deep-seated vascular malformations.

Conclusions

Computer-assisted stereotactic procedures continue to find new applications which will ultimately expand to all intra-axial intracranial procedures [3]. The precision, accuracy, and convenience provided by new instrumentation will render conventional free-hand techniques for the management of many lesions obsolete as more surgeons become 'stereotacticians'. Present and future advances in electronics, ultrasound, laser, computer, and robotics technologies can be interfaced to stereotactic instrumentation. These will continue to have great impact on the future development of stereotactic methodology.

References

1 Goerss, S.; Kelly, P.J.; Kall, B.; Alker, G.J., Jr.: A computed stereotactic adaptation system. Neurosurgery *10:0* 375–379 (1982).

2 Kall, B.A.; Kelly, P.J.; Goerss, S.: Interactive stereotactic surgical system for the removal of intracranial tumors utilizing the CO_2 laser and CT-derived data base. IEEE Trans. biomed. Enging *32:* 112–116 (1985).

3 Kelly, P.J.: Special article: Future possibilities in stereotactic neurosurgery. Surg. Neurol. *19:* 4–9 (1983).

4 Kelly, P.J.; Alker, G.J., Jr.: A stereotactic approach to deep-seated CNS neoplasms using the carbon dioxide laser. Surg. Neurol. *15:* 331–334 (1981).

5 Kelly, P.J.; Earnest, F.; Kall, B.A.; Goerss, S.J.; Scheithauer, B.: Surgical options for patients with deep-seated brain tumors: computer-assisted stereotactic biopsy. Mayo Clin. Proc. *6:* 223–229 (1985).

6 Kelly, P.J.; Kall, B.; Goerss, S.; Alker, G.J.: Precision resection of intra-axial CNS lesions by CT-based stereotactic craniotomy and computer monitored CO_2 laser. Acta neurochir. *68:* 1–9 (1983).

7 Kelly, P.J.; Kall, B.; Goerss, S.; Alker, G.J.: A method of CT-based stereotactic biopsy with arteriographic control. Neurosurgery *14:* 172–177 (1984).

8 Kelly, P.J.; Kall, B.; Goerss, S.: Transposition of volumetric information derived from CT scanning in stereotactic space. Surg. Neurol. *21:* 465–471 (1984).

9 Kelly, P.J.; Kall, B.A.; Goerss, S.: Computer simulation for the stereotactic placement of interstitial radionuclide sources into CT defined tumor volumes. Technical note. Neurosurgery *14:* 442–448 (1984).

Patrick J. Kelly, MD, Mayo Clinic, 200 S.W. First Street,
Rochester, MN 55905 (USA)

Proc. 9th Meeting World Soc. Stereotactic and Functional
Neurosurgery, Toronto 1985
Appl. Neurophysiol. *48:* 7–10 (1985)

Real-Time Three-Dimensional Graphic Reconstructions Using Brown-Roberts-Wells Frame Coordinates in a Microcomputer Environment

M. Peter Heilbrun, Russell A. Brown, Paul R. McDonald

Division of Neurosurgery, University of Utah Medical Center,
Salt Lake City, Utah, USA

Key Words. Computer tomography · Computer graphics · Stereotactic surgery

Abstract. A desktop microcomputer environment that utilizes Brown-Roberts-Wells (BRW) frame coordinates for creation of three-dimensional depiction of operator-defined intracranial structures has been developed. The system allows direct reading of Siemens CT scan images from a floppy disc, structural edge definition, and reconstruction of defined images. The system is used in the operating room to view scans, perform standard BRW stereotactic functions, and create three-dimensional graphics for such tasks as defining tumor margins, conceptualizing positional relationships of intracranial structures, and radiation planning.

Introduction

CT-guided stereotaxy is rapidly evolving into a standard neurosurgical tool for localization of intracranial structures and lesions. This evolution has been furthered by the design of stereotactic guidance systems, such as the Brown-Roberts-Wells (BRW) system, which efficiently transform two-dimensional image coordinates into three-dimensional stereotactic frame coordinates utilizing programmable calculators and portable microcomputers. In addition, the unique design of arc systems such as the BRW arc allows easy access to surface as well as deep structures [1].

Kelly et al. [2] have demonstrated the value of sophisticated three-dimensional graphics to enhance the ability of the neurosurgical operator to conceptualize both approaches to and configurations of intracranial structures.

Results

A microcomputer environment has been developed to display CT image data files utilizing BRW stereotactic frame coordinates to create three-dimensional outlines of intracranial structures. The hardware for this portable, relatively inexpensive microcomputer system includes a DEC VT103 based on the PDP 11/23 system, combined with the following peripherals: a dual 8-inch floppy disc drive and hard disc, a Peritek graphics processor and color monitor, and a Hawley mouse system. The latter allows the operator to move the computer cursor freely to mark specific points on a scan, to draw outlines on the scans, and to send specific commands to the computer. An inexpensive computer console instant camera system provides hard copy of the annotated images.

The Siemens company provided the appropriate software subroutines to read data stored on floppy discs, which made it possible to hand carry all of the CT scan data to the operating room for display. Subroutines were written to display images and adjust windows. The stereotactic routines for transformation of the two-dimensional CT scan data to three-dimensional BRW frame coordinates originally written by one of the authors *(R.A.B.)* were added. The display was formatted so that the entry point, azimuth and declination entries, calculated target point, and frame settings and probe distances were all displayed on the color monitor. With this software all of the necessary functions to utilize the BRW stereotactic guidance system without either the HP 41CV calculator or the Epson HX-20 microcomputer were present.

The system provides three-dimensional graphics which depict relative positions of intracranial structures. The initial step utilizes the mouse so that the operator can trace on the screen the outline of various structures such as tumor borders, ventricular systems, or major blood vessels. We found that with minimal practice an operator can rapidly trace out the required outlines in several scan slices.

Once each tracing is completed, each point or pixel in the tracing is transformed and saved in a data file as a BRW frame coordinate. The traces that are drawn on different scan slices can be selected and redisplayed on the same monitor in three-dimensional perspective. Each pixel in the three-dimensional display represents a specific BRW frame coordinate. This allows the operator to move a cursor to a specific point on the three-dimensional display to automatically define a BRW coordinate, a process which can be used for both solid modeling and establishing targets on the BRW phantom. The three-dimensional display can be rotated and transformed around the x, y, and z axes. Because of the limits of our computer memory, the rotations and transformations could be done at a satisfactory speed but not yet in real time. For this reason, we divided the computer console into four screens to view simultaneously the outlines in the following four configurations: (1) transaxially in the same plane as the CT scan; (2) rotated 15° off of the x axis; (3) rotated 15° off of the y axis, and (4) rotated to look down an operator defined probe track.

Utilizing this latter configuration of four simultaneous static displays in specified positions gives a comparative perspective which we found more useful than continuous rotation of outlines.

The graphic program is also utilized to enhance planning for interstitial radiation seed placement. We analyzed our means of determining probe tracks for seed placement and decided that, in mathematical terms, the simplest approach would be to define a central probe track which can be surrounded with parallel tracks. Once this central operator defined probe track is established, then the stored outline data points which are saved from scan slices are integrated to create new outlines configured orthogonally to the probe track. These orthogonal slices are created at 5- or 10-mm intervals through the tumor, placed in separate windows, and superimposed with a 10-mm spaced grid. Intersecting grid points can be chosen by the operator with the mouse cursor for seed placement. Different seed placement pattern configurations can be overlaid with isodose curves following which the dosages can be integrated to define a combined isodose curve related to the orthogonally defined tumor border. Optimal parallel probe tracks can be defined to hold the appropriate seeds efficiently.The afterloading catheters can then be easily placed utilizing the Wright grid adaptation to the BRW arc. We have found that the integration of the isodose curves outstrips the capabilities of our present computer and will require communication with a larger computer or use of a 32-bit microcomputer.

Manufacturers

Siemens Medical Systems Inc., 186 Wood Avenue South, Iselin, NJ 08830, USA; Digital Equipment Corp. 129 Main Street, Maynard, MA 01754, USA; Hewlett-Packard, 1000 Northeast Circle Boulevard, Corvallis, OR 97330, USA; Peritek Corp., 5550 Redwood Road, Oakland, CA 94619, USA; The Mouse House, A Division of Hawley Laboratories, 1741 8th Street, Berkeley, CA 94710, USA; Epson America, Inc., PO Box 2854, Torrance, CA 90509, USA; M.P. Heilbrun, MD, Division of Neurosurgery, University of Utah Medical Center, 50 North Medical Drive, Salt Lake City, UT 84132 (USA).

References

1 Heilbrun, M.P.; Roberts, T.S.; Apuzzo, M.L.J.; Wells, T.H.; Sabshin, J.K.: Preliminary experience with Brown-Roberts-Wells (BRW) computerized tomography stereotaxic guidance system. J. Neurosurg. *59:* 217–222 (1983).
2 Kelly, P.J.; Kall, B.; Goerss, S.: Preoperative computer determination of interstitial iridium-192 source placement into CNS tumor volumes. Acta neurochir. *33:* suppl., pp. 377–383 (1984).

M.P. Heilbrun, MD, Division of Neurosurgery,
University of Utah Medical Center,
50 North Medical Drive, Salt Lake City, Utah 84132 (USA)

Proc. 9th Meeting World Soc. Stereotactic and Functional
Neurosurgery, Toronto 1985
Appl. Neurophysiol. *48:* 11–17 (1985)

New CT-Guided Stereotactic Apparatus and Clinical Experience with Intracerebral Hematomas

Yoshio Tanizaki, Kenichiro Sugita, Toshihide Toriyama, Masanobu Hokama

Department of Neurosurgery, Kakeyu Hospital, Maruko, Tiisagata, Nagano, and Department of Neurosurgery, School of Medicine, Shinshu University, Matsumoto, Japan

Key Words. Computerized tomography · Stereotactic surgery · Intracerebral hematoma · CT stereotaxis

Abstract. The conventional Sugita stereotactic frame has been improved to perform CT-guided stereotactic surgery both in the CT and operating rooms. The development of our instrument and the software of the scanners' computer are presented. Newly designed equipment produced almost no artifacts on the CT image. Using the improved stereotactic frame, we have operated upon 44 intracerebral hematomas in the CT room. More than 80% of the cases had satisfactory results. Two complications were encountered, and 1 patient died from pneumonia. Our initial experience of the pre- and postoperative cerebral blood flow measurement with ^{133}Xe inhalation method and single photon emission CT is described.

Introduction

Different types of stereotactic systems have been developed to accurately probe deep-seated brain lesions [2, 4]. In order to perform the CT-guided stereotactic surgery both in CT and operating rooms, we have improved the conventional Sugita stereotactic frame [5].

Improvements of the Stereotactic Frame

We have improved the following points: (1) An adaptor was made to fix the stereotactic frame to the CT table and adjust the angle between the frame and table (fig. 1). (2) Carbon fiber and alumina-ce-

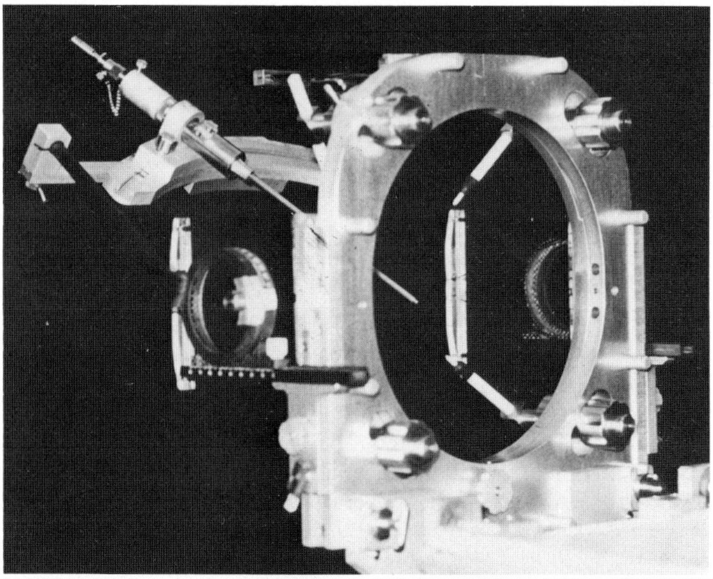
a

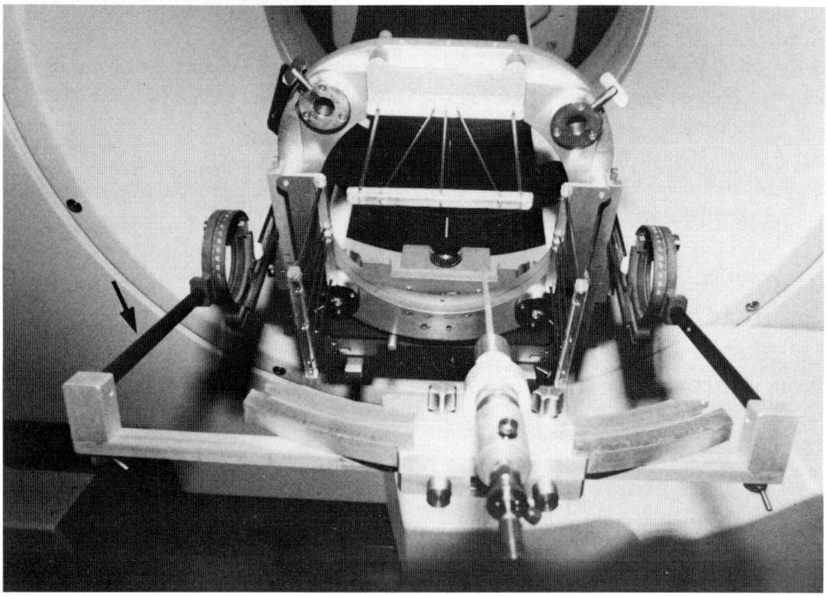
b

Fig. 1. a, b Our new CT-guided stereotactic frame fixed to CT table.

Table I. Intracerebral hematomas

Hematoma removal:	total 44 cases
Sex:	26 males, 18 females
Age:	35–81 years (mean 59.1)
Location:	putamen Hx 27 cases
	thalamus Hx 13 cases
	subcortical Hx 4 cases
Timing:	4–82 days (mean 19.7)
Complications:	2 cases
Died:	1 case

Table II. Cerebral blood flow measurements

CBF measurements	
^{133}Xe inhalation and single photon emission CT	10 cases
Sex:	6 males, 4 females
Age:	48–73 years (mean 56.2)
Location:	putamen Hx 11 cases
Timing:	11–82 days (mean 21.9)

ramic pins were made for fixation of the patient's head (fig. 2a). (3) A Z-axis marker and needle-holding frame (fig. 1) were made of carbon fiber and metal. (4) Two types of needles for hematoma evacuation were designed, one made of teflon and the other an Archimedes' water-screw type needle. The tip of the screw was made of alumina-ceramic (fig. 2b). New software was developed for the scanner computer (Toshiba Medical Systems) to calculate values of the target point and confirm the position of the needle within the lesion (fig. 2c).

Clinical Experience of Intracerebral Hematomas

We have operated on 44 intracerebral hematomas with the improved stereotactic frame (table I), each procedure taking 2 h. To evaluate the surgical effect, we measured pre- and postoperative cerebral blood flow (CBF) by the ^{133}Xe inhalation method and single photon emission CT (SPECT) in 10 cases (table II).

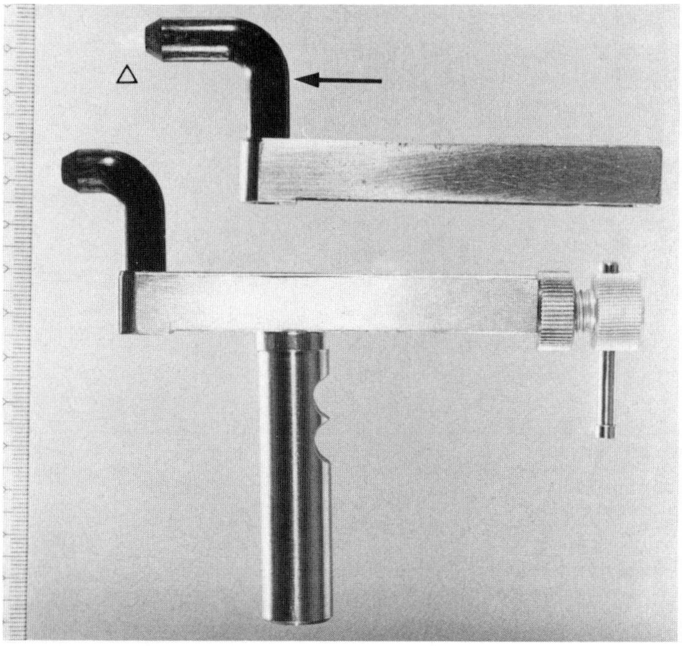

2a

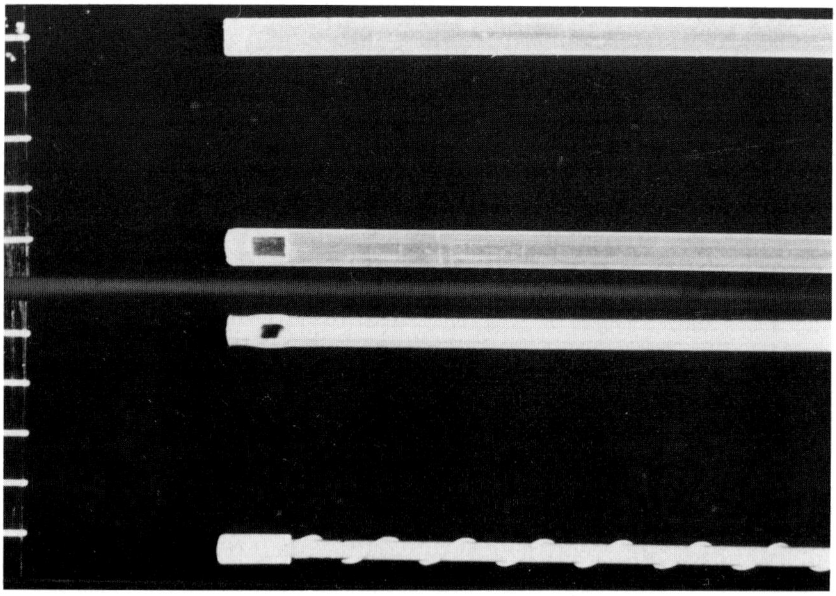

b

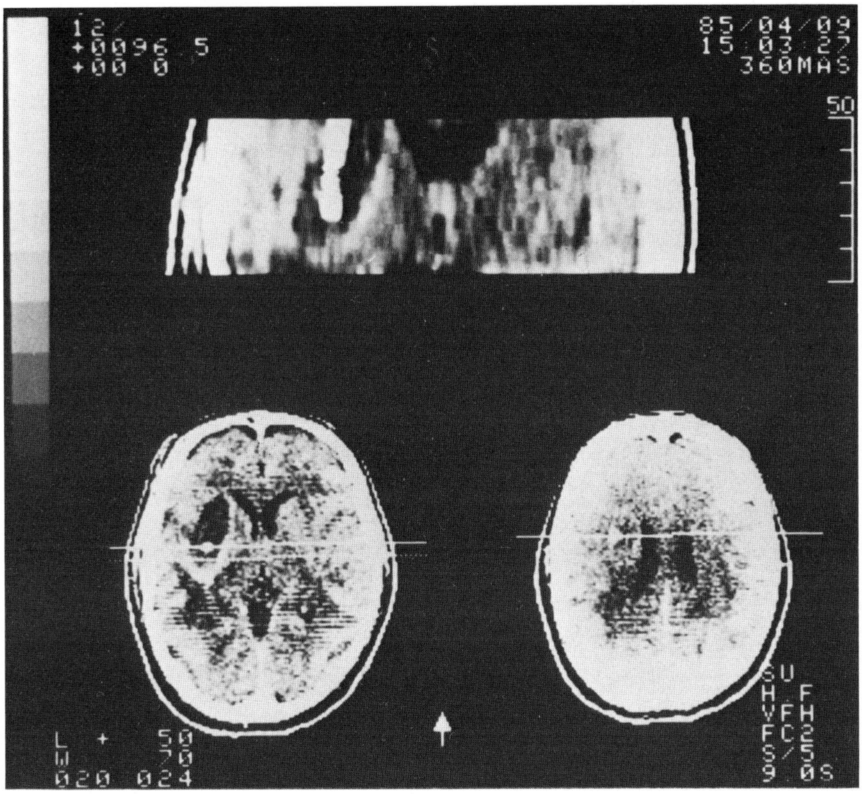

c

Fig. 2. **a** Head fixation pins made of carbon fiber STET and alumina-ceramic (arrowhead). **b** Needles for aspirating hematomas are 4 mm in outer diameter. The upper needle is made of teflon. The lower are a set of Archimedes' water-screw type needles. The tip of the screw is made of alumina-ceramic. **c** Intraoperative reconstruction.

Results

An almost artifact-free CT image can be obtained with our improved instrument. Figure 3 shows the CT scan for each step during hematoma evacuation. In our surgical results in stereotactic evacuation of intracerebral hematomas, more than 80% were satisfactory. Two complications were encountered. One patient with thalamic hemor-

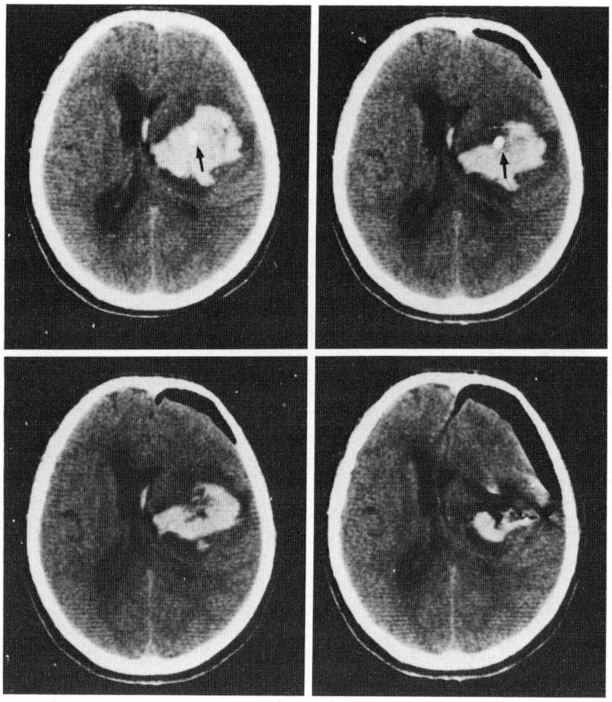

Fig. 3. CT image during each step of hematoma removal. The arrows indicate the tip of the needle within a hematoma.

rhage developed postoperative rebleeding due to hypertension. One patient with putaminal hemorrhage became worse after surgery due to therapeutically induced hypotension. The neurological deficits caused by the complication were fortunately transient. One case with putaminal hemorrhage died of pneumonia.

On the affected side, the CBF increased significantly in the region of the thalamus and basal ganglia and the anterior part of the territory of the middle cerebral artery. Even on the nonaffected side, a significant increase of CBF was observed in the region of the thalamus and basal ganglia.

Discussion

Different systems for CT-guided stereotactic surgery have been developed by various groups [2, 4]. *Brown* et al. [2] reported CT-guided stereotactic biopsy. *Perry* et al. [4] have developed an essentially artifact-free stereotactic frame for CT imaging and a computer program that spatially integrated the patient, stereotactic frame and scanner to calculate the potential trajectories.

Backlund et al. [2] reported an Archimedes' water-screw type of needle for evacuating hematomas. Our initial clinical experience of this type of needle is also favorable. *Matsumoto* et al. [3] reported that CT-guided stereotactic evacuation of hypertensive intracerebral hematoma had many advantages compared to hematoma removal by craniotomy, as is supported by our clinical results. CBF measurement indicated that the postoperative improvement in CBF could be obtained only by the CT-guided stereotactic hematoma evacuation.

References

1 Backlund, E.; Holst, H. von: Controlled subtotal evacuation of intracerebral hematomas by stereotactic technique. Surg. Neurol. *9:* 99–101 (1978).
2 Brown, R.A.; Roberts, T.; Osborn, A.G.: Simplified CT-guided stereotactic biopsy. Am. J. nucl. Radiol. *2:* 181–184 (1981).
3 Matumoto, K.; Hondo, H.: CT-guided stereotaxic evacuation of hypertensive intracerebral hematomas. J. Neurosurg. *61:* 440–448 (1984).
4 Perry, J.H.; Rosenbaum, A.E.; Lunsford, L.D.; Swink, C.A.; Zorub, D.S.: Computed tomography-guided stereotactic surgery: conception and development of a new stereotactic methodology. Neurosurgery *7:* 376–381 (1980).
5 Sugita, K.; Murata, K.: A stereotaxic apparatus for brain surgery and high frequency coagulator with automatic thermocontrol. Nagoya J. med. Sci. *28:* 126–141 (1966).

Dr. Yoshio Tanizaki, Department of Neurosurgery, Kakeyu Hospital, Maruko, Tiisagata, Nagano (Japan)

Proc. 9th Meeting World Soc. Stereotactic and Functional Neurosurgery, Toronto 1985
Appl. Neurophysiol. *48:* 18–21 (1985)

CT-Guided Ablative Stereotaxis without Ventriculography

Lauri V. Laitinen

Department of Neurosurgery, University Hospital, Umeå (Sweden)

Key Words. Computed tomography · Stereotactic surgery

Abstract. A new technique is described which permits all types of stereotactic surgery to be done without ventriculography, with CT guidance only. The present series consists of 42 patients who underwent thalamotomy, posteromedial hypothalamotomy, dentatotomy or anterior capsulotomy for movement disorders, chronic pain, spasmodic torticollis or psychiatric illness. Postoperative lesion control with repeated CT showed that the method was accurate. The clinical results were considered to be better than those after previous ventriculography-guided surgery. It is concluded that ventriculography is no longer needed for stereotactic neurosurgery.

The recent development of computed tomography (CT)-guided stereotaxis has opened a new era in morphological and functional stereotactic neurosurgery. The CT shows both intraventricular and extraventricular structures, whereas ventriculography only gives information on the interior of the ventricles, but nothing can be seen of the extraventricular structures, such as the internal capsule and the cisterna ambiens. Additionally, ventriculography and pneumoencephalography cause ventricular dilatation and displacement of other anatomical structures [1, 3, 4]. Headaches and nausea may increase the surgical morbidity. *Meyerson* et al. [3] were the first to use the CT study to localize the anterior internal capsule in patients undergoing anterior capsulotomy for obsessive-compulsive neurosis.

In Umeå, ventriculography was completely abandoned in stereotactic neurosurgery in March 1984 when a new CT adapter had been tested experimentally and clinically [2].

Table I. CT-guided ablative stereotaxis (June 1985)

Diagnosis	Cases, n	Target	Comments
Parkinson's disease	15	VL thal. 13	Tremor at CT: 1
		med. pall. 2	Tremor at CT: 1
Intention tremor	5	VIM thal.	
Deafferentation pain	10	pulv. 6, 1 bilat., CM 4	2 poor effects
Cancer pain	4	VPM 1, VPL 1, parafasc. 2	1 poor effect
Cerebral palsy	2	dentate bilat.	
Spasmodic torticollis	1	VOI thal.	
Schizophrenic aggressiveness	3	PM hypothal. bilat.	
Anxiety neurosis	1	ant. capsule bilat.	
Obsess-compulsive neurosis	1	ant. capsule bilat.	
Total	42		

Patients and Methods

Forty-two patients underwent functional stereotactic interventions without ventriculography, with a CT guidance only (table I). The CT study was carried out usually 1 day prior to surgery, or immediately before it if general anesthesia was needed for surgery (2 children with cerebral palsy and 2 schizophrenic patients). On average, the CT study lasted 12 min. The adapter was removed after the CT study. Two parkinsonian patients had a severe tremor during the CT study which had to be repeated because of movement artifacts. For surgery the adapter was remounted on a sitting patient and the base-ring of Laitinen's stereoguide around it was fixed rigidly to the skull under local anesthesia. In the 4 patients who required general anesthesia the adapter and the stereoguide were mounted in a semisitting position. In 9 patients, surgery was performed bilaterally in one session.

The x, y and z coordinates from the CT study were marked on the anteroposterior and lateral radiograms and projected onto the x and y axis of the stereoguide, which gave the stereotactic x, y and z coordinates. Before radiography, the spherical system of the stereoguide, consisting of two cylinder components and a semicircular arc with an electrode carrier, was so positioned around the adapter that the midpoint of the spherical system coincided with the CT target. The functional localization of the electrode introduction to the target was tested with impedance measurement and electrical stimulation.

The electrocoagulation lesions varied from 3 × 3 mm in diameter in the hypothalamus to 7 × 17 mm in the anterior internal capsule. Their site and size were verified with a postoperative CT study with the CT adapter remounted.

Short-Term Clinical Results

All patients tolerated the surgery without headaches, nausea, or fatigue and could have their luncheon a few hours postoperatively. They were discharged 1–4 days later. Two patients with medial pulvinotomy and 1 with parafascicular thalamotomy did not get any pain relief, or the relief was of a short duration. The latter patient had a slight diplopia and dizziness postoperatively. No other side effects were observed. The postoperative CT study showed a good correlation with the site of the lesion as compared with the preoperative target.

Discussion

The new CT adapter is noninvasive, quick and easy to mount on the patient's head and repeated mountings have a high degree of reproducibility [2]. A comparison of the CT and ventriculographic coordinates of the posterior commissure showed an average difference of 0.6 and 0.7 mm for the y and z coordinates, respectively, and a maximal difference of 0.5 mm for the x coordinate [2]. A recent modification of the adapter has further improved the reproducibility, and it is likely that the remaining sources of localization error depend on the inaccuracy of the CT machine, if the CT adapter has been adequately mounted.

The x, y and z coordinates of the CT study are easily transferred to stereotactic radiograms in the operating room. However, such a radiological transfer may not be necessary, because the CT study already contains all necessary data of the target. The spherical stereotactic system can be positioned around the brain in such a relation to the adapter that the midpoint of the spherical system coincides with the surgical target. Our preliminary studies indicate that radiology in the operating room may in fact increase the error risk.

The short-term clinical results of CT-guided stereotaxis seem to be better than those after previous ventriculography-guided surgery. A striking difference in favor of the CT-guided technique is the complete lack of headaches and nausea. Even elderly patients tolerate the interventions without stress. The CT study permits some visualization of the internal capsule and thus improves the chances to place the therapeutic probe close to the capsule in patients with parkinsonism and intention tremor. In posteromedial hypothalamotomy an accurate placement of the electrode, 2.5 mm lateral to the wall of the third ventricle, is easy with the CT, but difficult with ventriculography. I agree with *Meyerson* et al. [3] that anterior capsulotomy cannot be carried out accurately with ventriculographic localization. In posterior thalamotomies for chronic pain the CT technique is superior to ventriculography, because the medial and posterior margins of the pulvinar may vary greatly in relation to the posterior commissure and the midline of the third ventricle. All these factors may explain why CT-guided surgery seems to give better clinical results than earlier surgery based on ventriculography. I feel that ventriculography is no longer necessary in stereotactic neurosurgery.

References

1 Dieckmann, G.; Schmidt, K.; Prager, J.: Positional changes of intracranial structures after encephalography and during stereotaxic operations. Acta radiol. *5:* 644–653 (1966).
2 Laitinen, L.V.; Liliequist, B.; Fagerlund, M.; Eriksson, A.T.: An adapter for CT-guided stereotaxis. Surg. Neurol. *23:* 559–566 (1985).
3 Meyerson, B.A.; Bergström, M.; Greitz, T.: Target localization in stereotactic capsulotomy with the aid of computed tomography; in Hitchcock, Ballantine, Meyerson, Modern concepts in psychiatric surgery, pp. 217–224 (Elsevier/North-Holland, Amsterdam 1979).
4 Thulin, C.-A.; Essen, C. von; Zeuchner, E.: Displacements of brain due to positional changes during stereotactic operations. Confinia neurol. *34:* 348–354 (1972).

Lauri V. Laitinen, MD, PhD, Department of Neurosurgery, University Hospital, S-901 85 Umeå (Sweden)

Proc. 9th Meeting World Soc. Stereotactic and Functional
Neurosurgery, Toronto 1985
Appl. Neurophysiol. *48:* 22–29 (1985)

X-Ray and Magnetic Resonance Stereotaxy for Functional and Nonfunctional Neurosurgery

W. Birg, F. Mundinger, M. Mohadjer, K. Weigel, R. Fuermaier

Abteilung Stereotaxie und Neuronuklearmedizin, Neurochirurgische
Universitätsklinik, Freiburg i.Br., BRD

Key Words. Stereotactic surgery · Computer tomography · Magnetic resonance imaging · CT stereotaxis

Abstract. By means of new plastic stereotactic ring and head fixers, stereotactic procedures can be combined with MRI, with stereotactic coordinates obtained from the MRI images. The method was rechecked against CT stereotaxy and shows a good correspondence of the target coordinates. With MRI stereotaxy, structures near boney regions will be more accessible than with CT stereotaxy. Moreover, the MRI procedure seems to have advantages for functional therapy without the necessity of contrast ventriculography.

Introduction

1,200 successful CT stereotactic interventions have been performed in our department [2, 6]; it has therefore become the method of choice. In order to utilize the great diagnostic potential of magnetic resonance imaging (MRI) we developed a method to adapt the Riechert-Mundinger stereotactic device [9], including the computer compatible modification of *Birg and Mundinger* [1], for use with MRI. In principle, the method holds true for all the other stereotactic devices.

Materials and Methods

All parts of any stereotactic system exposed to the magnetic field of the MRI scanner must be made from a nonmetallic material, and yet the stability of the material should have the same good qualities as a special aluminium alloy device.

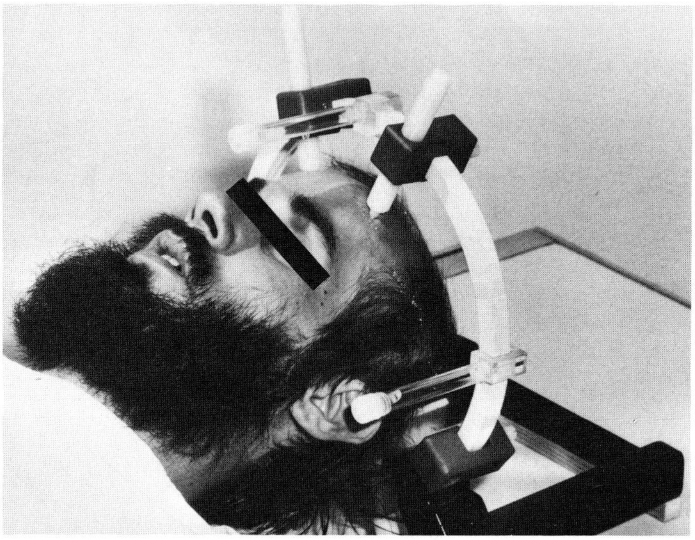

Fig. 1. MRI stereotaxy ring fixed to patient's head.

After having done several tests we chose a special plastic material whose torsion model and mechanical stability withstands the extreme forces and at the same time minimizes the artifacts in the MRI picture.

Figure 1 shows this plastic ring whose dimensions correspond exactly with the stereotactic ring made from metal, so all the additional equipment of our stereotactic device [1, 9] fit exactly. The patient's head is fixed by movable plastic attachments carrying the plastic screws tipped with sharp points made from quartz or steel. These points produce only small local artifacts in the MRI picture, so the image is not distorted. In addition, the plastic ring carries a small plastic tube filled with paramagnetic liquid. On the bottom of the sagittal and coronal MRI picture, this tube appears as a bright image which allows precise localization. In addition, there are four small plastic tubes orthogonally related to place the ring at 0, 90, 180 and 270°, so their midpoint is the zero point of the stereotactic ring and the diameters between them coincide with the X- and Y-axes. From these references and the MRI scanner software, we can measure the coordinates of all points of the brain. For the precise alignment of the ring in the MRI scanner, we used a special fixation unit made from solid plastic with the laser positioning light of the MRI scanner to assure a precise orthograde position of the stereotactic ring. The target determination requires an exact positioning. In the two cases in which we have used this method with different MRI scanners, we confirmed the accuracy of this procedure.

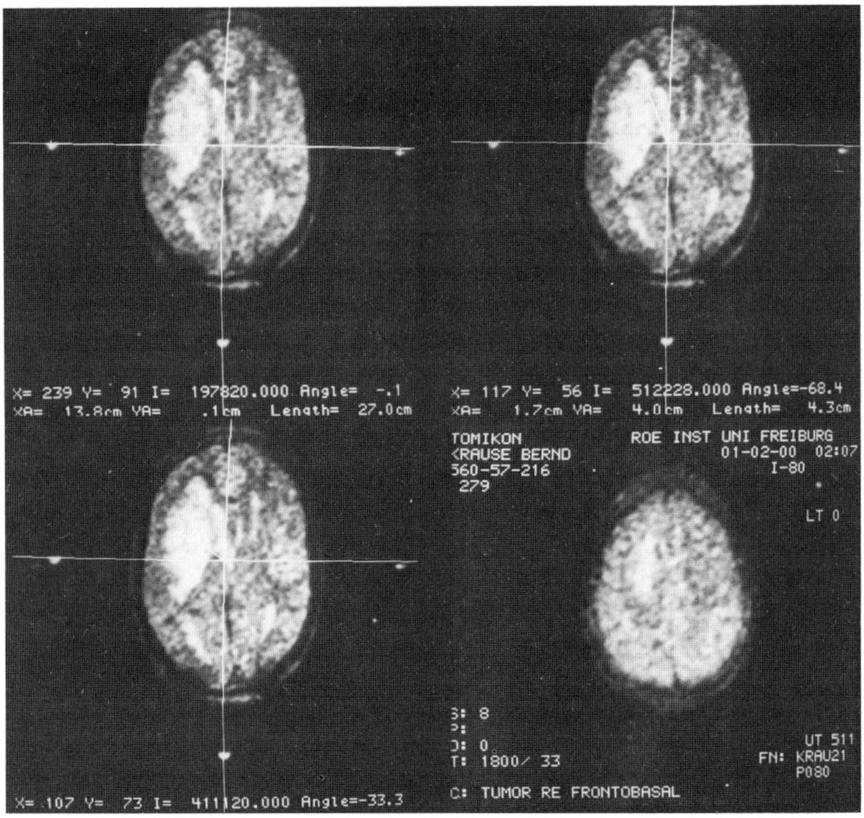

Fig. 2. MRI axial slice (Brucker) with tumor.

Evaluation

The patient with the ring fixed to his head is placed on the MRI table with the ring fixed to the holder. By means of the laser positioning lights, the first axial section is selected and the scan started. Figure 2 shows the axial images of the first patient scanned with the Brucker 0.23 tesla MRI Unit. Because of the diameter of the ring with the fixing screws, the normal body coil must be used, rather than the head coil, so the signal-to-noise ratio was not good and the pictures were rather fuzzy. We are presently constructing a special head-holder in which the MRI coil is integrated, with which we will get MRI stereotactic pic-

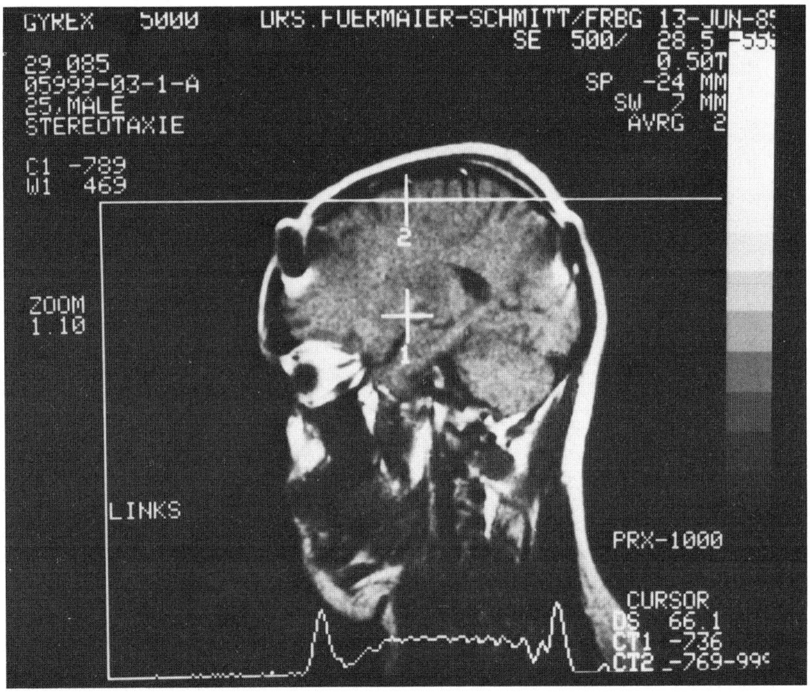

Fig. 3. MRI sagittal slice (Elscint Gyrex 5000).

tures of good quality. The coordinates of the tumor which can be seen in this MRI picture have been confirmed by CT stereotactic biopsy. Then we did a ^{125}I implantation [3–5, 7, 10] (fig. 6).

Our second case of a MRI stereotaxy has been done with a 0.5 tesla unit from Elscint. The signal-to-noise ratio is better because of the higher field strength, which allowed accurate determination of the tumor shape. The stereotactic coordinates are determined in the following way: Since the two small spots at the top of the picture correspond to the midsagittal section of the concentric tube on the inner side of the stereotactic ring, the line correcting these two points represents the Y–Z plane of the stereotactic system, and the midpoint of this line is the zero point. The coordinates of the tumor can be determined by the joystick feature of the MRI scanner (fig. 3). The x-coordinate is obtained from the coronal section in the same way (fig. 4). The height of

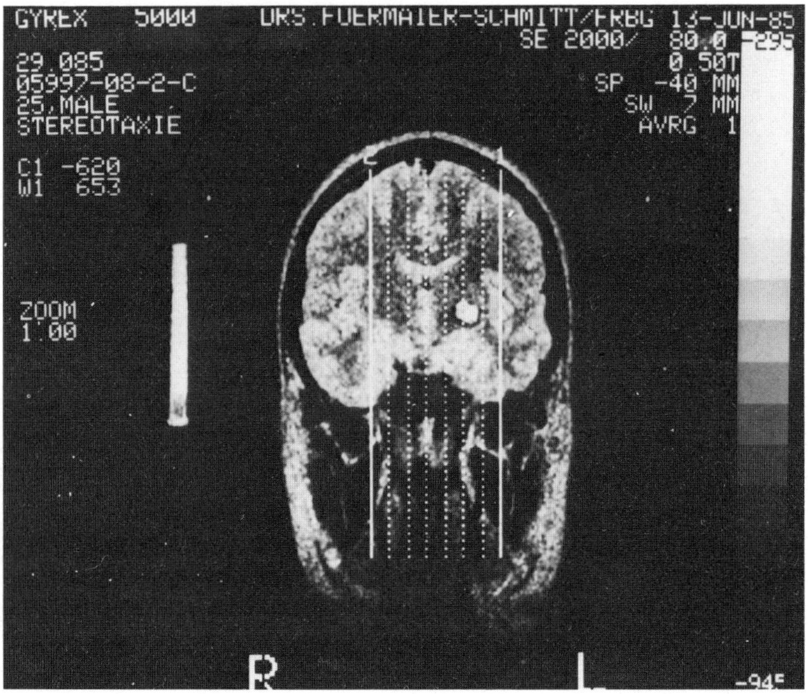

Fig. 4. MRI coronal picture.

the slice is the z-coordinate, and the x- and y-coordinates are measured by means of the joystick (fig. 5). The precision of this method was evaluated by comparing to the CT stereotactic procedure [3]. The correspondence of the z-values was satisfactory, and the x- and y-coordinates very good. The small difference of 2 mm in the z-direction could be taken into account by adjusting the MRI scanner.

Operation

The tumor coordinates taken from the MRI pictures are checked on the CT system and transferred to the X-rays. Then the optimal approach and the trephination point are determined. A metallic attachment block is used to fix the electrode holder on the plastic ring by clamp-mounting, to have a minimum of drill holes on the ring. In the

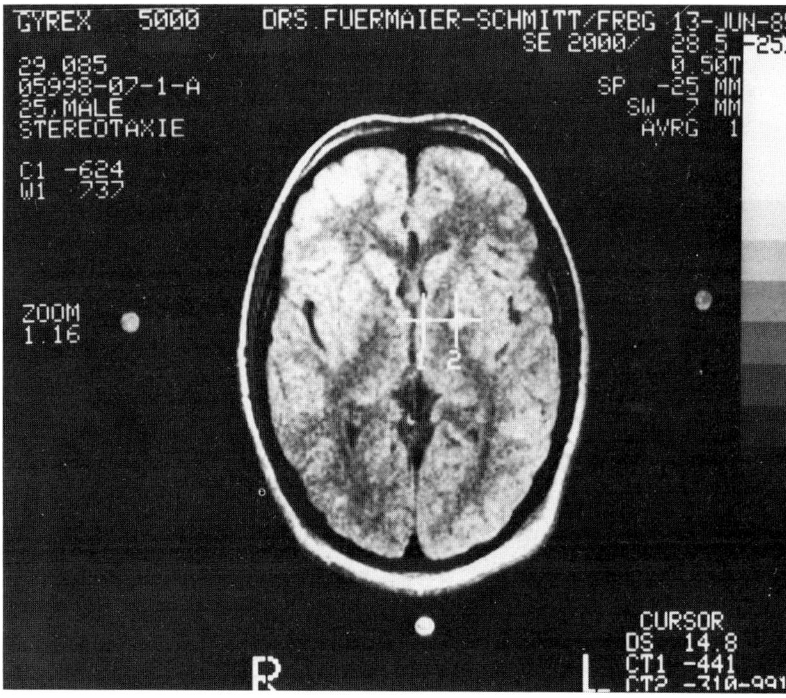

Fig. 5. Measurement on the MRI axial slice.

first case of MRI stereotaxy, the biopsy yielded an astrocytoma grade II. An ^{125}I seed was implanted with an accumulation dose of 9,000 cGy and a radius of 14 mm (fig. 6). In the second case, we did not obtain the diagnosis of tumor, so only a small silver clip was implanted. The conventional paraffin embedding revealed the diagnosis of a former hemorrhagic focus.

Functional Therapy

If we look at the sagittal and the coronal MRI slice it becomes clear that this method suits functional stereotaxy very well. The MRI scan taken from the midsagittal plane enables us to determine the necessary targets of the hypothalamus [8, 9], which is much better than can be obtained with CT scanning.

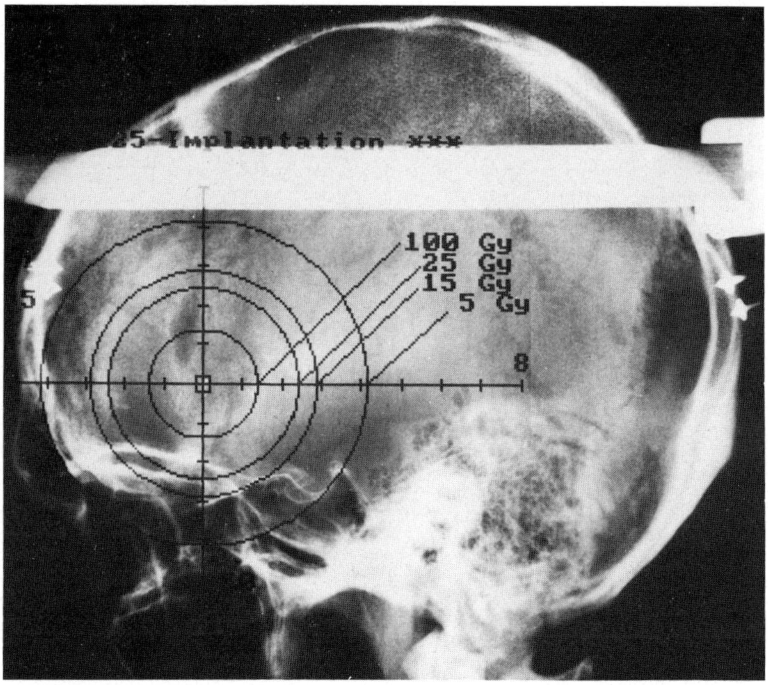

Fig. 6. X-ray with isodoses.

References

1 Birg, W.; Mundinger, F.: Computer calculations of target parameters for a stereotactic apparatus. Acta neurochir. *29:* 123–129 (1973).

2 Birg, W.; Mundinger, F.: Direct target point determination for stereotactic brain operations from CT data and the calculation of setting parameters for polar-coordinate stereotactic devices. Appl. Neurophysiol. *45:* 387–395 (1982).

3 Birg, W.; Schneider, J.; Bauer, S.; Mundinger, F.: An interactive program system for the stereotactic interstitial implantation of radionuclides in brain tumors; in Szikla, Stereotactic cerebral irradiation. Inserm Symposium No. 12, pp. 77–80 (Elsevier/North-Holland, Amsterdam 1979).

4 Mundinger, F.: Stereotaktische interstitielle Therapie nicht resezierbarer intracranieller Tumoren im Ir-192 und Jod-125; in Wannemacher, Schreiber, Gauwerky, Kombinierte chirurgische und radiologische Behandlung maligner Tumoren, pp. 90–112 (Urban & Schwarzenberg, München 1981).

5 Mundinger, F.: Implantation of radioisotopes; in Schalterbrand, Walker, Stereotaxy of the human brain, pp. 410–445 (Thieme, Stuttgart 1982).

6 Mundinger, F.: CT-stereotactic biopsy of brain tumors; in Voth, Gutjahr, Langmaid, Tumors of the central nervous system in infancy and childhood (Springer, Berlin 1982).

7 Mundinger, F.; Busam, B.; Birg, W.; Schildge, J.: Results of interstitial iridium-192 brachy-curietherapy and iridium-192 protracted long-term irradiation; in Szikla, Stereotactic cerebral irradiation. Inserm Symp. No. 12, pp. 303–320 (Elsevier/North-Holland, Amsterdam 1979).

8 Mundinger, F.: Stereotaktische Operationen am Gehirn. Grundlagen–Indikationen–Resultate (Hippokrates, Stuttgart 1975).

9 Riechert, T.; Mundinger, F.: Beschreibung und Anwendung eines Zielgerätes für stereotaktische Hirnoperationen (II. Modell). Acta neurochir. *3:* 308–337 (1956).

10 Szikla, G.; Pergut, J.C.: Irradiation interstitielle des gliomes; in Constans, Schlienger, Radiothérapie des tumeurs du système nerveux central de l'adulte. Neurochirurgie *21:* suppl. 2, pp. 187–228 (1975).

Dr. W. Birg, Abteilung Stereotaxie und Neuronuklearmedizin,
Neurochirurgische Universitätsklinik, D-7800 Freiburg i.Br. (FRG)

Proc. 9th Meeting World Soc. Stereotactic and Functional
Neurosurgery, Toronto 1985
Appl. Neurophysiol. *48:* 30–33 (1985)

Digital Image Processing to Handle Neuroanatomical Information and Neurophysiological Data

C. Giorgi[a], *U. Cerchiari*[b], *G. Broggi*[a], *P. Birk*[c], *A. Struppeler*[c]

[a] Division of Stereotactic Neurosurgery, Institute for Neurology, Milan, Italy,
[b] Division of Physics, INT, Milan, Italy;
[c] Neurologische Klinik der Technischen Universität, München, BRD

Key Words. Computer graphics · Stereotactic atlas · Neurofunctional data base

Abstract. An application of computer graphics technology to functional stereotactic neurosurgery is presented. Neuroanatomical images derived from a stereotactic atlas and information retrieved from a neurophysiological data base are drawn on a graphic monitor. The pictures are oriented and scaled according to appropriate landmarks. The aim of this work ist to add confidence in the surgeon's selection of the probe trajectory and to improve the knowledge of sensory and motor organization within the thalamus.

Introduction

Several workers have dealt with the localization of functional observations recorded during stereotactic operations [2, 3, 5–7], and a 3-dimensional atlas has been published based upon these observations [1]. The recent development of interactive graphic terminals and the introduction and diffusion of digital radiologic equipment has prompted us to write programs that run on relatively modest computational equipment, to use the power of computer graphics in stereotactic neurosurgery.

Materials and Method

We describe a program that runs on a graphic processor Tesak EGP 414 (Tesak, Florence, Italy), that drives two high-resolution graphic monitors Barco CDCT 3151 (Barco Industries, Kortrijk, Belgium). The management of a 20-Mbyte memory and the connection between work stations is done by a Digital PDP 11/23 computer (Digital

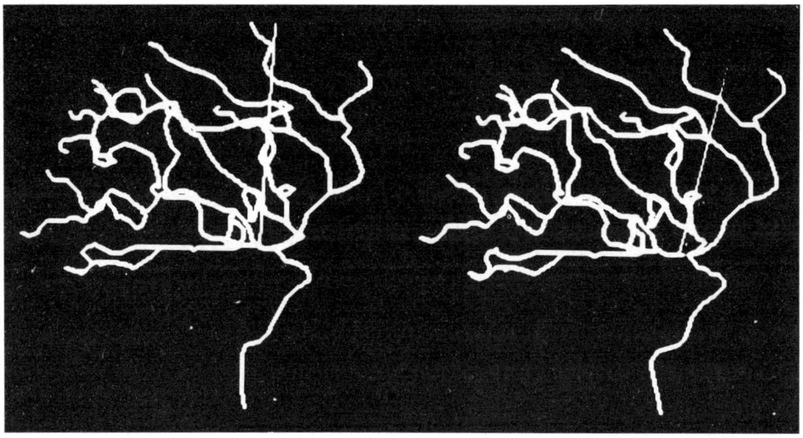

Fig. 1. Stereoscopic representation of arterial phase of cerebral vascular anatomy, with simulated position of probe.

Equipment Corp., Maynard, Mass.). The surgical procedure uses a BRW (Radionics, Burlington, Mass.) stereotactic frame, which has been modified for the acquisition of the cerebral vascular anatomy. Digital images obtained with computerized tomography (CT) and digital vascular imaging (DVI), are used to gather the necessary information to determine a 'safe' trajectory through a 3-dimensional representation of CT and vascular anatomy (fig. 1).

The selection of anatomical landmarks necessary to orient the anatomical frame of reference within the stereotactic apparatus is derived from stereotactic ventriculography with a digitizing tablet. The anatomical frame of reference is the intercommissural line, which is still better defined with this exam. The axes that appear at this point on the monitor represent the anatomical frame of reference; the length of the axes depends on the position of the landmarks selected in each individual case and determines the scale factor in the A-P (CA-CP distance) and vertical directions (floor of the lateral ventricle). Y axis length (mediolateral direction) can only be estimated by the position of the internal capsule, as indicated by CT.

The files of neuroanatomical and neurophysiological information, resident on the system memory, can be assessed via a menu. They contain all the structures illustrated on a stereotactic brain atlas [4] in a series of parallel frontal, sagittal and horizontal sections. Any structure can be individually displayed, with the scaling dictated by the length of the axes. Similarly, neurophysiological information recorded in previous procedures can be selected and displayed, according to the procedure which is going to be performed. These points are presented as clusters, colored according to a code that corresponds to different characteristics. Their position also undergoes the same scaling, as the anatomical structures, according to the length of the axes.

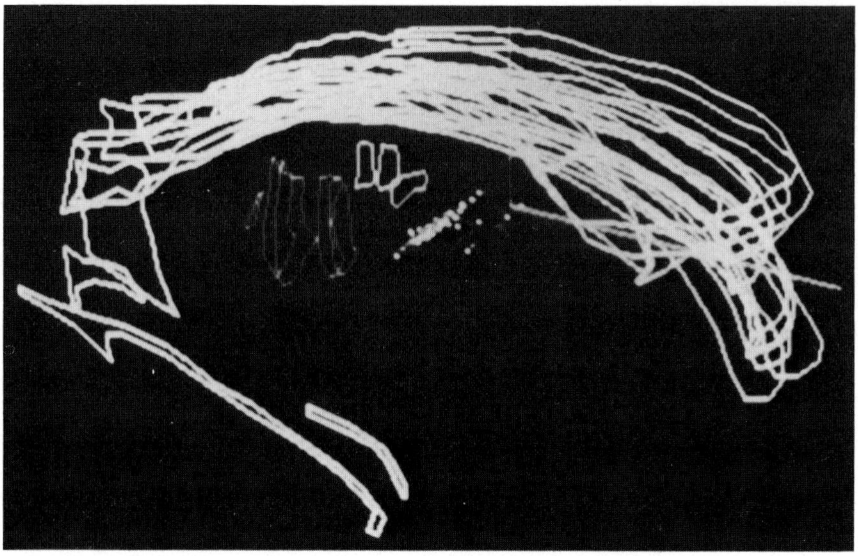

Fig. 2. Oblique projection of lateral ventricular and thalamic nuclei outlines, together with clusters of 'functional' points, within the atlas reference system.

The program allows for the rotation of the axes and the anatomical structures and functional points that have been selected, and a stereoscopic 3-dimensional display. The position of the probe is simulated on the monitor and can be modified to obtain a satisfactory trajectory. The angles and the depth corresponding to that trajectory are directly written within the reference system of the stereotactic frame (fig. 2).

All the information gathered along the probe trajectory can be filed while being observed via an interactive graphic date base that allows fast and simple access to the main memory.

Discussion

The system is being installed at the Division of Stereotactic and Functional Neurosurgery of the Istituto Neurologico, Milan, and at the Neurologische Klinik der Technischen Universität, Munich. It is important to start this work in different centers in order to gather rapidly a significant number of neurophysiological observations.

We do not have enough cases yet to demonstrate the clinical value of this approach. It is worth noting, however, that this is an updated version of a project that had been explored previously but failed to gain popularity due to the lack of a data acquisition system simple enough to use.

The weak point of the program is obviously the limited precision with which the data are 'adapted' to the anatomy of the single case. To reduce this disadvantage high-resolution diagnostic tools (CT and MRI) dedicated to stereotactic surgery are being developed.

References

1 Emers, R.; Tasker, R.R.: The human somesthesic thalamus with maps for physiologic target localization during stereotactic neurosurgery (Raven Press. New York 1975).

2 Hardy, T.L.: Computer display of the electrophysiological topography of the diencephalon during stereotactic surgery; MSc thesis McGill University (1975).

3 Hassler, R.: Functional anatomy of the thalamus. Physiol. med. Sci. *56:* 91 (1957/1958).

4 Shaltenbrand, G.; Wahren, W.: Atlas for stereotaxy of the human brain; 2nd ed. (Thieme, Stuttgart 1977).

5 Tasker, R.R.; Rowe, I.H.; Hawrylyshyn, P.; Organ, L.W.: Computer mapping of brain stem sensory centers in man. J. Neurosurg. *44:* 458–464 (1976).

6 Tasker, R.R.; Hawrylyshyn, P.; Organ, L.W.: Computerized graphic display of physiological data collected during human stereotactic surgery. Appl. Neurophysiol. *41:* 183–187 (1978).

7 Thompson, C.T.; Hardy, T.; Bertrand, G.: A system for anatomical and functional mapping of the human thalamus. Comp. biomed. Res. *10:* 9–24 (1977).

C. Giorgi, MD Divisione di Neurochirurgia Stereotassica e Funzionale,
Istituto Neurologico C. Besta, Via Celoria 11,
I-20133 Milano (Italy)

Proc. 9th Meeting World Soc. Stereotactic and Functional
Neurosurgery, Toronto 1985
Appl. Neurophysiol. *48:* 34–38 (1985)

A New Stereotactic Instrument for Use with Computerized Tomography and Magnetic Resonance Imaging

E. de A. Montagno, B.S. Nashold, Jr.

Division of Neurosurgery, Duke Medical Center, Durham, N.C., USA

Key Words. Computerized tomography guided operations · Magnetic resonance imaging · Stereotactic surgery · Computerized tomography scanning

Abstract. The new stereotactic instrument has the advantages of (1) use with computerized tomography (CT) or magnetic resonance imaging (MRI) without special adaptations of instruments, (2) brain targets transferred directly from CT or MRI to apparatus, and (3) use with conventional stereotactic techniques. The apparatus is designed to meet present demands of neurosurgical facilities of good standards and capabilities, encompassing present and future developments towards more efficient and less invasive brain operations.

Introduction

Stereotaxis has made it possible to reach deep target points in the brain without direct visualization. Computerized imaging techniques now permit broadening of stereotaxis to localize and reach any targets inside the skull with great precision [2]. The actual images of an individual brain with a neurological disease can be visualized using computerized tomography (CT) and magnetic resonance imaging (MRI). As CT and MRI become common diagnostic tests, new stereotactic instruments should be developed which are precise, simple to use, safe and affordable. A new stereotactic instrument has been developed which incorporates a set of properties for best spatial relationships that can be used with CT and MRI [3–5].

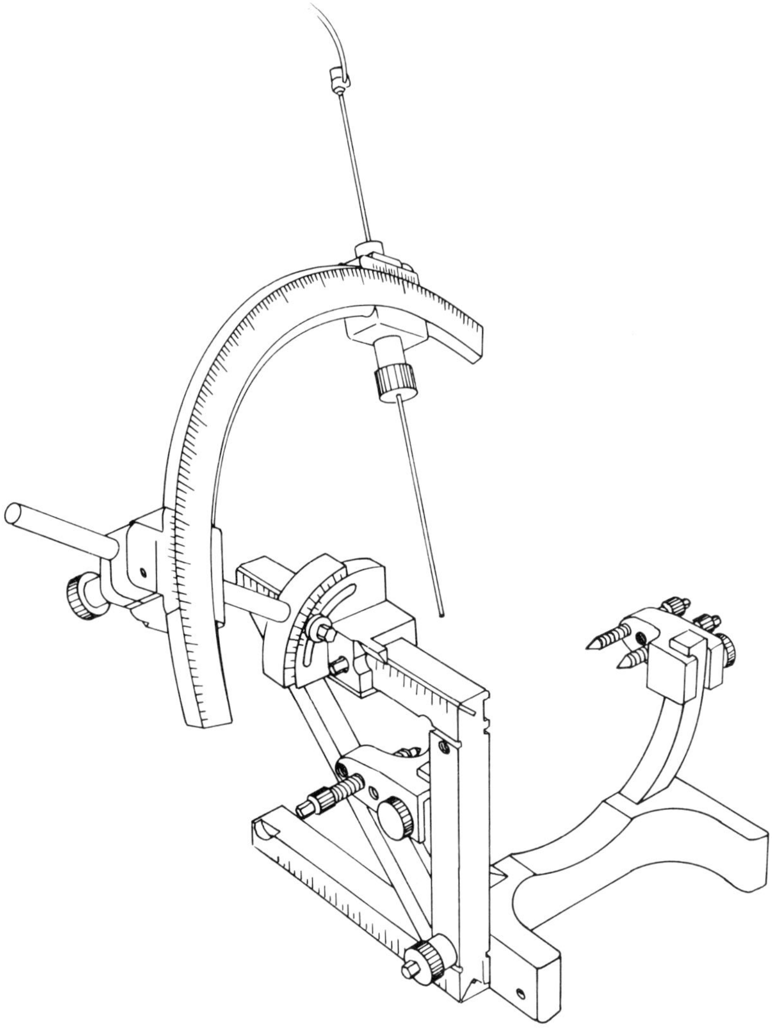

Fig. 1. Illustration of the stereotactic instrument.

Description and Theory

The stereotactic instrument consists of a base with head-holder, frame and probe-holder. An aluminum alloy which allows high precision, high resistance, low artifact and nonmagnetic construction was used (fig. 1).

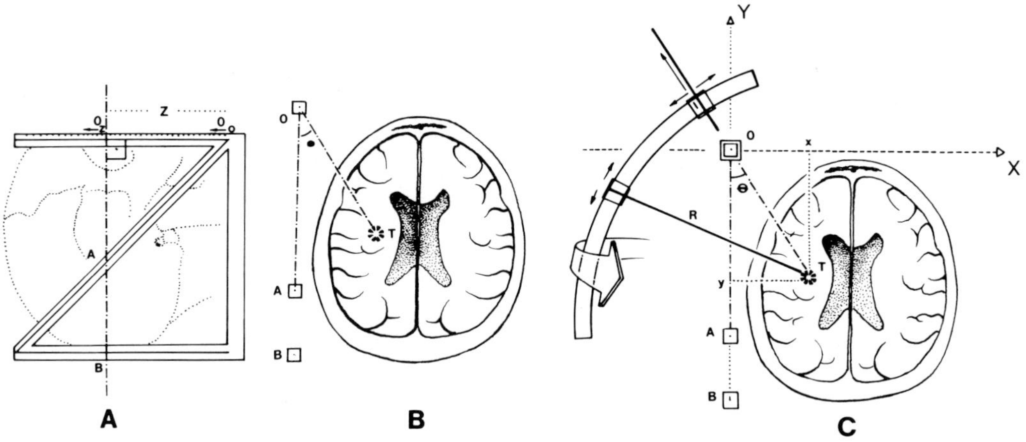

Fig. 2. A lateral view of the Z-shaped frame made for direct localization of CT planes along the frame's longitudinal axis (Z coordinate = distance OA = dist. 1). This is achieved by incorporating geometrical characteristics of right-angle isosceles triangles. **B** CT/MRI picture containing the target (T) and frame's reference points (O, A and B). Using the CT/MRI console facilities, a cylindrical coordinate system is depicted that makes use of two distances and one angle (distance 1 = OA, angle ∅ and distance 2 = OT). **C** Schematic vision of the cylindrical (for CT/MRI stereotaxis: OA, ∅, OT) and Cartesian (OX, OY) coordinates interacting with apparatus' mechanics. Probe-holder movements (arrows) form a spherical system centered in the target.

It can be used for standard computer tomography (CTS) and magnetic resonance stereotaxis. The apparatus includes the Cartesian system for conventional stereotaxis, but its advantages result from a combination of cylindrical and spherical systems. The target location depends on using two distances and one angle as coordinates to localize a point in space. The spherical probe-holder enables the neurosurgeon to choose from an infinity of directions along which to guide the probe to the target. This geometrical interaction in the apparatus' mechanical system allows the neurosurgeon the greatest ease and flexibility [4] (fig. 2).

From the practical point of view this coordinate system results (1) in *direct read-out* from screen or film and (2) in *direct setting* on the apparatus of the three coordinates, namely: (a) *distance 1*, (b) *angle* and (c) *distance 2* (fig. 3).

Fig. 3. The underlying theory is that three-dimensional space can be precisely assessed at each CT slice within the frame's built-in relationships. Two sides and an angle of a triangle are the coordinates to be read in the CT film or screen **(A)** and set on the apparatus **(B)** for target values: distance 1 (Z coordinate), angle and distance 2 (depth).

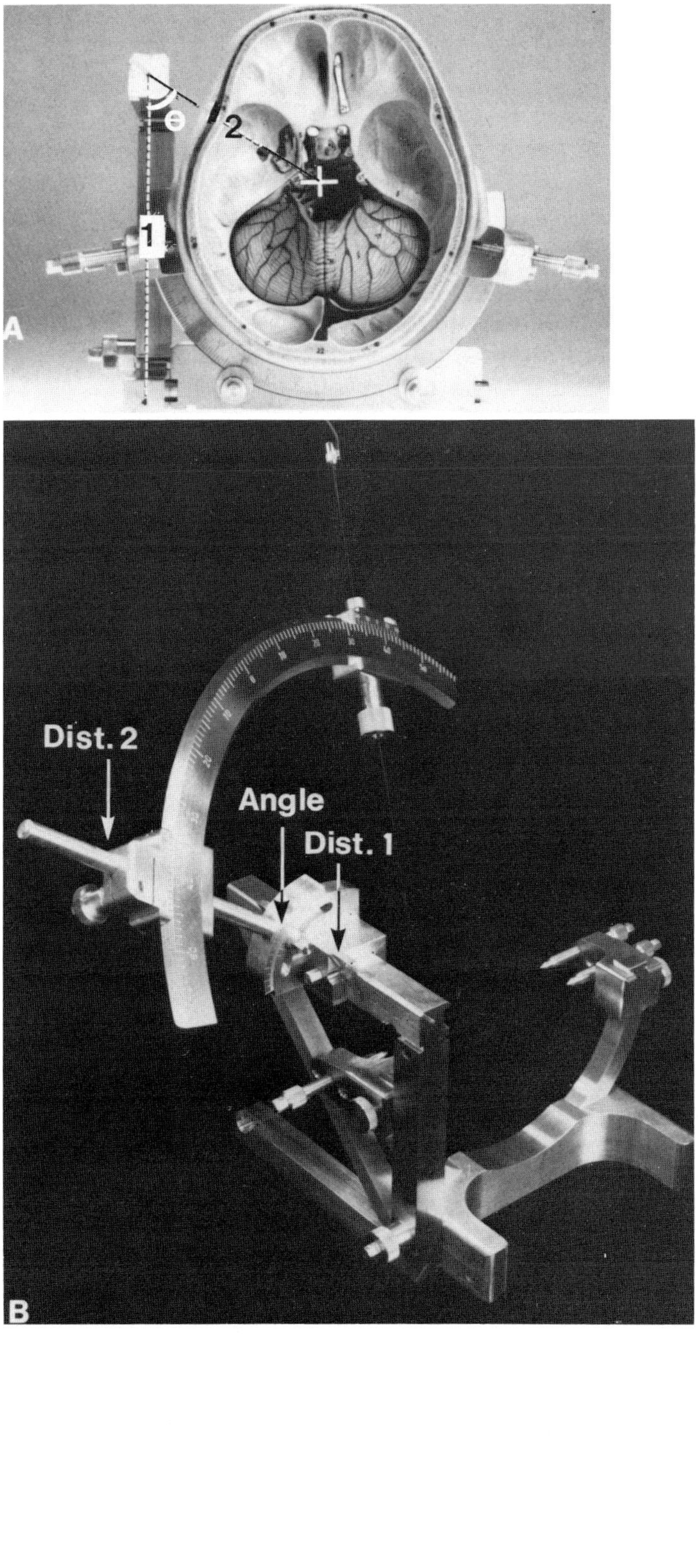
θ
2
1
A
Dist. 2
Angle
Dist. 1
B

The advantages of the apparatus are use with no target calculations, no phantoms, free choice of entry points, all CTs, MRIs, X-rays and probes. The economical design, with only few essential parts, make the instrument accurate and affordable.

Conclusion

CT-guided stereotaxis is a half-decade old innovation in neurosurgery. With increased use of stereotactic neurosurgery, new diagnostic and treatment methods will evolve in the future.

The present CTS apparatus is made with simplicity of concept and handling, observing all standards required by stereotaxis [1]. As we gain clinical experience using the instrument it may enable us to improve on some details. For instance, higher stability of the system's head instrument in managing patients with severe involuntary movements can perhaps be achieved by augmenting the distance between the screws of the tong-like bimastoid head-holder. This new device is prepared for entry point target freedom and multitarget guidance with a high degree of flexibility. The uncomplicated and precise handling make it suitable for functional stereotactic procedures, for biopsy and treatment of tumors and other inoperable lesions, for hematoma and abscess evacuation, etc.

References

1 Gildenberg, P.L., et al.: Performance requirement standard for cerebral stereotactic instruments, final draft (1980).
2 Gildenberg, P.L.: Computerized tomography and stereotactic surgery; in Spiegel, Guided brain operations, pp. 24–34 (Karger, Basel 1982).
3 Montagno, E. de A.: CT-Stereotaktische Hirnoperation: Entwicklung eines neuen Apparates; Diss. Freie Universität Berlin (1985).
4 Montagno, E. de A.; Römer, T.: Computertomographische Stereotaxie (CTS): Entwicklung eines neuen Systems, Teil I (in press, 1985).
5 Montagno, E. de A.; Römer, T.; Oppel, F.: Computertomographische Stereotaxie (CTS): Entwicklung eines neuen Systems, Teil II (in press, 1985).

E. de A. Montagno, Duke University Medical Center, Box 3807,
Division of Neurosurgery, Durham, NC 27710 (USA)

Proc. 9th Meeting World Soc. Stereotactic and Functional
Neurosurgery, Toronto 1985
Appl. Neurophysiol. *48:* 39–44 (1985)

Computer Tomography-Controlled Stereotactic Surgery

Keizo Matsumoto, Fumio Shichijo, Tsutomu Masuda, Hajime Miyake

Department of Neurological Surgery, School of Medicine, University of Tokushima, Japan

Key Words. Computed tomography · CT-stereotaxis · Hematoma evacuation · Hemorrhage, intracerebral · Stereotactic surgery

Abstract. In computed tomography (CT)-controlled stereotactic surgery, the coordinate system of the CT scanner is applied to determine the target depth and direction as well as for readjustment of final probe direction. This method can be used for all types of stereotactic surgery for the brain.

In computed tomography (CT)-controlled stereotactic surgery (fig. 1), a single coordinate system of the CT scanner is used to determine target and depth. The probe direction, which is directed to the target with primary information, is adjusted and corrected with information obtained from CT slices of the probe in the two opposing views before insertion of the probe, similar to X-ray control of stereotactic operations.

Logic of Stereotaxy

The three-dimensional coordinates were obtained as follows: values of X (left-right) and Y (fronto-occipital) axes are obtained by cursor numbers on the slice image. The value of the Z (vertex-basal) axis is obtained by indicator numbers of the sliding table on which the patient is lying.

First, in the axial slice of CT_0, coordinates of X_t and Y_t of the chosen target are obtained as cursor numbers. The value of the Z axis

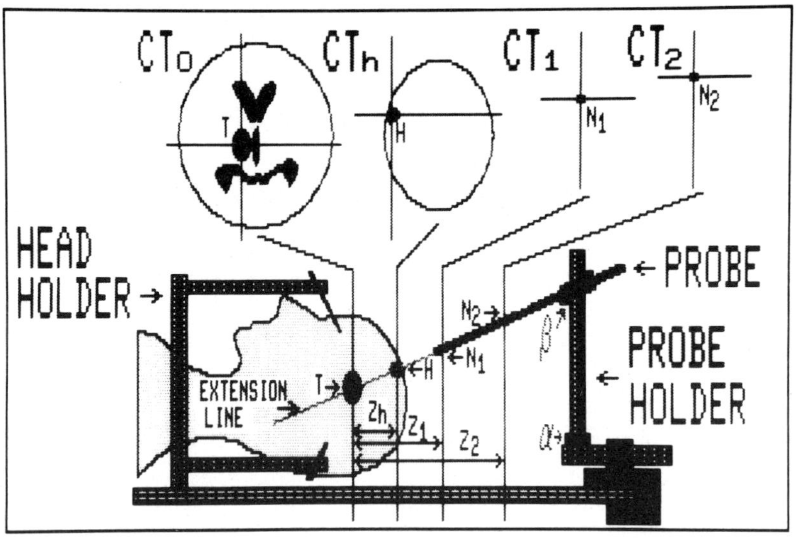

Fig. 1. Schematic representation of CT-controlled stereotactic operation. T = target point; H = burr hole; N_1 and N_2 = two different points of the probe; CT_0 = a slice through the point T; CT_0 = a slice through the point H; CT_1 and CT_2 = slices through the points N_1 and N_2; beta = angle of horizontal plane; alpha = angle of vertical plane; Z_h, Z_1 and Z_2 = distance of CT_h, CT_1 and CT_2 to the CT_0.

of this slice is set to zero (Z_0). In the slice CT_h, which passes through the center of the burr hole, values of X_h are also obtained as cursor numbers. The values of Z_h, the distance between Tn and CT_0, are obtained as a millimeter number.

The distance (D) and the direction of the angle in the horizontal plane and of the angle in the vertical plane are obtained from the following equation, provided the planes of axial slices are perpendicular to the Z axis (fig. 2a, b).

$$D = R^2[(X_t-X_h)^2+(Y_t-Y_h)^2]+Z_h^2 \quad (1)$$

$$= \tan^{-1}[R(X_h-X_t)/Z_h] \quad (2)$$

$$= \tan^{-1}[R(Y_h-Y_t)/R^2(X_h-X_t)^2+Z_h^2] \quad (3)$$

'R' is a derived ratio which transforms the cursor number to millimeter

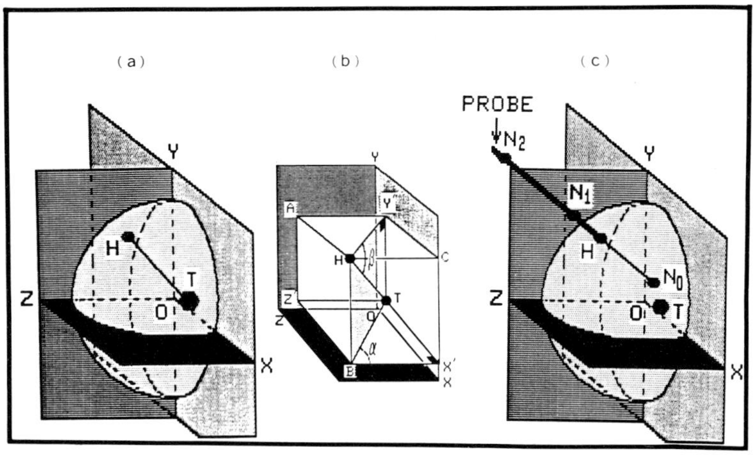

Fig. 2. Determination of probe trajectory of depth and direction to the target point. **a** Depth of the probe is calculated from the coordinates of H and T. **b** Direction of probe angle of beta and angle of alpha is calculated from coordinates of H and T. **c** Final correction of the direction of probe. Extension of straight line through the point of N_1 and N_2 will cross the plane XY at the point of N_0. The direction of the probe should be corrected until the point of N_0 is in concordance with the point of T.

length. In our CT scanner, the 240-mm scanning field is divided into a 320×320 matrix. Therefore,

$$R = 240/320 = 0.75$$

After setting the angles of the probe to the chosen target, the probe direction is adjusted and corrected again according to the values of cursor numbers in the two slices containing point N_1 (X_1, Y_1, Z_1) and N_2 (X_2, Y_2, Z_2). The coordinates of the aiming points (X_0, Y_0) of the probe in the CT_0 slice are calculated with the following equations (fig. 2c). In this equation, 'R' can be cancelled.

$$X_0 = (X_1Z_2 - X_2Z_1)/(Z_2 - Z_1) \quad (4)$$

$$Y_0 = (Y_1Z_2 - Y_2Z_1)/(Z_2 - Z_1) \quad (5)$$

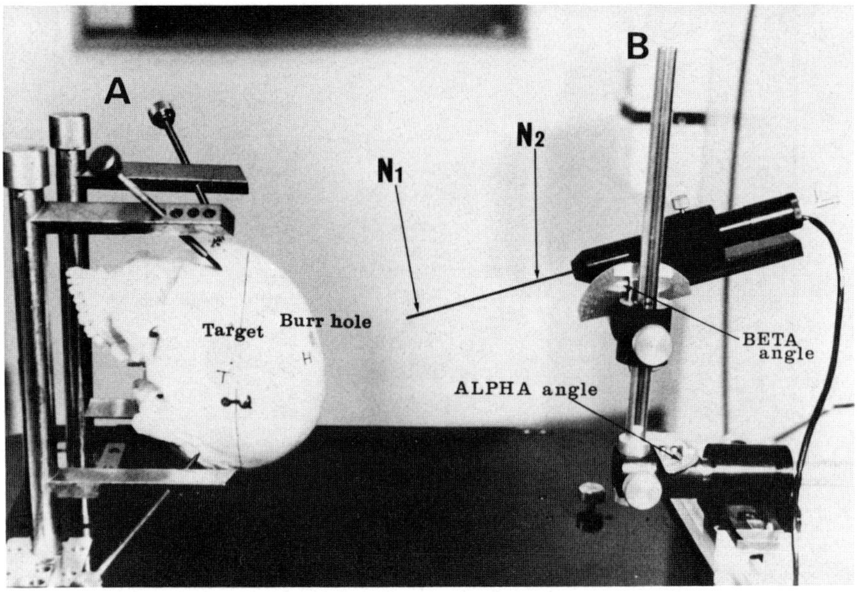

Fig. 3. Stereotactic apparatus. This apparatus consists of two functional components: a head holder (A) and a probe holder (B), and this system is fixed to the CT sliding table.

The probe direction should be corrected until the values of X_0 and Y_0 are in concordance with coordinates of the chosen target, X_t and Y_t, respectively. After the probe is inserted into the chosen target with predetermined depth (D), a slice of CT_0 should be made to confirm the location of the tip of the probe.

Stereotactic Apparatus

Our apparatus has a simple structure composed of two main parts, a hard plastic plate and aluminium pins, for fixation of the patient's head, and a probe guide, which has two scales for alpha and beta angles and a sliding probe holder with a millimeter scale (fig. 3).

Operative Procedures

A burr hole is made in the operating room, and the patient transferred to the CT room. The patient's head is fixed to the sliding table of the CT scanner and two slices of CT_0 and CT_h are made. The programs for equations 1, 2, and 3 should already be loaded into the hand-held computer, HC-20 (Epson Co. Ltd., Nagano, Japan), to obtain immediate answers of D, alpha and beta by direct input of the values of X_t, Y_t, X_h, Y_h and Z_h to this computer. The procedures for final correction of the direction of the probe are also done by this computer. From equations 4 and 5, which had been loaded into this computer, the answers of coordinates of X_0 and Y_0 are readily obtained by direct input of cursor numbers of X_1, Y_1, Z_1, X_2, Y_2 and Z_2. The range of error is 1.5 mm (two pixels) with 2 mm slice thickness. Scan time is 4.5 or 9 s. It takes about 40–50 min to hit the chosen target with this procedure.

Cases

15 acute cases of hypertensive thalamic and putaminal hemorrhages admitted to our service in 1984 were selected. An aspiration cannula was inserted into the center of the hematomas and they were evacuated successfully. The target accuracy was completely satisfactory in all cases.

We do not think very small hematomas should be evacuated. However, the patients we operated had apparent motor weakness as a neurological finding. We hope this condition may objectively demonstrate the surgical efficacy of hematoma evacuation in the acute stage. Two cases responded well and showed immediate recovery from their hemiplegic state after surgery.

Discussion

Procedures with similar logics of stereotaxy using the coordinate system of the CT scanner itself have been reported by *Koslow* et al. [2] and *Gildenberg* et al. [1]. However, *Koslow* et al. [2] did not use slices of the probe for correction of the trajectory and *Gildenberg* et al. [1] used a

Scout View to compute the coordinates of the CT scanner with that of the stereotactic apparatus.

In our method, the coordinates of the CT scanner are used fully for calculation of the target trajectory as well as precise control of the probe direction before insertion.

Conclusion

CT-controlled stereotactic surgery is a good practical method with high target accuracy. This method can be used for all types of stereotactic surgery, and we believe there is a possibility of automatic control of stereotactic surgery with further development of this method.

References

1 Gildenberg, P.L.; Kaufman, H.H.; Murthy, K.S.K.: Calculation of stereotactic coordinates from the computed tomographic scan. Neurosurgery *10:* 580–586 (1982).

2 Koslow, M.; Abele, M.G.; Griffith, R.C.; Mair, G.A.; Chase, N.E.: Stereotactic surgical system controlled by computed tomography. Neurosurgery *8:* 72–82 (1981).

Dr. K. Matsumoto, Department of Neurological Surgery, School of Medicine, University of Tokushima, Tokushima 770 (Japan)

Proc. 9th Meeting World Soc. Stereotactic and Functional
Neurosurgery, Toronto 1985
Appl. Neurophysiol. *48:* 45–49 (1985)

Experience in the First 100 Patients Undergoing Computerized Tomography-Guided Stereotactic Procedures Utilizing the Brown-Roberts-Wells Guidance System

Allan B. Levin

Division of Neurological Surgery, University of Wisconsin Hospital,
Madison, Wisc., USA

Key Words. Computerized tomography-guided stereotaxis · Brown-Robert-Wells guidance system · Stereotactic surgery

Abstract. A series of 100 patients undergoing CT-guided stereotactic procedures for biopsy and/or drainage (n = 87), deep brain electrode placement (n = 9), endoscopy (n = 1), and functional lesioning (n = 3) was reviewed. Only 1 patient required general anesthesia. There were 4 procedural related hematomas, only 1 of which was symptomatic. No other complications were encountered.

With an increasing interest in CT-guided stereotactic procedures and the development of numerous systems and methodologies, it is important to periodically review experiences with each of these systems.

From January 1982, through August 1984, 100 patients underwent 101 CT-guided stereotactic procedures utilizing the Brown-Roberts-Wells stereotactic system. The major indication for a CT-guided stereotaxy was biopsy for tissue differentiation of lesions. A complete list of the procedures performed is listed in table I.

Technique

The basic use of the Brown-Roberts-Wells stereotactic guidance system has been previously described [1, 2]. With the exception of the single thalamotomy for movement disorder, all procedures were performed under local anesthesia with a minimum amount of neuroleptic analgesia. The patients remained responsive throughout the procedure.

Table I. CT Stereotaxy

Patients: 100 in 30 months	
Biopsy/drainage/catheter placement	87
Electrode placement	9
Endoscopy	1
Functional	
Thalamotomy	1
Cingulotomy	2
Complications	
Hematomas	1
Symptomatic	
Asymptomatic	3
(one burr hole enlarged for control of cortical bleeding)	
Infections	0

At the time of CT scanning, the potential burr hole site was marked with a hypodermic needle and the location of the hypodermic needle as it entered the skull was used as one target and the potential biopsy, lesion, or electrode site as another target. Scanning was done either on a GE 8800 CT scanner or a Siemens Somatom DR3 scanner. The scan coordinates of each rod on the localizer ring and the target were entered into a HP-41CV hand-held computer which defined the AP, lateral, and vertical location of the targets in relation to the head ring. Using the location of the proposed burr hole site, as calculated, one could then calculate the appropriate angles on the arc system to allow the trajectory to the final target.

Biopsy/Drainage

A total of 88 biopsies or drainage procedures were performed in 87 patients. The primary purpose of biopsy was for tissue diagnosis to follow the therapeutic scheme as listed in table II. The biopsy consisted of multiple fragments comprising a core of tissue the diameter of the biopsy forceps (1 or 2.7 mm) times the length of the passage of the forceps through the tumor (10–20 mm). Frozen sections were performed on the initial specimens and, when definite tumor was identified, fur-

Table II. Therapy scheme

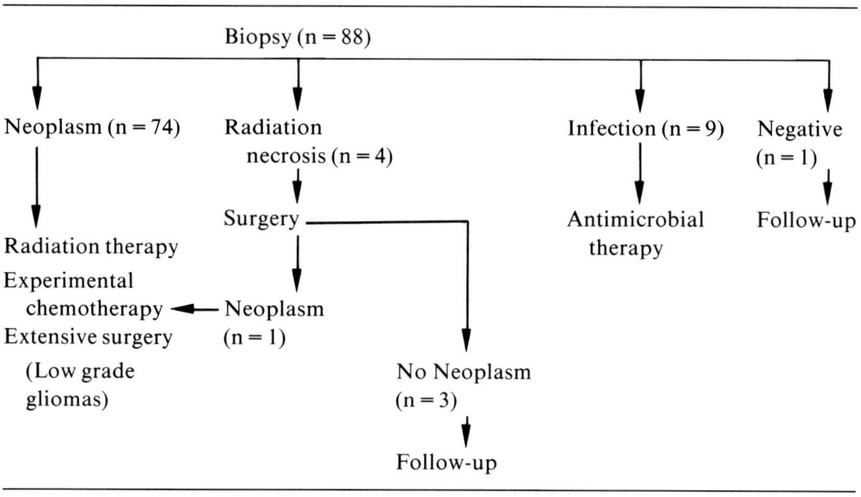

ther specimens were saved for permanent sections. When infection was suspected, a gram stain was immediately done and if organisms were seen, no biopsy taken. If organisms were not seen, then the walls of the cystic cavity were biopsied for possible tumor. It was important in cysts suspected to be tumors to biopsy first, so as to not change the target in relation to the burr hole. In the immediate postoperative period a CT scan was performed to document the location of the biopsy. In all cases, CT scan revealed that the biopsies were at the target. Only one nondiagnostic biopsy was performed. This was in the case of suspected metastatic disease. The CT done several months later revealed complete resolution of the lesions with steroid therapy.

The complications listed in table I occurred only in the patients who had undergone biopsies. Attempted removal of a pituitary tumor with a rotary dissector caused one of the hematomas which remained asymptomatic. Two additional asymptomatic hematomas involved lesions close to the cortex, and in both bleeding occurred from cortical vessels – one into a cystic cavity after fluid had been evacuated. Bleeding ceased spontaneously. In the second, bleeding required enlargement of the burr hole and coagulation of subcortical vessels. One additional patient with a deep lesion bled into the biopsy site. Postoperative CT scan revealed the hematoma; the patient remained alert through the procedure and postoperatively. The hematoma was evacuated at the time of more extensive surgery for a low grade glioma. The left upper extremity remained plegic from the hemorrhage and the surgery.

Endoscopy

Only one successful endoscopy has been performed in the case of tumor growing into the ventricle. The endoscopy is performed utilizing a 6.5 mm diameter Stortz operating hysteroscope with a straightforward telescope, and parallel viewing eyepiece. Both rigid and flexible instruments are used. It is best to have a laser available, either Argone or Nd:YAG. The endoscope is not efficient in the case of solid tumors within the brain, as one cannot discriminate tumor using the present system.

Electrode Placement

Table I lists 9 cases of bilateral electrode placement into orbitofrontal cortex, amygdala, and hippocampus through a bilateral frontal burr hole approach. The target points are located on the CT scan, which is performed using contrast to allow for visualization of the middle cerebral artery. The electrodes are then passed approximately 1 cm beyond the target point. There is some recoil as the electrode passer is withdrawn from the target. Postoperative CT scans have confirmed good electrode placement and there have been no surgical complications.

Functional Surgery

A thalamotomy was performed for an intractable movement disorder, very likely of vascular origin, in a patient with a midbrain AV malformation. This was the only procedure that had to be done under general anesthesia because of the severity of the dyskinesia. Although presenting as bilateral dyskinesia it had started initially on one side and was still worse on that side. Therefore, only a unilateral thalamotomy was performed. The target site selected was 9 mm anterior to the posterior commisure and 12 mm lateral to the midline and 8 mm above the intercommissural plane. The scanner was positioned to allow a cut through the intercommissural plane. A point 9 mm anterior to the posterior commissure was marked off using the cursor control on the CT scanner and the scanner was advanced to raise the target 8 mm above the intercommissural line. The target was then marked off 12 mm from the midline. A side outlet thermocouple stereotactic electrode with a 5×1.85 mm active tip was passed through the burr hole to the target site. Stimulation was carried out which showed driving of the tremor. With appropriate direction of the stereotactic electrode and use of the side outlet, there was no indication of contact with the internal capsule. The lesion was made over approximately a 6 mm path with complete control of tremor, which has persisted for well over a year. Two cingulotomies have also been performed for pain with good localization of the cingulotomy from postoperative CT scans.

Discussion

Initial experience with the Brown-Roberts-Wells CT stereotactic guidance system would indicate this to be a simple and accurate method of obtaining biopsies of deep neoplasms. The risk of hemorrhage appears to be very small and mainly confined to lesions which are close to the cortex where cortical vessels are involved. The tissue tension of the brain appears to provide enough pressure to control bleeding that may occur from small vessels. The procedure is also safe from the standpoint of infection and requires only a small sterile area and small incision. It is also much more cost effective than an open biopsy for tissue diagnosis.

References

1 Apuzzo, M.L.J.; Sabshin, J.K.: Computed tomographic guidance stereotaxis in the management of intracranial mass lesion. Neurosurgery *12:* 277–285 (1983).
2 Heilbrun, M.P.; Roberts, T.S.; Pauzzo, M.L.J.; Wells, T.H., Jr.; Sabshin, J.K.: Preliminary experience with the Brown-Roberts-Wells computerized tomographic stereotaxic guidance system. J. Neurosurg. *59:* 217–222 (1983).

Allan B. Levin, MD, University of Wisconsin Hospital, Division of Neurological Surgery, 600 Highland Avenue, Madison, WI 53792 (USA)

Proc. 9th Meeting World Soc. Stereotactic and Functional
Neurosurgery, Toronto 1985
Appl. Neurophysiol. *48:* 50–60 (1985)

A New Apparatus for CT-Guided Stereotactic Surgery

H. Iseki, K. Amano, H. Kawamura, T. Tanikawa, H. Kawabatake, M. Notani, T. Shiwaku, Y. Iwata, T. Taira, H. Nagao, Y. Umezawa, T. Shimizu, K. Kitamura

Department of Neurosurgery, Neurological Institute, Tokyo Women's Medical College, Shinjuku-ku, Tokyo, Japan

Key Words. Stereotactic surgery · Computed tomography · Magnetic resonance imaging · CT stereotaxis · Intracerebral hematoma

Abstract. Combining whole-body CT scan with a stereotactic system, the authors have developed and applied clinically an apparatus which readily provides intraoperative CT images, making it possible to confirm the location of the target point and ascertain the intraoperative environment. It takes about 9 s to obtain a CT image. Our purpose is to make stereotactic surgery, a kind of blind surgery, as safe and reliable as a visualized procedure by intraoperative CT scanning. By the method, in which there is very little invasion under local anesthesia, evacuation of deep-seated intracerebral hematomas as well as brain abscesses and also biopsy or brachytherapy of brain tumors in the brain can be done with safety and reliability.

Introduction

In 1947, *Spiegel and Wycis* [18] presented the first stereotactic apparatus for operation on the human brain. Since then, several stereotactic systems have been devised and stereotactic surgery has been established as the main surgical therapy for such brain functions as intractable pain [1–4], involuntary movement and epilepsy.

Recently, however, since *L*-dopa was developed, medical therapy has been predominant in areas such as Parkinson's disease. Moreover, there are fewer and fewer cases of involuntary movement or intractable pain in which the usual neuroablative stereotactic therapy is needed. On the other hand, a CT scanner, which provides a precise reference to intracranial morbid anatomy, has made remarkable progress during the past few years. It has also been applied to stereotactic operations for cerebral tumors, intracerebral hematomas, cerebral abscess and others which previously could not be treated surgically because of their deep location. CT-guided stereotactic surgery is now becoming the foremost method of surgery.

There are two kinds of CT-guided stereotaxis: (1) CT used just for measuring in order to define the target point, which is otherwise not very different from the former stereotactic surgery practiced in an operating room [5–11, 14]; (2) the use of an apparatus improved or newly developed for CT to perform an operation in a CT room, confirming by CT during operation the relative locations of the needle point and such deep-seated lesions as hematomas. Ours belongs to the latter kind [12, 13, 17].

First, we improved the Todd-Wells apparatus so it might be suitable for CT. We reduced the artifacts displayed on CT, to enable viewing of the lesion accurately by CT with the head fixed to the apparatus. However, if we want to insert the needle into the target point by use of Todd-Wells, it is necessary to move the head from side to side and back and forth, and thus the head cannot be positioned in the center of the CT gantry at all times. Consequently we were unable to use a smaller scanning field, which was needed in order to improve the accuracy of measurement. Therefore, a new apparatus was devised, by use of which the lesion can be approached by three-dimensional movement of the needle inserter, with the head being fixed in the center of the CT gantry (fig. 1).

We applied the use of this apparatus and an Archimedes' screw in the operation for evacuation of deep intracerebral hematomas of 67 cases with satisfactory results.

Outline of the Apparatus

Head Frame

In order to minimize the artifact as much as possible, the metal head frame was replaced by a carbon fiber one. The forehead and parieto-occipital region were fixed by either a carbon fiber rod with an embedded artificial ruby pin as necessary, to prevent inclination of the head. The head frame itself was attached to the carbon fiber base, to reduce artifacts displaced on the CT (fig. 1). Moreover, it was designed so that the angles of incidence and depression could be varied by about 6°

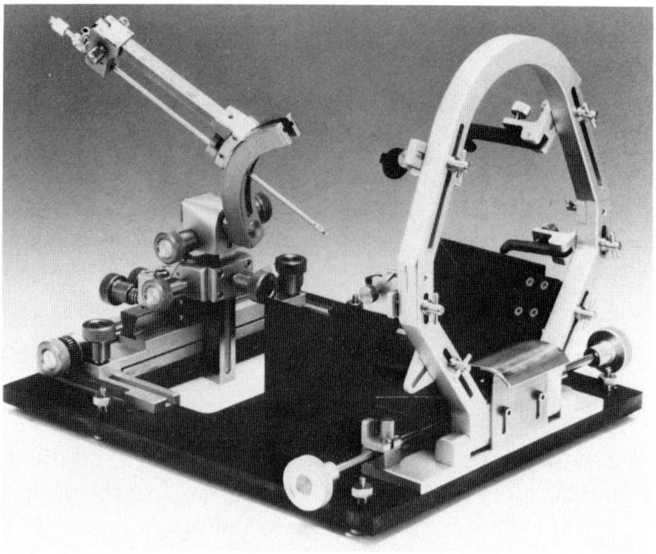

Fig. 1. An apparatus for CT-guided stereotactic surgery.

with the head fixed, so we were able to choose freely the safest trajectory during operation. As a result, the region of interest was extended for operations on deep brain lesions.

Needle Inserter

Attached to the carbon fiber base is a support allowing three-dimensional movement from the origin: 50 mm on the X axis (right and left), 90 mm on the Y axis (fronto-occipital), and 90 mm on the Z axis (rostrocaudal). A semicircular arm is attached to the vertical degrees in the X–Y plane, along which the needle inserter may traverse through 90°.

Target Measuring Markers

Metallic tubes with a diameter of 0.5 mm were used to measure the target during surgery. The midline marker showing the origin of the X coordinate was embedded along the center line of the carbon fiber base. The horizontal marker showing the origin of the Z coordinate (a leaden rod 10 mm in length) were set on a carbon fiber plate mounted in the X–Z plane bilaterally.

a

b

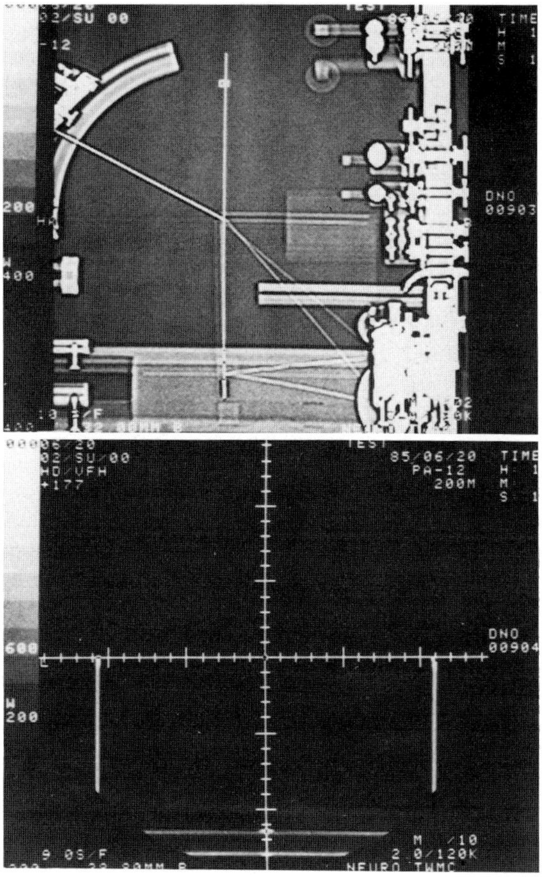

Fig. 2. Phantom lateral scanogram **(a)** and CT image **(b)** at 0 point.

Measuring Method for CT-Guided Stereotactic Surgery

Determination of the Position of the Z Axis

A lateral scanogram is photographed using the whole-body CT scan (Toshiba TCT 60A). Thus the head is scanned on the basis of the obtained scanogram, when the base line for scanning is set in accordance with the origin of the Z axis with the aid of ROI (region of interest). The optimal number of scanning slices is determined; consecutive CT scans are carried out with 10-mm wide slices. Use of 2- or 5-mm slice widths will, of course, result in increased accuracy in the Z axis.

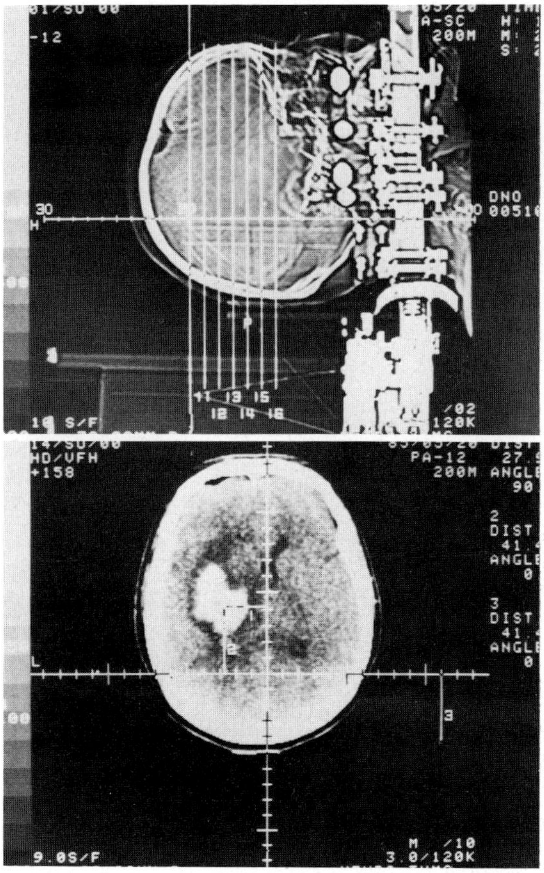

a

b

Fig. 3. Lateral scanogram **(a)** and CT image **(b)** of the target.

The slice of the CT scan containing the target is determined, that is, if the fifth slice from the origin contains the target point and each slice is 10 mm wide, then 50 mm is the distance to the target point. After the distance of the Z axis is measured in this way, the X and Y coordinates are determined (fig. 2).

Determination of the X and Y Coordinates

On the basis of the CT scan image on the determined Z axis, the distances from the origins of the X and Y coordinates to the target point are measured in the same way as the Z axis. The support for the needle inserter is moved according to the measurements in the X, Y and Z coordinates. In this apparatus the distance between the center of the globe formed by the semicircular arm and the zero point of the needle inserter is kept constant at 285 mm. Therefore the distance to the final target point is calculated by subtracting the effective length of the needle from 285 mm (fig. 2).

Method of Operation

A frontal burr hole is made in the operating room. The patient is moved to the CT room and his head is fixed to the stereotactic apparatus, which is already attached to the CT bed. During operation under neuroleptanalgesia (NLA), the blood pressure is kept at a maximum of about 80% of the normal systolic pressure, trimethaphan being used if necessary.

A lateral scanogram is photographed, the optimal slice number from the marker of the Z axis is determined, and a serial CT scan is performed (fig. 3a). One CT image is chosen as the target. With the origin markers of the X–Y coordinates referred to, the intersecting point of the cross is located on the TV display by the use of ROI, and the distance to the target point (X_T, Y_T) is determined (fig. 3b). The distance from the origin of the Z axis (Z_T) is that between the zero point and the slice containing the target. Subsequently, the effective real length of the screw for aspiration of hematoma is measured (external diameter 4 mm). The distance of insertion to the target point (D_T) is found by subtracting this from 285 mm, which is between the target point and the zero point of the needle inserter. According to the obtained values (X_T, Y_T, Z_T), the support for the needle inserter is moved left and right, back and forth, and up and down. The screw for aspiration of hematoma is inserted through the previously made burr hole and advanced to the target (D_T). A lateral scanogram is taken for confirmation by photographing three CT slices: the slice with the target point in it, plus the preceding and succeeding ones (each 10 mm width).

The lateral scanogram (fig. 4a) shows that the screw points coincide with the target slice. The artifact in the center of the hematoma is the screw point (fig. 4b). Figure 4c was taken after the 22-ml hematoma was aspirated. As the CT scan is performed intraoperatively, it is possible to confirm the aspiration of the hematoma. Figure 5c shows the CT

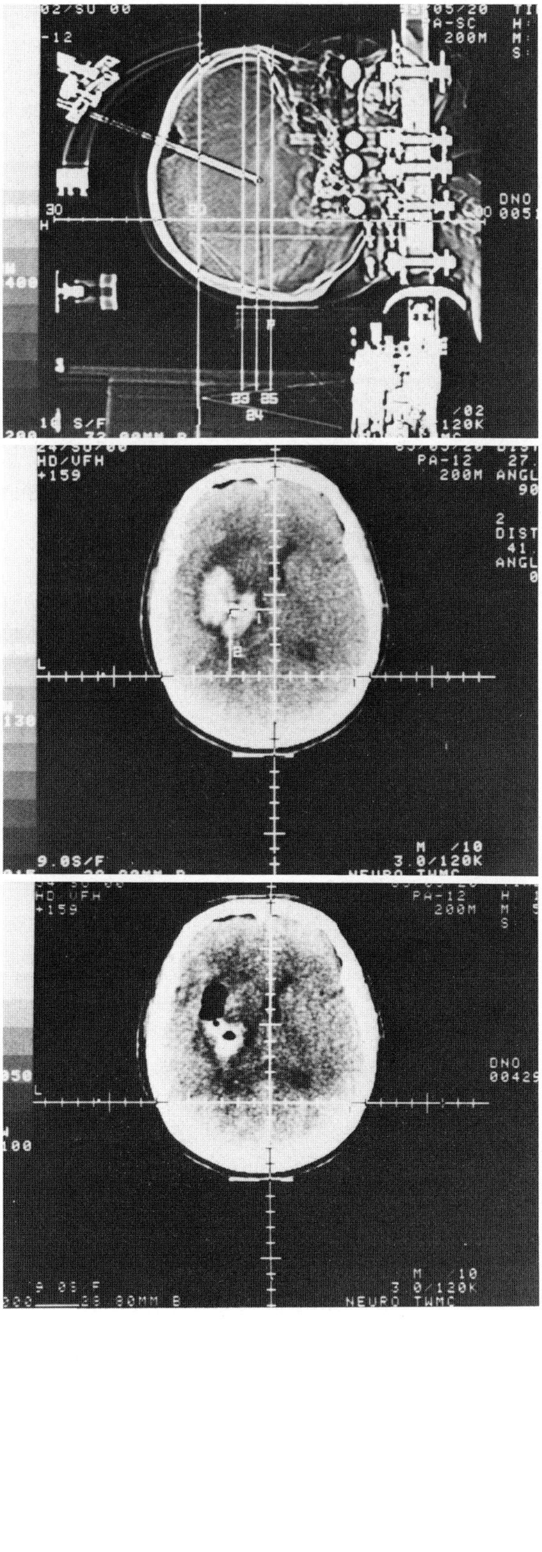

a

b

c

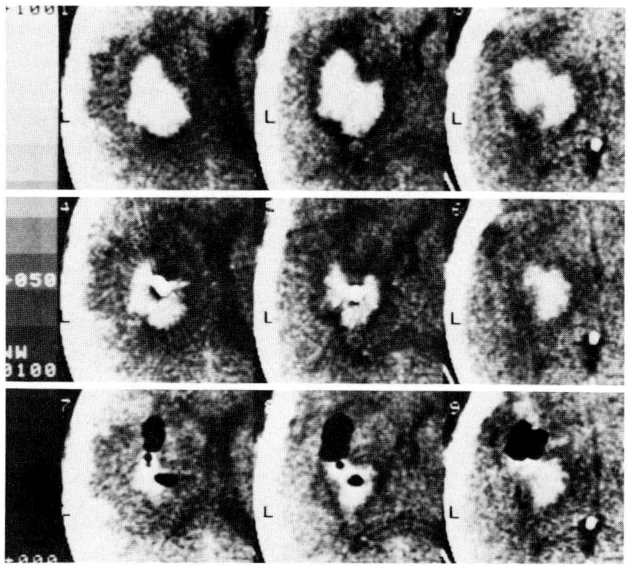

a

b

c

Fig. 5. Serial CT images: **(a)** preoperative state; **(b)** intraoperative state; **(c)** post-operative state.

images just after operation. Compared with the upper scans, it is clearly seen how the hematoma has been aspirated and the displacement of the ventricular system has been improved. The dissolved component of the hematoma can be removed just by aspiration, but the clot is hard to remove. The drain may be left in the hematoma cavity after aspiration of the dissolved component to irrigate with urokinase [9, 16], but it is necessary for several days to prevent the drain from moving and guard against infection caused by releasing the drain. A method of aspiration using a motor driving at a constant pressure is also reported [14]. To aspirate the clot component of hematoma more safely and easily, the use of an Archimedes' screw is effective. Based on the report of *Higgins* et al. [11] and our own experience, it is possible to prevent the clot from plugging up the screw, and the clot can also be

---

Fig. 4. Intraoperative lateral scanogram **(a)** and postoperative CT image **(b)** at the target point. **(c)** CT scan taken after the 22-ml hematoma was aspirated.

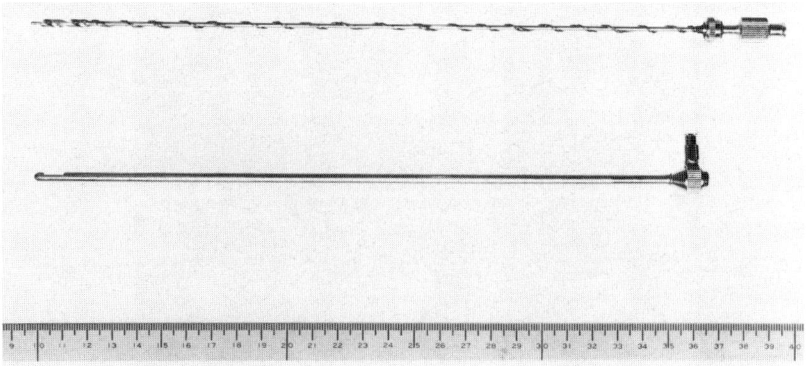

Fig. 6. A new type of Archimedes' screw.

aspirated more safely and effectively if it is irrigated with normal saline solution.

We have designed a new type of Archimedes' screw which is capable of both aspiration and irrigation at the same time. The middle of the screw is made of a tube, so that the normal saline solution can be injected. There are four side holes at the tip of the pipe. It looks like a twist drill as the wire is wound spirally around its outer circumference (fig. 6). By utilizing this apparatus, many surgical treatments can be performed with safety and reliability in evacuation of the deep-seated intracerebral hematoma as well as brain abscess and also biopsy or brachytherapy of brain tumors.

Discussion

In comparison with the ordinary craniotomy, by which an operation is performed under general anesthesia, stereotactic brain surgery can be performed under local anesthesia, resulting in much less invasion and may be applied even to poor risk patients. It is, however, still blind surgery. Therefore it is important to check the intraoperative state indirectly as often as possible. The usual stereotactic surgery is performed on the basis of ventriculography. Stereotactic surgery, which is performed in a CT room and guided by CT provides more information about the intraoperative state because of intraoperative CT scanning.

The MRI stereotactic frame relates to MRI images [15], which are different from CT images. Correspondingly, we are also examining the clinical application of MRI CT-guided stereotactic apparatus.

The treatment for hypertensive intracerebral hematoma is broadly divided into two categories – a conservative therapy and a surgical operation. Our method of aspiration of hematomas by stereotactic surgery lies between these two. Accordingly, the indications for stereotactic surgery differ from the usual criteria of operative intervention for hematomas. It also applies to the patient group which would ordinarily be treated by conservative therapy because of the high risk of surgery. One must think anew of improvement in functional prognosis. Thus it is considered useful to aspirate a small hematoma by our method with minimum invasion, for by doing so the secondary change caused by the mass effect of hematoma pressing on local tissue is prevented.

Acknowledgements

This work was awarded of the Japan Medical Association Grant-in-Aid for 1983 and the Ministry of Education, Science and Culture Grant-in-Aid for 1983–1984.

References

1 Amano, K.; Tanikawa, T.; Iseki, H., et al.: Single neuron analysis of the human midbrain tegmentum. Rostral mesencephalic reticulotomy for pain relief. Appl. Neurophysiol. *41:* 66–78 (1978).

2 Amano, K.; Notani, M.; Iseki, H., et al.: Homovanillic acid concentration of third ventricular CSF before and after electrical stimulation of the midbrain central gray and the periventricular gray in human; in Hitchcock, Modern concepts in psychiatric surgery (Elsevier, Amsterdam 1979).

3 Amano, K.; Kitamura, K.; Kawamura, H.; Tanikawa, T.; Kawabatake, H.; Notani, M.; Iseki, H.; Shiwaku, T.; Suda, T.; Demura, H.: Alterations of immunoreactive beta-endorphin in the third ventricular fluid in response to electrical stimulation of the human periaqueductal gray matter. Appl. Neurophysiol. *43:* 150–158 (1980).

4 Amano, K.; Tanikawa, T.; Kawamura, H., et al.: Endorphins and pain relief. Further observations on electrical stimulation of the lateral part of the periaqueductal gray matter during rostral mesencephalic reticulotomy for pain relief. Appl. Neurophysiol. *45:* 123–135 (1982).

5 Backlund, E.O.; Holst, H. von: Controlled subtotal evacuation of intracerebral hematomas by stereotactic technique. Surg. Neurol. *9:* 99–101 (1978).
6 Boëthius, J.; Bergström, M.; Greits, T.: Stereotaxic computerized tomography with a GE 8800 scanner. J. Neurosurg. *50:* 715–720 (1979).
7 Broseta, J.; Gonzalez-Darder, J.; Barcia-Salorio, J.L.: Stereotactic evacuation of intracerebral hematomas. Appl. Neurophysiol. *45:* 443–448 (1982).
8 Brown, R.A.: A computerized tomography-computer graphics approach to stereotaxic localization. J. Neurosurg. *50:* 715–720 (1979).
9 Doi, E.; Moriwaki, H.; Komai, N.; Iwamoto, M.: Stereotactic evacuation of intracerebral hematomas. Neurol. med. Chir., Tokyo *22:* 461–467 (1979).
10 Gildenberg, P.L.; Kaufman, H.H.; Murthy, K.S.K.: Calculation of stereotactic coordinates from the computed tomographic scan. Appl. Neurophysiol. *45:* 443–448 (1982).
11 Higgins, A.C.; Nashold, B.S.; Cosman, E.: Stereotactic evacuation of primary intracerebral hematomas; new instrumentation. Appl. Neurophysiol. *45:* 438–442 (1982).
12 Iseki, H.: CT-guided stereotactic surgery – application to evacuation of intracerebral hematoma. Neurol. Surg., Tokyo *12:* 663–672 (1984).
13 Iseki, H.; Amano, K.: CT-guided stereotactic surgery in combination with intraoperative monitoring by sector type ultrasonography. Asian med. J. *28:* 157–167 (1985).
14 Kandel, E.I.; Peresedov, V.V.: Stereotaxic evacuation of spontaneous intracerebral hematomas. J. Neurosurg. *62:* 206–213 (1985).
15 Leksell, L.; Leksell, D.; Schwebel, J.: Stereotaxis and nuclear magnetic resonance. J. Neurol. Neurosurg. Psychiat. *48:* 14–18 (1985).
16 Matsumoto, K.; Hondo, H.: CT-guided stereotaxic evaluation of hypertensive intracerebral hematomas. J. Neurosurg. *61:* 440–448 (1984).
17 Perry, J.H.; Rosenbaum, A.E.; Lunsford, L.D.; Swink, C.A.; Zorub, D.S.: Computed tomography-guided stereotactic surgery; conception and development of a new stereotactic methodology. Neurosurgery *7:* 376–381 (1980).
18 Spiegel, E.A.; Wycis, H.T.; Marks, M.; Lee, A.: Stereotaxic apparatus for operations on the human brain. Science *106:* 349–350 (1947).

H. Iseki, Department of Neurosurgery, Neurological Institute, Tokyo Women's Medical College, Kawada-cho 10, Shinjuku-ku, Tokyo (Japan)

Proc. 9th Meeting World Soc. Stereotactic and Functional
Neurosurgery, Toronto 1985
Appl. Neurophysiol. *48:* 61–68 (1985)

Use of the Brown-Roberts-Wells Stereotactic Frame for Functional Neurosurgery

Mark N. Hadley, Andrew G. Shetter, M. Rob Amos

Divisions of Neurological Surgery and Neuroradiology, Barrow Neurological Institute, Phoenix, Ariz., USA

Key Words. Stereotactic surgery

Abstract. The Brown-Roberts-Wells (BRW) stereotactic unit has proven itself to be a highly accurate instrument for biopsying or locating pathologic intracranial lesions based on CT scan information. We utilized the BRW frame to select 18 target sites in 12 patients undergoing functional stereotactic procedures. Two patients had bilateral cingulumotomies, 5 had thalamotomies for movement disorders, and 5 underwent electrode implantations for the treatment of chronic pain. Stereotactic frame settings were determined using a positive contrast ventriculogram, orthogonal radiographs, and a computer program provided with the BRW system. In addition, attempts were made to select targets based on CT scan landmarks alone, and these were compared to those derived using ventriculography.

We found the BRW frame to be a satisfactory device for performing functional neurosurgical procedures based on ventriculographic landmarks. Coordinates derived from CT scans were similar to those obtained with ventriculography, but were not accurate enough to permit the use of CT scanning as the sole means of target identification. Although future improvements in imaging techniques and computer software are likely to occur, our experience supports ventriculography as the current method of choice for the precise localization of functional targets with the BRW stereotactic system.

Introduction

The Brown-Roberts-Wells (BRW) stereotactic system has become well established as an effective device for accurately directing an instrument, biopsy needle or cannula into a brain target selected on a computerized tomographic (CT) scan image. Less well known and less extensively documented is the ability of this system to perform functional stereotactic surgery utilizing conventional radiographs and posi-

Table I. Functional neurosurgical procedures performed in 14 patients

Patients	Target	Number
1 EJ	cingulum	2
2 NP	cingulum	2
3 EF	VL thalamus (R)	1
4 JK	VL thalamus (L)	1
5 KJ	VL thalamus (R)	1
	zona inserta (R)	1
6 VT	VL thalamus (R)	1
	zona inserta (R)	1
7 DC	VL thalamus (R)	1
	zona inserta (R)	1
8 BV	VL thalamus (R)	1
	zona inserta (L)	1
9 MH	PVG (R)	1
10 JL	PVG	2
11 JT	PVG (R)	1
12 CT	PVG (L)	1
13 WM	PVG (R)	1
14 MB	SST (R)	1
	Total	21

tive contrast ventriculography. We report our experience over a 3-year interval using a BRW frame in a group of patients undergoing functional stereotactic procedures. Lesioning or stimulating electrodes were inserted using coordinates derived from ventriculographic anatomy and the Schaltenbrand atlas [4]. In addition, identical targets were independently selected from CT scan anatomy alone and attempts were made to compare the results obtained with the two methods.

Methods

Our series comprised 21 separate target points in 14 patients (table I). Two patients had bilateral cingulumotomies for a pain syndrome and obsessive-compulsive behavior respectively, 6 patients had radiofrequency lesioning of the zona inserta and/or ventro-

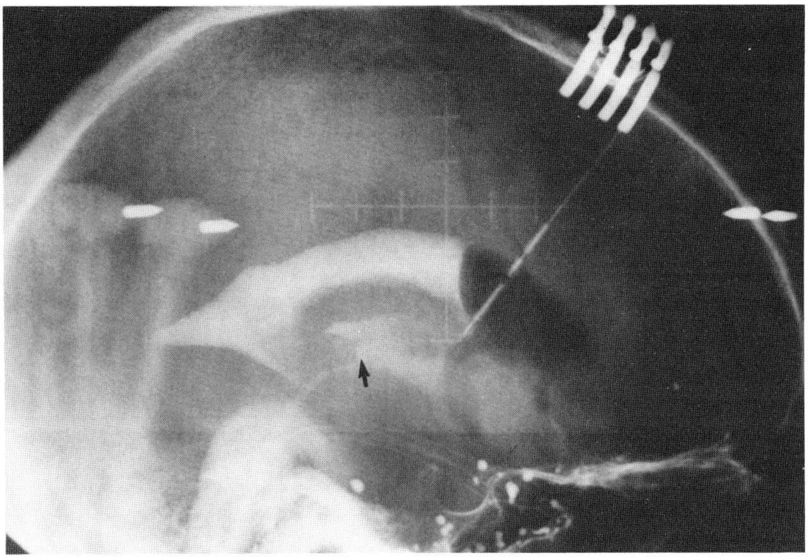

Fig. 1. Positive contrast ventriculogram (lateral projection) demonstrating ventricular anatomy. Periventricular gray electrode target site (black arrow).

lateral thalamus for movement disorders, and 6 patients underwent placement of stimulating electrodes in the periventricular gray or somatosensory thalamus for the treatment of chronic pain.

The BRW frame was applied and utilized in accord with the manufacturer's instructions [3]. An air or metrizamide ventriculogram was performed and a desired target point was selected on AP and lateral radiographs (fig. 1). The distance between the target and a reference reticule on the frame was measured in millimeters in the AP, lateral, and vertical planes, and this information was entered into a hand-held computer programmed with the 'BRWF' software package. AP, lateral, and vertical stereotactic target coordinates were generated, defining a discrete point in stereotactic space within an imaginary cylinder surrounding the patient's head. An entry point on the scalp was then selected and additional computer calculations were made to derive the arc assembly settings necessary to pass a probe to the desired brain target through the entry point. The remainder of the operation was carried out in standard fashion, including the use of physiologic monitoring before final electrode placement of radiofrequency lesioning.

In 10 patients, CT scans were performed prior to ventriculography with the BRW localizer assembly in place. This information was stored on computer tape, and at a later date an attempt was made to select a target site on an appropriate CT slice that was identical to the target selected from ventriculographic anatomy. The targets were chosen by careful study of the CT images in axial and reconstructed sagittal planes with particular reference to the location of the anterior and posterior commissures for thalamic targets

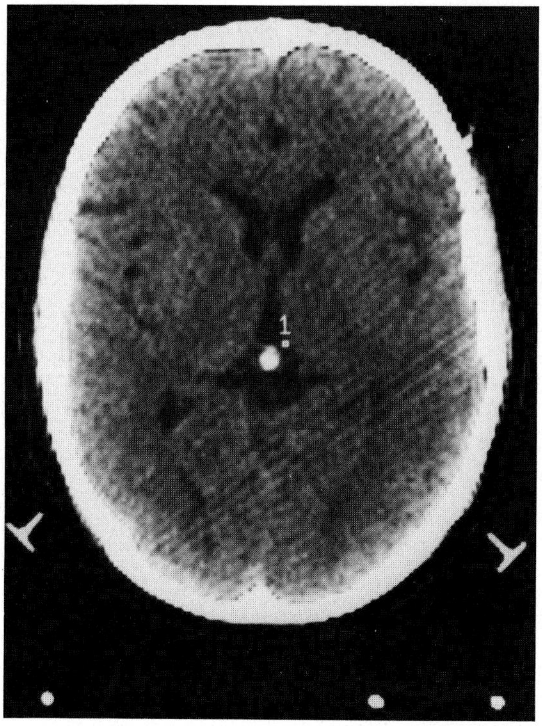

Fig. 2. CT scan depicting PVG electrode target site localization (1), lateral to the third ventricle just anterior to the posterior commissure.

and the frontal horns of the lateral ventricles for cingulum targets (fig. 2). Anteroposterior, lateral, and vertical stereotactic coordinates were calculated for the CT scan selected target using the 'BRWT' software program [1, 2]. A point in stereotactic space was thereby defined which could be directly compared to a similar point derived from ventriculographic anatomy.

Results

Functional stereotactic surgery using the BRW frame and positive contrast ventriculography was successfully completed in all instances. It was possible to consistently place an electrode with 1 mm accuracy into any designated location. Our prior experience had been with the

Table II. Target localization comparison between ventriculogram and CT scan techniques

Procedure		Ventriculogram		CT scan	CT vs. ventriculogram (mm)	
Cingulumotomy	1	AP	- 5.6	-12.8	posterior by	7.2
		LAT	- 8.4	- 8.2	medial by	0.2
		VERT	23.4	15.5	inferior by	7.9
	2	AP	- 5.6	-13.3	posterior by	7.7
		LAT	5.6	1.9	medial by	3.7
		VERT	23.4	15.9	inferior by	7.5
Ventrolateral thalamotomy	1	AP	17.6	-17.6	posterior by	0.2
		LAT	10.6	12.2	medial by	1.6
		VERT	-18.5	-13.3	superior by	5.2
	2	AP	-18.5	-16.7	anterior by	1.8
		LAT	13.2	17.3	lateral by	4.1
		VERT	-34.6	-32.5	superior by	2.1
	3	AP	-19.8	-18.0	anterior by	1.8
		LAT	-12.7	-13.7	lateral by	1.0
		VERT	-12.0	-11.3	superior by	0.7
Zona inserta lesions	1	AP	-23.6	-23.9	posterior by	0.3
		LAT	10.8	12.1	lateral by	1.3
		VERT	-20.6	-17.4	superior by	3.2
	2	AP	-25.4	-25.4	–	
		LAT	12.7	16.4	lateral by	3.7
		VERT	-40.2	-35.3	superior by	4.9
	3	AP	-24.9	-25.9	posterior by	1.0
		LAT	-10.8	-12.0	lateral by	1.0
		VERT	-18.9	-15.5	superior by	3.4
PVG electrode implants	1	AP	-18.8	-17.9	anterior by	0.8
		LAT	- 2.3	- 1.9	medial by	0.4
		VERT	-30.6	-31.7	inferior by	1.1
	2	AP	-11.6	-11.6	–	
		LAT	- 6.5	- 5.1	medial by	1.4
		VERT	-10.2	- 9.3	superior by	0.9

Table II (continued)

Procedure	Ventriculogram			CT scan	CT vs. ventriculogram (mm)	
PVG electrode implants	3	AP	-15.7	-17.0	posterior by	1.3
		LAT	0.9	1.5	lateral by	0.6
		VERT	- 4.6	- 1.5	superior by	3.1
	4	AP	-30.0	-28.2	anterior by	1.8
		LAT	0.0	2.4	lateral by	2.4
		VERT	7.4	9.8	superior by	2.4
	5	AP	-12.5	-14.9	posterior by	2.4
		LAT	0.0	0.5	lateral by	0.5
		VERT	-12.9	-13.4	inferior by	0.5

Todd-Wells instrument, and we found the BRW frame to be equally simple and rapid to use.

The BRW system can also be utilized in conjunction with the CT scanner, making it feasible to compare target points selected from both CT scan and ventriculographic anatomy. This was done for 13 targets, and the results are summarized in table II.

For cingulumotomy target localization, the coordinates we derived from CT scan images were on average 7.3 mm posterior, 2.0 mm medial and 7.7 mm inferior to the targets derived from the positive contrast ventriculograms. The ventrolateral thalamotomy targets derived from CT images were on average 1.1 mm anterior, 2.2 mm lateral and 2.6 mm superior to the targets selected based on ventriculographic anatomy. CT determined zona inserta targets were 0.4 mm posterior, 2.1 mm lateral and 3.4 mm superior to corresponding targets determined by standard ventriculographic means. Lastly, periventricular gray target coordinates derived from CT images were 0.5 mm posterior, 0.7 mm lateral and 1.0 mm superior to the ventriculogram targets.

Discussion

Numerous stereotactic frames are available that permit accurate placement of an electrode into the brain guided by orthogonal radiographs and ventriculography. Our experience indicates that the BRW stereotactic unit is another device capable of yielding satisfactory results using this standard technique. Newer stereotactic systems, including the BRW device, can also direct an electrode to a brain target selected by CT scan imaging alone, thus raising the possibility that functional stereotactic surgery could be performed without resorting to ventriculography.

CT scan guided functional stereotaxis might have certain advantages over the conventional method. It would avoid the small risk of hemorrhage associated with insertion of a ventricular catheter, and it would obviate the need for injecting air or an iodinated contrast material which may distort ventricular anatomy and produce side effects of meningismus or seizures. Perhaps more importantly, CT scans directly image relevant neural structures in an individual patient while the ventriculographic method relies on indirect means to identify neural targets which are based on statistical averages. CT scans, however, may lack sufficient resolution to locate very small targets due to the effects of volume averaging. This is particularly true with thicker CT scan slices. In addition, it can be difficult to precisely identify the location of the desired neural target since standard reference points such as the anterior and posterior commissures may not be present together on a single CT scan slice and since stereotactic atlases based on CT scan anatomy are not widely available.

Functional stereotactic surgery using ventriculographic landmarks is a proven technique which has been refined over several decades of use. We felt it was important to compare this approach with CT scan directed stereotaxis in a critical fashion before considering its abandonment for a newer method. Thirteen target points were selected using both techniques, and although the final results were similar, there were certain discrepancies (table II). The correlations between the two methods were closest for PVG electrode implantation where the target was near a readily identifiable landmark (the posterior commissure) which could be seen on a single CT scan slice. Ventriculographic and CT derived coordinates were most divergent for cingulumotomy lesions due to our inability to accurately define the most anterior and superior aspects of the frontal horns of the lateral ventricles and then display that data on one CT scan image. The application of three-dimensional CT scan software and the development of atlases referenced to extraventricular structures which could be seen on CT scan images might help with these problems.

It is important to keep in mind that our comparisons involved stereotactic target points rather than the ultimate clinical outcome that would have occurred using either method. All lesions and electrode placements were performed during ventriculographic guidance (modified by physiologic monitoring if necessary), and it is possible that the CT scan selected targets might have given equal or superior results. Nevertheless, our experience suggests caution in utilizing CT scanning as the sole means of target identification and we continue to employ ventriculography as the current method of choice for performing functional stereotactic surgery with the BRW system. It seems likely, however, that additional experience and technical advances will ultimately eliminate the need for ventriculography. MRI scanning appears particularly promising in this regard since it provides excellent differentiation between gray and white matter structures and can obtain images in any plane without loss of resolution. A modified BRW frame for use with the MRI scanner is being developed, and should provide an opportunity for future research in this area.

References

1 Apuzzo, M.L.; Sabshin, J.K.: Computed tomographic guidance stereotaxis in the management of intracranial mass lesions. Neurosurgery *12:* 277–285 (1983).

2 Heilbrun, M.P.; Roberts, T.S.; Apuzzo, M.L.J.; Wells, T.H., Jr.; Sabshin, J.K.: Preliminary experience with Brown-Roberts-Wells (BRW) computerized tomography stereotaxic guidance system. J. Neurosurg. *59:* 217–222 (1983).

3 Heilbrun, M.P.; Roberts, T.S.; Wells, T.H., Jr.; Ball, R.E.; Cosman, E.R.: Instruction manual for the BRW Brown-Roberts-Wells CT stereotaxic system (Radionics, Burlington, Mass. 1983).

4 Schaltenbrand, G.; Wahren, W.: Atlas for stereotaxy of the human brain; 2nd ed. (Thieme, Stuttgart 1977).

Mark N. Hadley, MD, Division of Neurosurgery, Barrow Neurological Institute, 350 W. Thomas Road, Phoenix, AZ 85013 (USA)

Proc. 9th Meeting World Soc. Stereotactic and Functional
Neurosurgery, Toronto 1985
Appl. Neurophysiol. *48:* 69–72 (1985)

A True 'Advanced Imaging Assisted' Skull-Mounted Stereotactic System

Mark Carol

Bassett Hospital, Divison of Neurosurgery, Cooperstown, NY, USA

Key Words. CT stereotaxis · Stereotactic surgery

Abstract. A stereotactic system has been designed based upon a series of interlocking discs secured to the skull with self-tapping screws. Unlike previous skull-mounted systems, this system is a true, advanced imaging based stereotactic device with the capabilities and accuracy of more traditional, frame based devices. It has been used in a range of applications, from simple biopsies to interstitial radiation implant procedures. Well tolerated by the patient, it allows reaccess to the intracranial target without rescanning. It is convenient for the physician to utilize, both mechanically and timewise, is adaptable to MRI, DSA, and conventional X-ray techniques without modification, and is affordable.

With the precison in CNS imaging which has occurred as a result of CT, MRI, DSO and because of its inherent low mortality, morbidity, and hospital stay, stereotactic surgical procedures are fast becoming the diagnostic and therapeutic procedures of choice for many disorders involving the intracranial cavity. Unfortunately, a wide variety of factors, including system cost and complexity, have limited the use of stereotactic surgical procedures in private neurosurgical practices, a fact which may cause patients unnecessary risk and harm by subjecting them to more traditional procedures which may not be in their best interest.

A system has been designed with these concerns in mind, based upon the skull-mounted approaches of the early 50s. The resultant approach, which allows for true 2-coordinate imaging space to 3-coordinate stereotactic space data transfer, is compact, easy to use, precise, reappliable without the need for coordinate recalculation, relatively inexpensive, and portable.

The system, manufactured by MEDCO, consists of three main

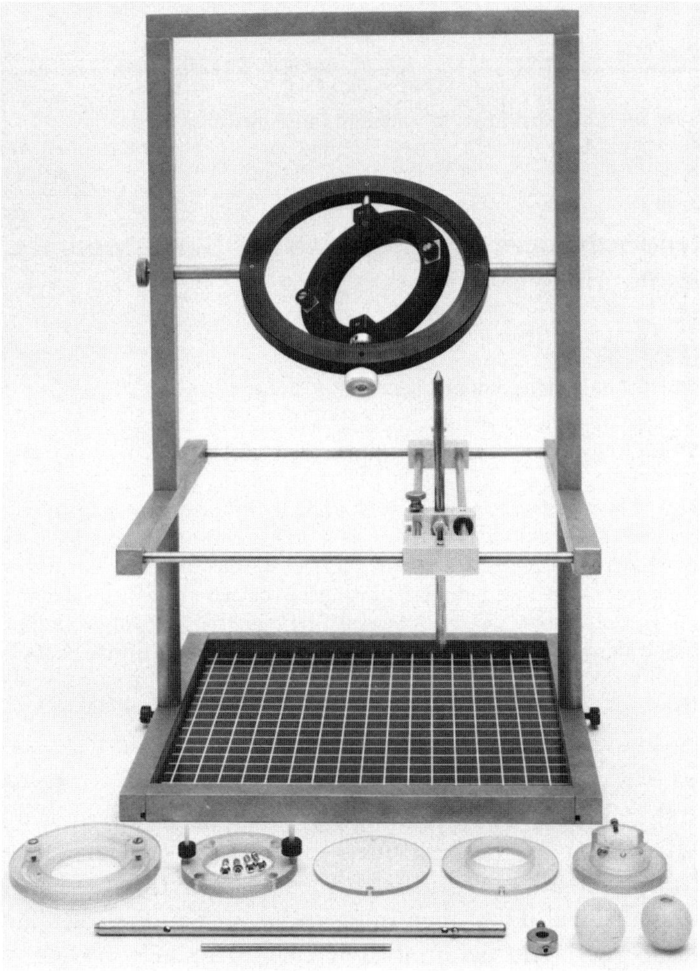

Fig. 1. Phote of gyrantom and skull mount pieces.

components; a skull set, a modified phantom-type device called a gyrantom, and a table mount (fig. 1). The single patient use skull set consists of a series of 2½ inch lexan discs. The primary disc blank is secured to the skull, and a secondary disc, with an arm extending from a ball and socket unit, can be secured to either the primary disc or the gyrantom (fig. 2). The gyrantom, in addition to having the ability to move a target around in three-dimensional space common to all stereotactic phantoms, has the unique ability, through two rotatable rings, to duplicate the slope of the skull at the site of skull set attachment.

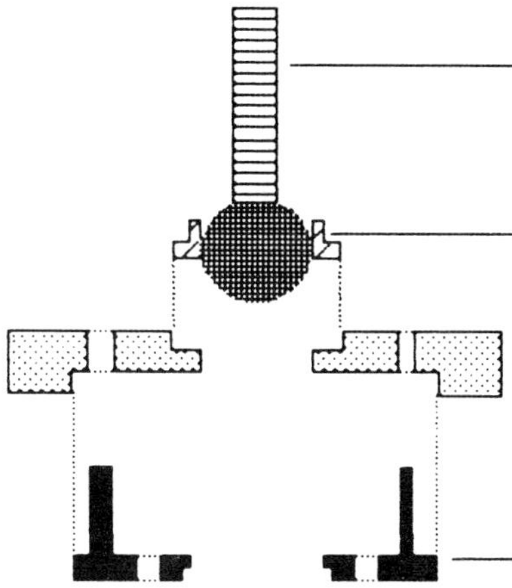

Fig. 2. Blowup of skull mount.

Briefly, the skull set is secured to the skull under local anesthesia by two self-tapping cancellous bone screws, and the secondary plate is applied over the primary plate. The patient is then secured to the imaging table via the table mount. The mating of the guide rod with the table mount insures that the skull set arm is orthogonal to the table. The patient is imaged, and the relative location of the target with respect to the position of the skull set as seen on the images is generated by the imager after appropriate cursor placement. The x and y offsets are read directly off the screen; the z offset is equal to the table displacement for the target slice minus the table displacement for the marker slice, values listed on the appropriate slices. The secondary plate is then transferred to the phantom where the arm is brought to lie orthogonal to the plane of the phantom by rotation of the rings. Target location is simulated on phantom, and the trajectory and depth for target intersection through the rotatable ball is determined. The ball is locked in position, a depth stop on the probe set appropriately, and the secondary plate, after sterilization, is transferred back to the skull. Surgery is performed by drilling a hole in the skull using the ball as a guide and then passing the appropriate biopsy instrument to the predetermined depth.

The system, rather than imposing a fixed frame external to the skull to establish the coordinate frame of reference, reproduces on the phantom an arbitrary relationship between the skull and the imaging table. This arbitrary orthogonal relationship is established by bringing the arm of the skull set into the plane of the table and locking it there. It is reproduced on the phantom by virtue of the rotating planes, which allow the skull set to be rotated until it can mate orthogonally with the phantom itself. It is reestablished on the patient by transferring the secondary plate, with its locked ball indicating trajectory, back to the skull. What this in essence accomplishes is the replacement of the imaging table to the phantom, maintaining at all times the orientation of the skull set on the skull to the target.

The system has several desirable characteristics. It can be used in CT, MRI or DSA with minor modifications and will support supra- or infratentorial approaches. Spinal cord applications are also possible. Computer programs or imaging equipment modifications are not required for target coordinate generation. The imaging suite and OR do not need to be tied up for extended periods of time. We apply the skull set in the outpatient department for 5 min, scan the patient, and then take the patient back to OPC for a 5 to 10 min biopsy procedure. In instances where delays or emergencies arise, the actual procedure can be done either later in the day or on a separate day altogether. Because the target trajectory is retained by the locked position of the ball in the secondary plate, which is a single patient item, the skull set can be removed and reapplied at a later date. Phantom testing has shown a reproducible accurary of 1 mm, suggesting that sensitive areas can be biopsied and interval access accomplished without reimaging. An accessory has been developed, which replaces the ball in order to allow lineal movement along the x and y axes, providing volume access and parallel trajectory access to intracranial lesions for biopsying tumor removal or radiation implants without redetermining coordinates. It also supports stereotactic-guided craniotomy Finally, the portability of the system makes it easy to use in a variety of settings.

Based upon our initial experience with this system, it appears that it may be a useful alternative to more complicated systems in settings where an accuracy of not less than 1 mm is required. Our hope is that less complicated and less expensive systems such as this may allow a greater number of patients and physicians alike to benefit from the low risk, high yield procedures which have resulted from the marriage of advanced imaging systems and stereotaxis.

M. Carol, Bassett Hospital, Division of Neurosurgery,
Cooperstown, NY, 13326 (USA)

Proc. 9th Meeting World Soc. Stereotactic and Functional
Neurosurgery, Toronto 1985
Appl. Neurophysiol. *48:* 73–76 (1985)

An Applicability Study on a CT-Guided Stereotactic Technique for Functional Neurosurgery

T. Asakura, K. Uetsuhara, R. Kanemaru, K. Hirahara

Department of Neurosurgery, Faculty of Medicine, Kagoshima University,
Usuki-cho, Kagoshima City, Japan

Key Words. Biopsy · CT-guided stereotaxy · Functional neurosurgery · Stereotactic surgery

Abstract. When a CT-guided stereotactic technique for functional neurosurgery is adopted, extremely precise targeting is needed to obtain satisfactory surgical results. In this study the authors have investigated the accuracy of the target points determined by CT-guided techniques and compared with those of conventional roentgenographically controlled stereotactic procedures.

Stereotactic surgery, employing the Brown-Roberts-Wells (BRW) system, was performed contemporarily 26 times in 23 patients, that is, 9 times in 8 patients for functional neurosurgery using with the roentgenographic method, and 17 times in 15 patients with the CT-guided method only for intracranial neoplasm biopsy. As a result, there were no problems of accuracy of determining the target points by CT-guided stereotactic surgery with the BRW system. When applying this technique for functional neurosurgery, it should be pointed out that there could be a discrepancy within 2 mm from the conventional target determination.

Introduction

Recent advances in technology have provided a technique for CT-guided stereotactic procedures which is already widely applied for intracranial neoplasm biopsy and hematoma evacuation. When this technique is used for functional neurosurgery, an extremely precise targeting is needed to obtain a satisfactory surgical result and to avoid surgical complications. The authors have investigated the accuracy of the target points determined by CT-guided techniques and compared them with those of conventional roentgenographically controlled stereotactic procedures.

Table I. Summary of the cases who underwent stereotactic operation (1984–1985)

Method	Case	Operation
Rentogenographic	8	9
CT-guided	15	17
Total	23	26

Material and Method

Method

A Brown-Roberts-Wells (BRW) apparatus was employed with a GE 8800 whole-body CT scanner. The BRW system includes two calculating programs: one is for CT-guided stereotactic surgery and the other is for functional surgery. A head ring is first applied to the patient's head under local anesthesia and then a localizer ring is attached to it. The coordinates of the target point and the nine carbon rods of the localizer ring are calculated, recorded and displayed on the CT screen. A line through the anterior and posterior commissures and a target point, determined on a lateral projection film taken after positive contrast thin ventriculography with metrizamide, are referred to the image scales. Finally, the angles and the depths of the probe insertion to the target point through the cranial the cranial entry point are calculated for both programs.

In both the conventional and CT-guided method, the target points, that is, the location of the tip of the probe, should be set up and confirmed with the arc system mounted on the phantom base ring before application to the patient's brain. When the conventional method is applied, the zero point of the phantom base corresponds to the intersecting point of the reticulated scale.

Material

Stereotactic surgery employing the BRW system was performed 26 times in 23 patients, that is, 9 times in 8 patients for functional neurosurgery along with the roentgenographic method, and 17 times in 15 patients with the CT-guided method only for intracranial neoplasm biopsy (table I).

Results

(1) CT-guided stereotactic biopsy for intracranial neoplasm: For neoplasm biopsy, there have been no problems in accuracy and no complications in the surgical procedures.

(2) Functional neurosurgery with roentgenographic control: In 8 cases, for 9 functional neurosurgical procedures, both conventional

and CT-guided methods were carried out coincidentally and compared with each other:

(a) *Axial CT images:* When comparing the two methods, it is important to get a horizontal CT image presenting the AC-PC line. Therefore, the authors have studied the angle of the scan by comparing the X-ray film taken with conventional radiography with the ScoutView of the CT scan. The study led us to adopt the angle of 11 + 1° to Reid's baseline. Thus, when the CT scan is performed at 5-mm intervals at this angle, the AC-PC line will be shown at least in one slice.

(b) *The thickness of the slices:* Although 6 consecutive scans of 5-mm slices were made at first, it was reformatted at 2 mm to acquire a scan accurately including the AC-PC line for the determination of the target point.

(c) *The CT-guided target point versus the conventional method:* The CT-guided point was later actually calculated by determination with conventional ventriculographic control. It seemed to be almost identical in most cases.

(d) *The discrepancy between target points determined by two methods:* There is little discrepancy of target points in a few cases, usually less than 2 mm.

Discussion

Despite the attempt at accuracy in the determination of target points in both conventional and CT-guided methods, there can be a little discrepancy between the points calculated with each method, because of (1) the thickness of CT slices; (2) partial volume phenomena in CT images, and (3) pathoanatomical factors of brains.

Some attempts were made to avoid the discrepancy and improve accuracy: (1) AC-PC line reconstruction: Although reformatted, sagittal images were obtained from 12 horizontal scans at 2 mm, the resolution of which is apparently less than that of conventional ventriculograms. (2) Using MR imaging for the AC-PC line is not yet possible because of the problem of metal frames.

The remaining discrepancy of 2 mm could be improved technically by employing (1) micromanipulation, (2) electrophysiological identification stimulation, (3) a curved tip or looped electrode, and (4) coagulation of a 2 mm diameter or greater.

Conclusion

(1) There were no problems of accuracy to determine the target point by CT-guided stereotactic surgery with the BRW system. (2) It was found that the AC-PC line crossed Reis baseline at an angle of 11 + 1°, and therefore it is important to obtain at CT image including the AC-PC line at this angle. (3) When applying the CT-guided stereotactic procedure for functional surgery, it should be pointed out that there could be a discrepancy of up to 2 mm from the conventional target determination.

Dr. T. Askura, Department of Neurosurgery, Faculty of Medicine, Kagoshima University, 1208 1 Usuki-Cho, Kagoshima-Shi 890 (Japan)

Proc. 9th Meeting World Soc. Stereotactic and Functional
Neurosurgery, Toronto 1985
Appl. Neurophysiol. *48:* 77–78 (1985)

Simultaneous Recordings in the Human Thalamus and Cortex of an Early Evoked Component

D. Albe-Fessard, R.R. Tasker, K. Yamashiro, J. Chodakiewitz, J. Dostrovsky

Key Words. Evoked potentials · Stereotactic surgery · Thalamus · Cortex

Abstract. Evoked potentials have been simultaneously recorded in 9 patients at thalamic and scalp cortical levels. The similarity of wave characteristics at both levels seems to demonstrate the origin in a thalamic near-field of the P14–16 cortical wave. A thalamic origin of at least a part of N18–20 is also indicated.

It has been stated that the cortical positive potential evoked by radial nerve stimulation and having a peak latency of 14–16 ms has its origin in a near-field potential from the thalamic ventral posterior nucleus [1, 2].

Evoked thalamic potentials were recorded in 9 patients during stereotactic surgery performed for the relief of abnormal movements or pain syndromes. They were compared to the scalp evoked activities recorded during operation. In 4 of these patients, electrodes were left in place at the ventralis posterior level for subsequent therapeutic stimulation, and both cortical and thalamic events were observed during different states of alertness. Such a recording is presented in figure 1.

In all the studied cases, the thalamic evoked potential had the same peak latency as the cortical one (fig. 1). The potential onset latencies were also similar, with the cortical often slightly preceding the other (0.2–0.5 ms). Progressive increases in nerve stimulation have shown similar thresholds and amplitude evolutions of both cortical and thalamic events. All these facts support the P14–16 cortical event being produced by a thalamic field.

Some questions are still open: The thalamic evoked activity had in general a longer duration than the associated cortical one. Are there

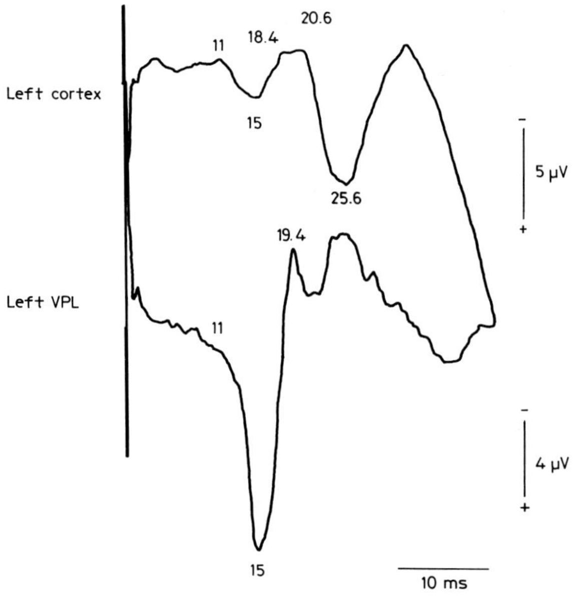

Fig. 1. Responses recorded on scalp (left-hand area) and in left ventralis posterior after right median nerve stimulation. Mean responses to 100 successive stimulations given once every second. Reference electrode for cortex and thalamus on the left ear lobe. Latencies of main events noted in milliseconds.

corresponding cortical components to these late thalamic activities? In particular, at the thalamic level (recordings always being made with reference to a distant electrode), a negative wave follows the positive (fig. 1). Its latency is in the range of the negative events present in cortical hand area (N18–20). In consequence, this last wave must have a part of its origin in a thalamic near-field.

References

1 Mauguière, F.; Brunon, A.M.; Echallier, J.F.; Courjon, J.: Early somatosensory evoked potentials in thalamo-cortical lesions of the lemniscal pathways in humans; in Courjon, Mauguière, Revol, Advances in neurology, vol. 32, pp. 321–338 (Raven Press, New York 1982).
2 Tsuji, S.; Shibasaki, S.; Kato, M.; Kurowa, Y.; Shima, F.: Subcortical thalamic and cortical somatosensory evoked potentials to median nerve stimulation. Electroenceph. clin. Neurophysiol. *59:* 465–476 (1984).

Proc. 9th Meeting World Soc. Stereotactic and Functional
Neurosurgery, Toronto 1985
Appl. Neurophysiol. *48:* 79–80 (1985)

Advantages of Computerized Tomography-Assisted Interaction during Stereotactic Procedures Using Computer-Generated Graphics

Roy A.E. Bakay, James C. Hoffman, Michael Rhodes

Emory University Clinic, Atlanta, Ga., USA

Key Words. Stereotactic procedures · Brain biopsy · Image reconstructions · Three-dimensional assessment

In most CT-stereotactic procedures, the patient is taken to the scanner suite where coordinates are obtained, and then returned immediately to the operating room. While this is most advantageous for a variety of complex procedures, simple procedures such as biopsies and implantations can be readily performed in the CT suite with the advantage of persistent CT interaction capabilities.

We use a Multiplanar stereotactic frame (Howland Ind.) and software to produce simultaneous axial, coronal, and sagittal reconstructions allowing a three-dimensional assessment of the target image. A simulated stereotactic trajectory can then follow the proposed pathway millimeter by millimeter from entry point to target and project that point in all three projections simultaneously. This insures that vital structures are not injured during the procedures. High dose contrast immediately prior to scanning distinctively outlines the main vascular structures. Improperly selected trajectories are readily identified in the CT suite and appropriate correction can be made preoperatively.

In addition to biopsies, a variety of implantations for epilepsy localization, deep brain stimulation, and brachytherapy have been performed. The reconstructions give excellent tumor geometry in relationship to catheter probes for calculation of dosimetric curves. The demonstration of normal neuroanatomic resolution is so good that electrodes can be placed in mesial temporal structures without the need for contrast in the temporal horns. CT scanning after placement of implanted devices allows for immediate anatomical confirmation and correction of aberrant trajectories intraoperatively and without subjecting the patient to a second procedure.

As CT-assisted procedures get more complex, the need for image manipulations becomes greater. The CT contribution to stereotaxis is the high anatomical resolution of the lesion, and the ability to accurately reproduce target location. CT image manipulation and transformation is the next logial step to use the sophisticated computer software to perform increasingly complex procedures safely, rapidly, and precisely.

R.A.E. Bakay, MD, Emory University Clinic, 1365 Clifton Road, N.E., Atlanta, GA 30322 (USA)

Proc. 9th Meeting World Soc. Stereotactic and Functional Neurosurgery, Toronto 1985
Appl. Neurophysiol. *48:* 81–82 (1985)

X-Ray Photogrammetry and Floating Line Concept Applied to Cerebral Probes Implantation

L. Cloutier[a], *D.N. Nguyen*[a], *P. Labissonnière*[a], *S.K. Ghosh*[b], *M. Boulianne*[b], *G. Bouvier*[c], *R. Béique*[c]

Departments of [a] Mechanical Engineering and [b] Photogrammetry, Laval University, Quebec, and [c] Hôpital Notre-Dame, Montréal, P.Q., Canada

Key Words. Floating line · Stereoscopy · X-ray photogrammetry · Three-dimensional viewing

This new apparatus can greatly help the neurosurgeon in such functional neurosurgical procedures as stereotactic biopsies, interstitial irradiation, chronic depth electrodes, surgery for abnormal movements, implantation of neurostimulator and implantation of canulae for drug injection. Its greatest advantages are accurate and reliable positioning of the probe and thus reduction of hemorrhages, opportunity to reach any cerebral zone from any convenient direction, easier determination of the potential path for introduction of probes, and compatibility with CT and NMR.

The method is based on the application of stereophotogrammetric techniques to radiographic images [1, 2]. The greatest novelty is a new device (fig. 1) allowing the simultaneous stereoscopic perception of the blood network with a movable pseudo-probe: the 'floating line'. An accuracy of around ±0.1 mm (SD) for each coordinate of any point on the object is obtainable. It permits accurate determination of a safe path for a probe implantation.

Control points on the stereotactic frame are visible on two stereoscopic angiographs. An optical system allows 3-D viewing of the arteries and veins. The probe simulator permits movement of the 'floating line', and an adequate path is identified for the probe. Appropriate

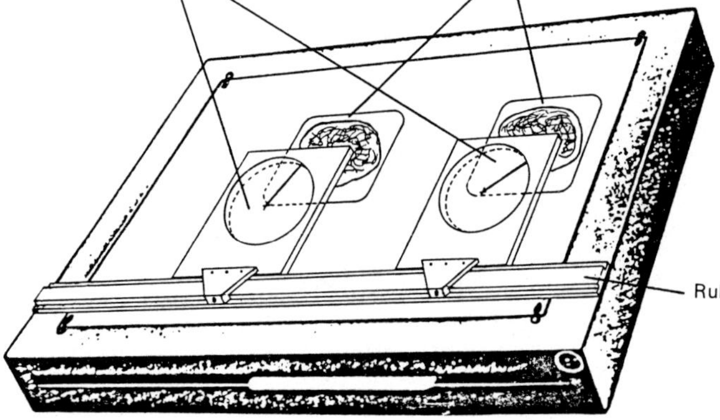

Fig. 1. Floating line device (prototype).

measurements and mathematical operations on the computer define the parameters to be set on the stereotactic frame for a given direction and length of the probe into the brain. That mathematical operation is rigorous and can lead to a standard error of less than ± 0.3 mm in regard to the probe position.

References

1 Boulianne, M.: Transformation d'une salle de radiographie conventionnelle en appareil de mesure; thèse Université Laval (1983).
2 Marcotte, P.: Elaboration d'une méthode de mesure spatiale à partir d'un principe photogrammétrique adapté aux rayons-X; thèse Université Laval (1984).

L. Cloutier, MD, Mechanical Engineering Department, Laval University, P.Q. Quebec, G1K 7P4 (Canada)

Proc. 9th Meeting World Soc. Stereotactic and Functional
Neurosurgery, Toronto 1985
Appl. Neurophysiol. *48:* 83–84 (1985)

The Modified Gouda Frame Interfaced with GE 8800 CT Scanner Used for Stereotactic Brain Surgery

Stephen R. Freidberg, Kasim Gouda, Carl Larsen, Richard Baker, Mark Silverman

Departments of Neurosurgery, Diagnostic Radiology and Pathology, Lahey Clinic Medical Center, Burlington, Mass., USA

Key Words. Gouda frame · CT scanner · Stereotactic brain surgery · Stereotactic thalamotomy

The original Gouda stereotactic frame [J. Neurosurg. *53:* 256, 1980] had been modified to adapt it to computed tomography (CT) guidance rather than ventriculography [Neurosurgery *13:* 176, 1983]. The present work describes a new frame based on the principles of the original but designed specifically to interface with CT. The principle of a movable arc whose target is the center of a sphere with an infinite number of radii is retained. A zero CT reference plane in all three axes, which corresponds to the zero plane on the frame, is established. A target point in the X, Y, and Z axes is chosen and its coordinates printed directly in millimeters directly on the CT screen. The coordinates can then be transferred directly to the frame and the biopsy made through a convenient burr hole. Mathematical calculations, atlases, or diagrams are not needed. The basic CT computer programs provide all of the necessary information with software modification. A model system has demonstrated that the frame is accurate to 1 mm.

We have performed 31 stereotactic biopsies since May 1981. Sixteen have been for gliomas in surgically inaccessible portions of the brain, deep hemisphere and corpus callosum. Three patients have had metastatic tumors. One patient thought clinically to have a glioma had a reticulum cell sarcoma. The biopsy on 1 patient revealed inflammatory tissue, a sterile abscess associated with Behçet's syndrome. On patient had infarction, 1 demyelination and 1 intraparenchymal sarcoid.

In 7 patients nondiagnostic cerebral tissue was present in the biopsy specimen. In 2 a tumor was found at craniotomy, a grade 2 astrocytoma and a glioblastoma. One patient with a small deep thalamic tumor had a prior V-P shunt and had brain collapse when the dura was opened thereby shifting the target. One patient's CT lesion subsequently cleared and she has been left with dementia. Presumably she had an inflammatory or vascular problem. In 3 patients the clinical and CT picture progressed without diagnosis. Two clinically had glioma and 1 metastatic disease. We have performed one stereotactic thalamotomy with the Gouda frame.

Stephen R. Freidberg, MD, Department of Neurosurgery, Lahey Clinic Medical Center, Burlington, MA 01805 (USA)

Proc. 9th Meeting World Soc. Stereotactic and Functional Neurosurgery, Toronto 1985
Appl. Neurophysiol. *48:* 85 (1985)

An Interactive Stereotactic Machine

Stephan J. Goerss, Patrick J. Kelly, Bruce Kall
Mayo Clinic, Rochester, Minn., USA

The stereotactic interactive machine is based on the arc-quadrant principle. The position, size, and orientation of the target are determined from CT and MRI scans. The head, fixed in a stereotactic headholder, is moved in three dimensions to bring the target to the focal point of the stereotactic arc-quadrant by activating servomotors mounted on each axis. The stereotactic position on each axis is determined by linear encoders providing a digital readout.

Two doubled gimballed arcs are used to orient all the instrumentation to the focal point. A 135-mm arc directs biopsy forceps, electrodes, and lesioning probes to targets selected from CT and MRI scans. It may also be used to implant radionuclide source carriers for interstitial radiation. A 400-mm arc orients a laser and surgical microscope to the focal point. An interactive joystick controls the motion of the laser beam and transmits its position to the operating room computer. The position of the laser is displayed on the operating room graphics monitor which guides the surgeon in the removal of deep-seated tumors.

S.J. Goerss, MD, Mayo Clinic, 200 First Street S.W., Rochester, MN 55 905 (USA)

Proc. 9th Meeting World Soc. Stereotactic and Functional
Neurosurgery, Toronto 1985
Appl. Neurophysiol. *48:* 86–88 (1985)

Open Stereotactic Excisional Surgery

E.R. Hitchcock

Department of Neurosurgery, University of Birmingham, Midland Center for Neurosurgery, Smethwick, Warley, Birmingham, UK

Key Words. Stereotactic imaging · Excision · Tumor · Angioma

The interface of stereotactic instrumentation with the CAT scan has facilitated tumour localization and subsequent management including cyst aspiration and tumour biopsy.

In recent years attempts have also been made to remove small gliomas by laser incorporated into the stereotactic instrumentation and using precise coordinates obtained by CAT scan. A number of attachments are available which are fixed after the stereotactic instrument has been applied in theatre and the patient transferred, with stereotactic instrument attached, to the scanning room. There are difficulties in arranging scan and theatre time and contamination of the stereotactic apparatus introduces the risk of infection (fig. 1, 2).

A stereotactic CAT scan interface device (SCID) has been designed to avoid these difficulties and has been used successfully over the past 3 years. Accurate lesion siting is possible and the instrument can be reapplied with exactitude. A variety of cysts and tumours have been aspirated and biopsied.

The simplicity of the method has also encouraged its use for the removal of small discrete lesions such as metastatic tumours from dangerous sites such as internal capsule or dominant hemisphere. After

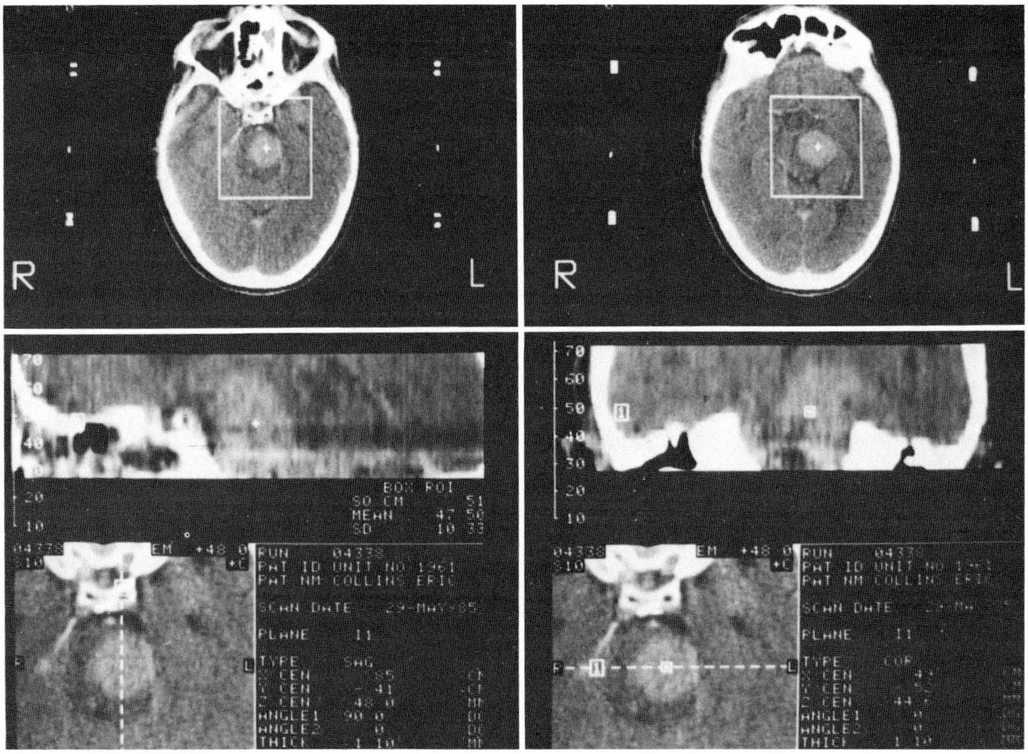

Fig. 1. The lesion is reconstructured in coronal and sagaital phases.

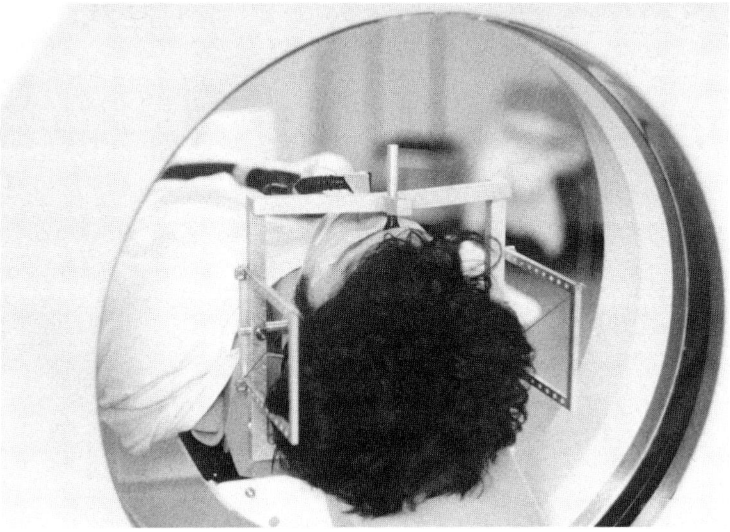

Fig. 2. The SCID applied to a patient during CAT scan.

the lesion has been localized using the SCID its coordinates can be found by simple arithmetic without need of computer or calculator. Subsequently these coordinates are used to localize the tumour which is approached via a small craniotomy or trephine. Tissue displacement is minimal and tumour identification is positive. Examples are given of its use for the removal of colloid cysts, gliomas, metastatic lesions and ventricular meningiomas.

E. Hitchcock, MD, Department of Neurosurgery;
Midland Centre, Holly Lane, Smethwick, B61 7JX Warley, (UK)

Proc. 9th Meeting World Soc. Stereotactic and Functional Neurosurgery, Toronto 1985
Appl. Neurophysiol. *48:* 89–90 (1985)

The Computer as a Stereotactic Surgical Instrument

Bruce A. Kall, Patrick J. Kelly, Stephan Goerss, Franklin Earnest
Mayo Clinic, Rochester, Minn., USA

Key Words. Computer-assisted surgery · Multimodality data base · Stereotactic software

We have developed the methodology and stereotactic software for an operating room computer system. This is useful to provide rapid transformation of pre- and intraoperative information into a form useful to the surgeon for treatment planning and interactively monitored and controlled neurologic surgery. This method replaces cumbersome mathematical and graphical methods for transposition of computed tomographic (CT), magnetic resonance (MR) and digital angiographic (DA) data into stereotactic space.

Patients undergo CT, MR and DA scanning with their heads fixed in a CT/MR/DA-compatible head-holder. Imaging compatible fiducial localization systems attach to the head-holder when each study is performed. This enables computer transposition of two-dimensional image coordinates into the three-dimensional stereotactic coordinate system of our custom arc-quadrant operating table. These imaging data are archived onto magnetic tape and transferred to our IPDC computer system adjacent to the operating room.

At the computer display console, the surgeon digitizes target points on CT and MR slices, confirms avascular trajectories on DA images and geometrically aligns substructures from a computer-resident stereotactic atlas within radiologically defined anatomical boundaries. In addition, contours of CNS lesions are circumscribed on serial CT and MR slices and are suspended by computer into a common three-dimensional image matrix. Intermediate contours are interpolated and all digitized and interpolated CT and MR contours are filled with 1-mm cubes to produce a composite solid volume. Every cube is encoded as originating from CT, MR or common to both modalities.

During surgery the computer rapidly reformats and displays cross sections of the computer-resident three-dimensional stereotactic data base on a graphics monitor in the operating room. The computer also monitors the position of stereotactically directed surgical instruments intraoperatively.

Two hundred and sixty computer-assisted stereotactic procedures have been performed at Mayo Clinic between July 1984 and June 1985. These include 154 biopsies, 71 CO_2 laser craniotomies, 6 third ventriculostomies, 5 ^{192}Ir interstitial implants, 5 Ommaya reservoir placements, 2 internal cyst diversions and 8 thalamotomies. Over 400 computer-assisted stereotactic procedures have been performed since January 1980.

Bruce A. Kall, MS, Section of Information Processing and Systems, Mayo Clinic, Rochester, MN 55905 (USA)

Proc. 9th Meeting World Soc. Stereotactic and Functional
Neurosurgery, Toronto 1985
Appl. Neurophysiol. *48:* 91–92 (1985)

Project of a Whole-Body Computerized Stereotactic Device

P. Nádvorník, J. Bolf, P. Mauerová

Department of Neurosurgery, Comenius University, Bratislava, CSSR

Key Words. Whole-body device · Stereotactic surgery

The programmed whole-body stereotactic device connected with the computer tomography enlarges the efficacy of stereotaxy for the need of other medical branches.

The contemporary trend to connect the stereotactic technique with investigation on the computer tomograph led to the idea of constructing a whole-body stereotactic device. The projected apparatus should meet the requirement of hitting accurately the determined target in the body along the chosen trajectory. The basic part of the device is a contrast bar, parallel with the plane of the body on its dorsal or ventral side. The bar is fixed in three points to the skeleton (alae ilica and sternum or processus spinosus C7) and carries a sliding bow-shaped segment with a holder of the probe. It is possible to slide the holder on the bow-shaped segment, so that it controls the whole cylindric space of the body (fig. 1). In addition, the holder can be deviated according the angles β, ψ and φ (fig. 2). The position of the probe is calculated by means of a special computer program.

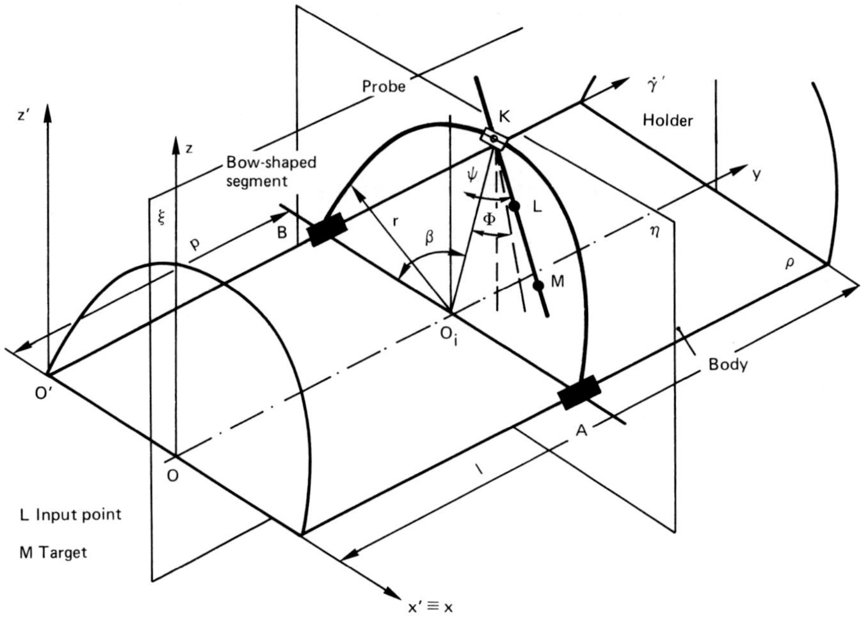

Fig. 1. Activity of the device.

$$\cos \beta = \frac{x_K}{\sqrt{x_K^2 + z_K^2}}$$

$$\beta = \text{arc} \cos (\cos \beta).$$

$$\cos \Psi = \frac{x_K(x_M - x_L) + z_K(z_M - z_L)}{\sqrt{x_K^2 + {}_K^2} \cdot \sqrt{(x_M - x_L)^2 + (z_M - z_L)^2}}$$

$$\Psi = \text{arc} \cos (\cos \Psi).$$

$$\cos \varphi = \frac{z_M - z_L}{\sqrt{(y_M - y_L)^2 + (z_M - z_L)^2}}$$

$$\varphi = \text{arc} \cos (\cos \varphi).$$

Fig. 2. Calculation of the angles.

P. Nadvornik, Department of Neurosurgery, Limbova 5, Bratislava 83305 (CSSR)

Proc. 9th Meeting World Soc. Stereotactic and Functional Neurosurgery, Toronto 1985
Appl. Neurophysiol. *48:* 93 (1985)

Functional Stereotactic Neurosurgery with Computerized Tomographic Guidance Using the Brown-Roberts-Wells Apparatus

I.M. Turnbull, D. Graeb, V. DaSilva

Divisions of Neurosurgery and Neuroradiology, University of British Columbia and Vancouver General Hospital, Vancouver, Canada

Key Words. Computed tomography · Sterotactic surgery

Using a Brown-Roberts-Wells stereotactic apparatus and a General Electric 9800 scanner, we have been able to use conventional ventricular landmarks as well as anatomical structures not visible on ventriculography for localization in functional neurosurgery. The subarachnoid space at the base of the brain provides a boundary that is not visible on plain X-ray images as does the internal capsule. The pineal gland becomes a key landmark once its size, shape and position have been visualized on a reformatted midsagittal image, likewise the aqueduct of Sylvius. Once the plane of the original CT cuts has been identified in relation to the intercommissural line, one may screen successive cuts, note anatomical details which label each slice and choose a cut that is judged to pass through the target, or one may reformat the intercommissural plane. If the plane of the scan is approximately parallel to the intercommissural plane, one may deposit a marker on a screened CT slice that identifies the X and Y coordinates and keep the marker in position while another slice with a different Z coordinate is screened.

The abundance of landmarks more than compensates for the fact that a particular structure, such as the anterior commissure, may not be sharply or unambiguously defined. The validity of this technique is illustrated with postoperative scans which show the size and location of stereotactic lesions and location of an implanted electrode's tip.

I.M. Turnbull, MD, FRCS, 700 West 10th Avenue, C Floor, Room 305, Vancouver, BC V5Z 4E5 (Canada)

Proc. 9th Meeting World Soc. Stereotactic and Functional Neurosurgery, Toronto 1985
Appl. Neurophysiol. *48:* 94–96 (1985)

Stereotactic System and Apparatus for Use with Magnetic Resonance Imaging, Computerized Tomography, and Digital Subtraction Imaging

A. Olivier, T. Peters, G. Bertrand

Montreal Neurological Institute and Hospital, Montreal, Que., Canada

Key Words. Stereotactic surgery · Digital subtraction angiography · Magnetic resonance imaging · Epilepsy · Brain tumors · CT stereotaxis · CT scanning

Abstract. A light-weight nonmagnetic, nonconductive instrument has been devised for use with magnetic resonance imaging, computerized tomography, and digital subtraction imaging for work in the field of epilepsy, brain tumors and vascular lesions. The apparatus' main characteristic is its ability to use optionally either the lateral orthogonal or the spherical-radial approach.

Introduction

Magnetic resonance imaging (MRI), computerized tomography (CT) and digital subtraction angiography (DSA) can all be used in the stereotactic management of seizure disorders and brain tumors as long as the stereotactic apparatus is versatile enough to handle this combined digitized information and to provide coordinates and various approaches to predetermined targets by the use of user-friendly computer programs. For several years we have tried to combine all these characteristics in a single apparatus and system [2–6].

Descripition of Apparatus

The apparatus is made of aluminum and plastic and is lightweight, nonmagnetic and nonconductive. Its main characteristic is the ability to use optionally either the lateral orthogonal approach of the

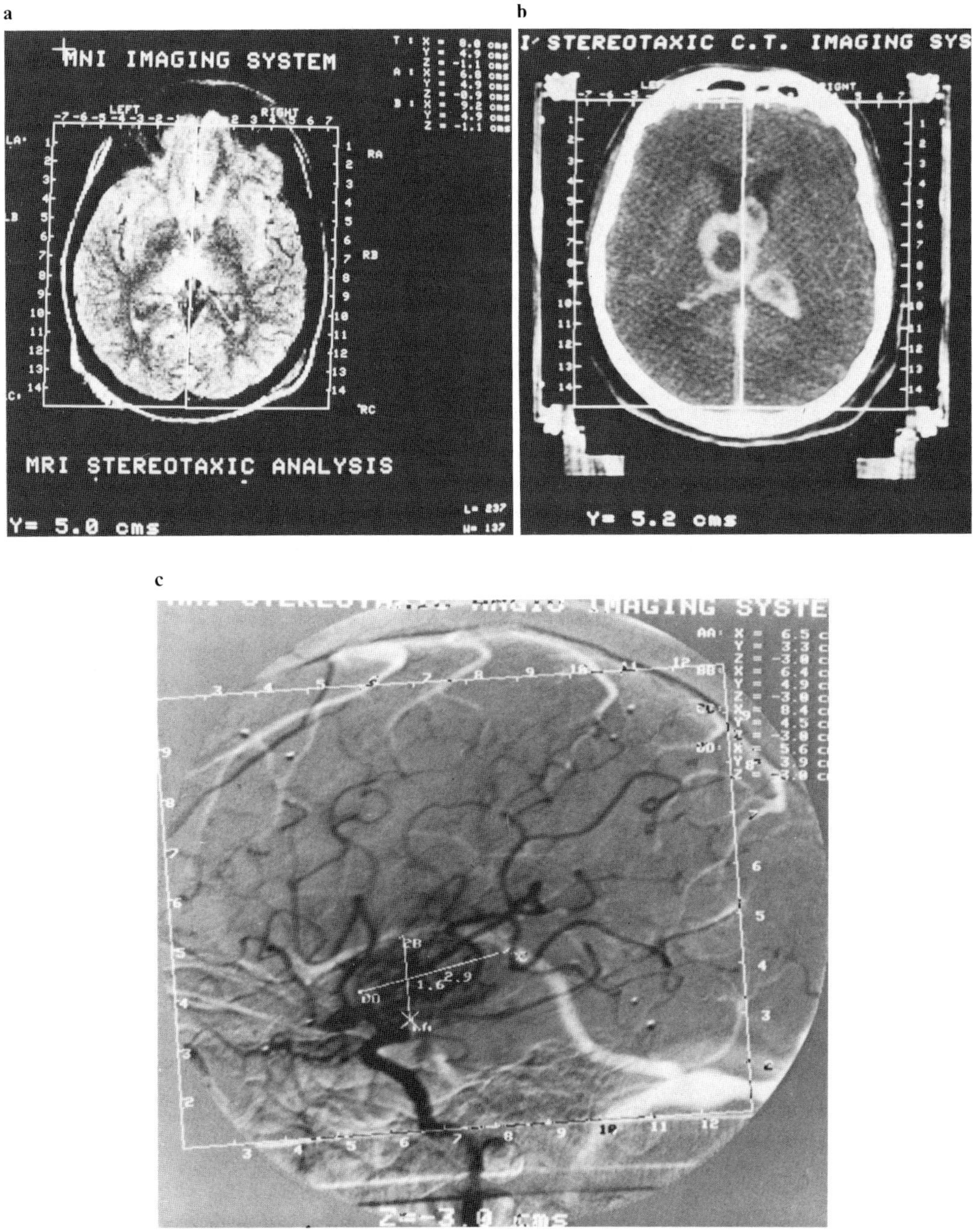

Fig. 1. Stereotactic studies with **(a)** MRI, **(b)** CT and **(c)** DSA.

Talairach system or the radial-sphere approach of Leksell. The lateral approach, which is more convenient for placement of multiple depth electrodes in epilepsy and for the management of brain tumors, is facilitated by the use of an orthogonal carrier.

The apparatus frame is equipped with interchangeable fiducial markers for MRI, CT and DSA. The plastic vertical posts and carbon fixation pins do not interfere with CT scanning. Its aluminum plastic construction makes it a nonmagnetic, nonconductive structure appropriate for MRI. Finally, its base bridges makes it possible to use markers for DSA.

It is thus possible with a single instrument to superimpose and correlate in various planes images of MRI, CT and both arterial and venous phases of the subtracted angiogram with user-friendly software programs (fig. 1). The frame can be replaced easily in the same position when used for a two-stage procedure, such as depth electrode placement. Finally, the frame characteristics make it compatible for radiotherapy of brain tumors and vascular lesions with a linear accelerator after *Betti's* [6] principle.

References

1 Betti, O.; Derechinsky, V.: Irradiation stéréotaxique multifaisceaux. Neurochirurgie *29:* 295–298 (1983).

2 Olivier, A.; Peters, T.M.; Bertrand, G.: Stereotaxic system for use with CT, DSA and MRI. Can J. neurol. Sci. (in press, 1985).

3 Olivier, A.; Peters, T.M.; Bertrand, G.; Vanier, M.; Feindel, W.; Ethier, R.: The role of MRI in stereotaxic surgery. Proc. Ass. Neurochirurgiens de la Province de Québec, Montreal 1985.

4 Olivier, A.; Peters, T.; Clark, J.; Mawko, G.; Winfield, J.: The role of digital angiography in stereotaxy. Proc. Réunion de l'Assoc. des Neurochirurgiens de Langue Française, Paris 1984.

5 Peters, T.M.; Olivier, A.: CT-aided stereotaxy for depth electrode implantation and biopsy. Can. J. neurol. Sci. (in press, 1985).

6 Peters, T.M.; Olivier, A.; Bertrand, G.: The role of computed tomographic and digital radiographic techniques in stereotactic procedures for electrodes implantation and mapping and lesion localization. Proc. Am. Soc. Stereotactic and Functional Neurosurgery, Durham 1983. Appl. Neurophysiol. *46:* 200–205 (1983).

A. Olivier, PhD, Montreal Neurological Institute and Hospital,
3801 University Street, Montreal, Que. H3A 2B4 (Canada)

Session II: Spasticity

Proc. 9th Meeting World Soc. Stereotactic and Functional
Neurosurgery, Toronto 1985
Appl. Neurophysiol. *48:* 97–104 (1985)

Microsurgical Selective Procedures in Peripheral Nerves and the Posterior Root-Spinal Cord Junction for Spasticity

Marc Sindou, Benaïssa Abdennebi, Paul Sharkey

Department of Neurosurgery, Hôpital Neurologique and UER Grange Blanche, University of Lyon, France; Department of Clinical Neurophysiology and Vivian L. Smith Foundation for Restorative Neurology, Institute for Rehabilitation and Research, Houston, Tex., USA

Key Words. Dorsal root entry zone lesions · Pain · Selective peripheral neurotomy · Selective posterior rhizotomy · Spasticity

Abstract. This review deals with the long-term results of selective peripheral neurotomy (SPN) of the tibial nerve and selective posterior rhizotomy (SPR) in 123 cases of severe spastic syndromes in the limbs. The microtechniques and peroperative electrostimulation for identification of the nervous structures responsible for the spastic components give to these methods an advantage of a substantial reduction of the harmful spasticity, without suppressing the useful muscle tone and impairing the residual motor and sensory functions. The results were effective, with a 1- to 13-year follow-up, in 89% of 47 SPN of the tibial nerve for spastic foot, in 92% of 53 SPR for paraplegia and in 87% of 23 SPR for hemiplegia.

Introduction

When spasticity in the limbs becomes severe and harmful in spite of physical and medical therapy, one can have recourse to functional neurosurgery. In such spastic disorders, on the condition that they are localized, a definite improvement can be achieved with microsurgical selective procedures applied to the corresponding peripheral nerves or posterior roots at their junction with the spinal cord, without suppressing the useful muscle tone or impairing the residual motor and sensory functions.

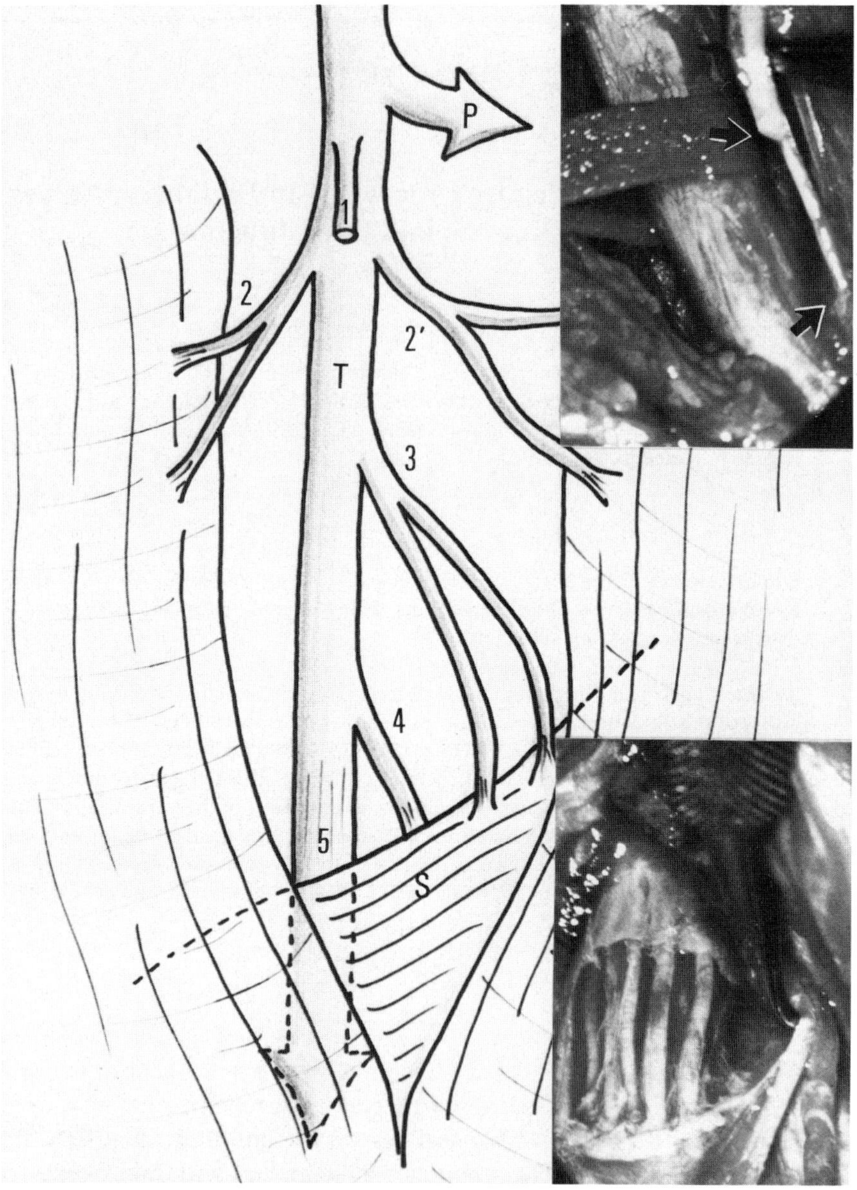

Fig. 1. Selective neurotomy of the tibial nerve. Exposure of the tibial nerve (T), from the peroneal nerve (P) down to the soleus (S) arcade. Identification of its collaterals: the sensory sural nerve (1), the internal (2) and external (2′) gastrocnemius branches, the soleus nerve (3), the posterior tibialis nerve (4). The flexor fascicles (5) of the toes are

Procedures in the Peripheral Nerves: Selective Peripheral Neurotomies (SPN)

Recently, the antiquated methods of peripheral neurotomies have been made more selective by using microsurgical techniques and intraoperative electrostimulation, which make it possible to dissect, identify and interrupt very precisely each nerve (or fascicle) corresponding to the hyperspastic muscles [3]. Among all the various sites of SPN applications, the tibial nerve level is used for the so-called spastic foot.

Technique

After exposure of the tibial nerve from the popliteal region down to the soleus muscular arcade, under general anesthesia without curarization, all its branches are individualized and identified one by one using the operating microscope and bipolar stimulation. Each branch (or fascicle) considered to contribute to the harmful spasticity is partially resected over a 5 mm length, in order to prevent regrowth of fibers. Conservation of one fifth of the fibers of each branch is sufficient to avoid loss of motor function and amyotrophy. A comparative stimulation of the distal and proximal parts of the resected fibers is useful to control the effects of section on the muscular contraction in the operated territory.

The branches to be operated on are determined preoperatively according to the components of the spastic disorders (fig. 1). Equinus deformity and/or ankle clonus require section of the soleus nerve (S), and if necessary of the two gastrocnemius branches. Varus deformity necessitates interruption of the posterior tibial nerve. Tonic flexion of the toes needs section of the flexor fascicles situated inside the distal trunk of the tibial nerve. Their precise identification, apart from the sensory fascicles, is of paramount importance to avoid hypo- and dysesthetic disturbances, as well as trophic lesions of the plantar skin.

Material and Operative Results

47 operations (31 uni- and 8 bilateral) were performed in 39 patients whose age ranged from 6 to 68 years (35 on average) and were evaluated with a follow-up lasting from 1 to 9 years (4 on average). The results were most often (89%) excellent and long-lasting, as illustrated in table I.

---

dissected inside the distal part of the tibial nerve trunk just above the soleus arcade, using bipolar electrical stimulation for identification. Upper operative view: resection, over a 5 mm length, of four fifths of the soleus nerve (arrows). Lower operative view: microsurgical dissection of the fascicles inside the distal trunk of the tibial nerve.

Table I. Selective tibial neurotomy effects in a series of 47 operations (31 uni- and 8 bilateral) in 39 patients, affected with a spinal cord (14 times) and a brain (25 times) lesion: evaluation after a 1- to 9-year follow-up (4 years average)

On spasticity
Complete suppression of all spastic components in 42 procedures and fair improvement in 5 more (i.e. 89% excellent results)

On voluntary movement
Improvement in 38, no change in 8 and mild aggravation in 1.

On preoperative pain
Complete relief in 40 (of 43 cases) and no effect in 3 cases.

Complications
Transient plantar hyperesthesia: 3
Transient plantar hypoesthesia: 2
Permanent plantar hypoesthesia with plantar ulcer: 2

Procedures in the Posterior Root-Spinal Cord Junction: Selective Posterior Rhizotomy (SPR)

In 1972, in order to treat some kinds of painful and/or spastic syndromes, we proposed a surgical procedure whose target was the posterior root-spinal cord junction, i.e., the so-called dorsal root entry zone. This method aims at selectively interrupting the small nociceptive and the myotatic fibers (situated laterally and centrally), while sparing the large lemniscal fibers (regrouped medially), and at enhancing the inhibitory mechanisms of Lissauer's tract and the dorsal horn.

Technique

SPR, which has been detailed elsewhere with regard to its anatomical bases [7, 8, 11, 12] and techniques [7, 9, 10] is illustrated in figure 2. For paraplegia, the L2-S2 spinal cord segments are approached through a T10-L2 laminectomy, while for the upper limb in hemiplegic patients, a C4-C7 hemi-laminectomy with conservation of the spinous processes is sufficient to reach the C5-T1 segments.

Identification of the accurate metameric levels, i.e., those selected as supporting the harmful tonic mechanisms and corresponding to the painful territories, is achieved by studying the muscle responses to bipolar electrical stimulation of the accessible anterior and/or posterior roots. Then under the microscope, the lateral aspect of the posterior root-spinal cord junction is exposed by retracting backwards all the rootlets of each se-

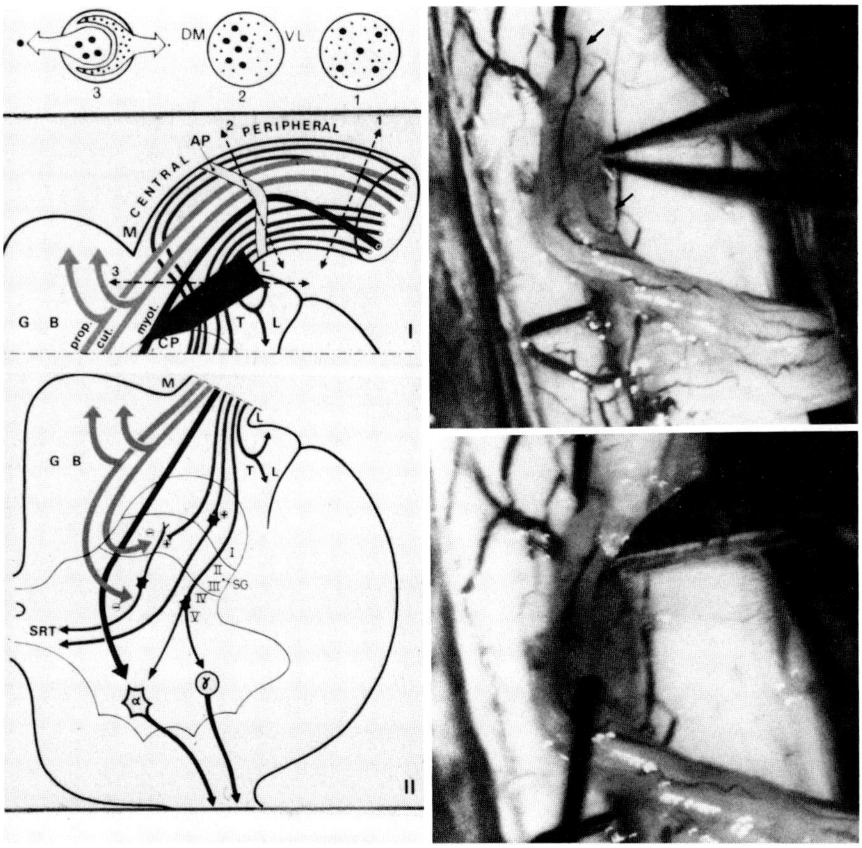

Fig. 2. Left: organization of fibers at the DREZ in man. Each rootlet comprises a peripheral and a central segment. The junction between the two constitutes the pial ring (AP). Peripherally the fibers have no organization. In the neighborhood of the pial ring, the small fibers are situated under the rootlet surface, predominantly on its lateral side. Then in the central segment, they regroup laterally to enter the tract of Lissauer (TL). The large fibers are situated centrally for the myotatic fibers and medially for the lemniscal ones. The black triangle shows the proposed extent of the SPR lesion, i.e., the lateral and central bundles formed by the nociceptive and myotatic fibers, as well as the excitatory (according to Denny-Brown) internal part of the TL. Right: technique of SPR. Example in the cervical area through a right cervical hemilaminectomy (the procedure for the lumbosacral roots is approximately the same). The right C6 posterior root (which has 6 rootlets) has been retracted toward the inside to make the ventrolateral region of the spinal cord-rootlet junction accessible (arrows). A continuous coagulation is made with a sharp bipolar microforceps along the lateral edge of the posterolateral sulcus, which is the site of small pial vessels (upper operative view). Then the incisions performed into the DREZ using a small piece of razor blade (lower operative view). This incision is 1–2 mm deep in Lissauer's tract and makes a 45° angle with the posterior plane of the dorsal column.

Table II.

SPR in spastic hemiplegia (23 cases)		SPR in spastic paraplegia (53 cases)	
Etiology			
Trauma (13), vascular (8), miscellaneous (2)		multiple sclerosis (28), trauma (14), miscellaneous (11)	
Clinical status			
Hyperspasticity		hyperspasticity	
Abnormal flexion postures		abnormal flexion (or hyperextension) postures	
Pain		pain	
Results			
1- to 12-year follow-up	87% effective	1- to 13-year follow-up	92% effective
(1) Upper limb group success in 17 of 19 cases		(1) hyperflexion group success in 46 of 50 cases	
(2) Lower limb group success in 3 of 4 cases		(2) hyperextension group success in 3 of 3 cases	
Complications			
Death (0)		death due to pulmonary insufficiency (2)	
Wound infection (0)		wound infection (2)	
Motor aggravation (1), paresthesias (1)		motor aggravation (2)	

lected root. The procedure consists of a continuous coagulation of the lateral edge of the posterolateral sulcus using a sharp bipolar microforceps and afterwards a 1–2 mm deep incision with a microbistoury oriented at a 45° angle into the lateral part of the DREZ and Lissauer's trct.

Material and Operative Results

53 operations were performed on both sides for hyperspastic paraplegia with abnormal postures in triple flexion and adduction (50 times) or hyperextension (3 times), whilst 23 hemiplegic patients underwent the procedure for hyperspasticity with irreducible flexion either in the upper (19 cases) or the lower limb (4 cases). Severe painful manifestations were present 22 times in the paraplegic and 15 times in the hemiplegic group. The patients age ranged from 11 to 66 years, 41 on average.

After a 1- to 13-year follow-up, 5.1 on average, as shown in table II, the results were judged as effective on the harmful spasticity, abnormal postures and pain in 92% of the paraplegic and in 87% of the hemiplegic patients. In addition, in 30 patients there was reappearance of or improvement in some useful motility.

General Conclusions

As demonstrated in these series and shown by others using SPN, SPR or some kindred procedures [1-6], these methods, provided that patient selection is correct, revealed most often useful (1) in suppressing the excess spasticity, (2) in correcting the abnormal postures and the flexion spasms when present (with complementary lengthening of tendons and capsulolysis of joints, if they were irreducibly retracted), and (3) in relieving the frequently associated pain.

In the most severe situations (so-called 'comfort' indications), these effects allow nursing and kinestherapy to be resumed and sometimes reappearance of some useful voluntary movements. In the less affected patients (so-called 'functional' indications), correction of the localized harmful spasticity facilitates the persistent functional capacities.

References

1 Fasano, V.A.; Barolat-Romana, G.; Ivaldi, A.; Sguazzi, A.: La radicotomie postérieure fonctionnelle dans le traitement de la spasticité cérébrale. Neurochirurgie *22:* 23-34 (1976).

2 Fraioli, B.; Guidetti, B.: Posterior partial rootlet section in the treatment of spasticity. J. Neurosurg. *46:* 618-626 (1977).

3 Gros, C.: Spasticity. Clinical classification and surgical treatment; in Krayenbühl, Advances and technical standards in neurosurgery, vol. 6, pp. 55-97 (Springer, Vienna 1979).

4 Laitinen, L.; Nilsson, S.; Fugl-Meyer, A.: Selective posterior rhizotomy for treatment of spasticity. J. Neurosurg. *58:* 895-899 (1983).

5 Ouaknine, G.E.: Le traitement chirurgical de la spasticité. Un. Méd. Can. *109:* 1424-1444 (1980).

6 Siegfried, J.; Hood, T.: Current status of functional neurosurgery; in Krayenbühl, Advances and technical standards in neurosurgery, vol. 10, pp. 19-66 (Springer, Vienna 1983).

7 Sindou, M.: Etude de la jonction radiculo-médullaire postérieure. La radicellotomie postérieure sélective dans la chirurgie de la douleur; MD thesis No. 173, Lyon (1972).

8 Sindou, M.; Fischer, G.; Goutelle, A.; Schott, B.; Mansuy, L.: La radicellotomie postérieure sélective dans le traitement de la spasticité. Revue neurol. *130:* 201-215 (1974).
9 Sindou, M.; Fischer, G.; Mansuy, L.: Posterior spinal rhizotomy and selective posterior rhizidiotomy. Prog. neurol. Surg., vol. 7, pp. 201-250 (Karger, Basel 1976).
10 Sindou, M.; Goutelle, A.: Surgical posterior rhizotomies for the treatment of pain; in Krayenbühl, Advances and technical standards in neurosurgery, vol. 10, pp. 147-185 (Springer, Vienna 1983).
11 Sindou, M.; Millet, M.F.; Mortamais, J.; Eyssette, M.: Results of selective posterior rhizotomy in the treatment of painful and spastic paraplegia secondary to multiple sclerosis. Appl. Neurophysiol. *45:* 335-340 (1982).
12 Sindou, M.; Quoex, C.; Baleydier, C.: Fiber organization at the posterior spinal cord-rootlet junction in man. J. comp. Neurol. *153:* 15-26 (1974).

M. Sindou, MD, Hôpital Neurologique, 59, Boulevard Pinel,
F-69003 Lyon (France)

Proc. 9th Meeting World Soc. Stereotactic and Functional
Neurosurgery, Toronto 1985
Appl. Neurophysiol. *48:* 105 (1985)

Spinal Cord Stimulation for the Treatment of Muscle Hypertonia in Patients with Chronic Spinal Cord Injury

P.C. Sharkey[a], *M.R. Dimitrijevic*[a], *K. Nakajima*[b], *A.M. Sherwood*[a]

[a] Department of Clinical Neurophysiology, Institute for Rehabilitation and Research and Department of Rehabilitation, Baylor College of Medicine, Houston, Tex., USA; [b] Department of Neurosurgery, Juntendo University School of Medicine, Tokyo, Japan

Sixty patients with muscle hypertonia after spinal cord injury have undergone spinal cord stimulation (SCS). These patients had spinal cord injuries (SCI) ranging from C2 to T12. Electrodes were placed above, below or above and below the lesion in the posterior epidural space for a period of at least 3 days during which time stimulation pulses, typically of 3–5 Ma amplitude and of 0.2 ms duration at 30 Hz were applied. The effects of SCS were monitored by recording motor unit activity with surface electrodes over leg muscles during an examination of segmental and suprasegmental spinal cord activity, in addition to patient reports and neurological evaluations. The results of spinal cord stimulation can be divided into four distinct categories. In group I, consisting of 17 patients, or 28% of the entire group, the effect was characterized by marked suppression of muscle hypertonia and so-called spontaneous spasms. In group II, the effect of spinal cord stimulation on muscle hypertonia was moderate, as evidenced by the suppression of the tonic but not phasic features of spasticity. This was observed in 20 patients, or 33% of the total. In group III, neurological and neurophysiological evaluations revealed only a marginal effect. The condition of this group of 9 patients (15%) did not improve significantly. In group IV, consisting of 14 patients (23%), there was no effect.

P.C. Sharkey, MD, Department of Clinical Neurophysiology,
The Institute for Rehabilitation and Research, Baylor College of Medicine,
1333 Moursund Avenue, Houston, TX 77030 (USA)

Proc. 9th Meeting World Soc. Stereotactic and Functional
Neurosurgery, Toronto 1985
Appl. Neurophysiol. *48:* 106–110 (1985)

Characteristics of the Tonic Stretch Reflex in Spastic Spinal Cord and Head-Injured Patients

Philip L. Gildenberg[a], *Robert J. Campos*[b], *Milan R. Dimitrijevic*[b]

[a] University of Texas Medical School, and [b] Institute for Rehabilitation and Research, Houston, Tex., USA

Key Words. Spasticity · Head injury · Spinal cord injury · Stretch reflex

Abstract. Spasticity is a known sequelae of spinal cord injury and head injury. We sought to examine whether there were any significant differences in the characterstics or underlying mechanisms of spasticity in these two groups in the chronic period which may be related to the level of injury of the neuraxis.The response to vibration applied to the muscle, or the tonic vibratory reflex, has been shown to be related to the degree of spasticity, and was therefore studied along with phasic reflexes and passive movements. These studies were carried out on cooperative, stabilized patients who were otherwise healthy, 5 with head injuries, and 5 with spinal cord injuries. The patients were examined in a supine position while surface EMG recordings were made of quadriceps and triceps surae muscles bilaterally. Tendon jerk responses, passive and volitional movements, and responses to a powerful vibratory stimulator were measured. In both head injury and spinal cord injury patient groups, a large EMG response was elicited by passive maneuvers, and tendon jerks were exaggerated. The tonic vibratory response, previously shown to be dependent upon brain influence, was present in both groups. These observations suggest that similar suprasegmental mechanisms may be responsible for hypertonia in both head-injured and spinal cord-injured patients.

Introduction

Generally, spasticity is looked upon as a single entity, whether it is caused by a head or spinal cord injury. However, which pathways are interrupted and the completeness of interruption is much different in these two types of injury.

A physiologic comparison was done in a group of patients in each group with a clinical diagnosis of spasticity, to shed light on the pathophysiology of spasticity, and perhaps lead to design of management protocols suited more specifically to each group.

SPINAL CORD INJURED				HEAD INJURED			
60 DEG/SEC	INJURY LEVEL	VOLIT. SPASM ACT.	TENDON TAPS	60 DEG/SEC	AMBULAT.	VOLIT. SPASM ACT.	TENDON TAPS
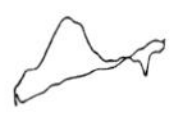	C2	++	+++	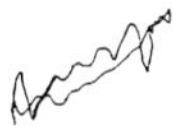	YES	–	+
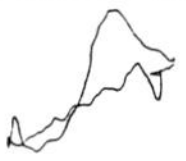	C5	–	+	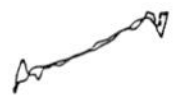	YES	+	+
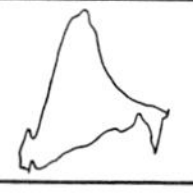	C6	–	+++	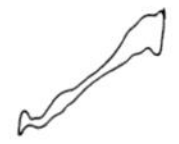	NO	+	+
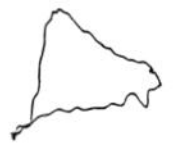	C6	–	+++	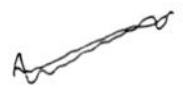	YES	–	+
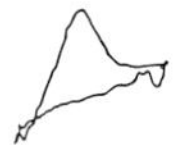	T8	+	+++	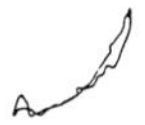	NO	–	+

Fig. 1. Cybex isokinetic dynamometry presents a different tracing in patients with spinal cord injury versus patients with head injury with manifestations of spasticity. Volit. spasm act. = volitional activation of spasms. Tendon taps: + = slightly increased; +++ = markedly increased.

Materials and Methods

Five patients with spasticity following spinal cord injury and 5 patients following head injury were selected. No attempt was made to develop homogeneous groups beyond those criteria, in order to sample a broad group of patients for the inital phase of the study.

Two patients with head injuries were wheelchair bound and 3 were ambulatory. One head-injured patient had a left frontal epidural and small subdural hematoma with contusion of the underlying brain. Another patient had a right temporoparietal contusion and intracerebral hematoma. A third had a gunshot wound of the left frontal area and remains aphasic and quadraparetic. The fourth patient had bilateral subdural hygromas and is the only patient who demonstrated cranial nerve palsy, a right lower facial weakness and occasional double vision. The fifth patient had a left subdural hematoma and has remained aphasic with quadraparesis. All have impairment of mentation and speech. All show the clinical picture of spasticity severe enough in 3 of the patients to

Table I. Patients tested for spasticity

Spinal cord-injured group

			Injury				Clinical description				
PEMG	Init.	Sex	level	onset	age years	dur. months	etiology com/inc	taps	bab.	spasm	amb.
1345	E.L.	F	C2	11–80	55	55	Fall-inc	+++	+	+++	no
1301	R.S.	M	C5	07–83	28	19	Diving-com	+++	+	+++	no
1344	R.D.	M	C6	06–84	15	14	MVA-inc	+++	+	+++	no
1277	D.S.	M	C6	10–82	19	27	MVA-inc	+++	+	+++	no
1298	P.R.	M	T8	11–83	17	15	MVA-com	+++	+	+++	no

Head-injured group

			type	onset	age years	dur. months	etiology, coma dur. (days)	cogn. funct. deficit	taps	spasm	amb.
1292	P.S.	M	closed	11–84	18	2	MVA 15	SMTP	+	–	yes
1316	R.M.	M	closed	06–80	18	54	MVA 120	S	+	–	yes
0997	L.T.	M	penit.	05–83	17	6	GSW 0	SM	+	+	no
1375	B.M.	M	closed	03–85	15	3	MVA 3	SM	+	+	yes
1221	B.R.	M	closed	03–80	19	54	MVA 180	SMTP	+	+	no

cause contractures. All of the patients required management of spasticity, which was generally not greatly successful. All had moderately increased deep tendon reflexes on clinical testing and 2 had ankle clonus.

The 5 patients with spinal cord injuries had closed injuries at the levels indicated in figure 1. All except 1 had complete loss of function below the lesion, with marked spasticity on clinical examination. Four patients had markedly increased deep tendon reflexes, which were moderately increased in the fifth patient.

Polyelectromyography (table I)

Polyelectromyography (PEMG) was used for recording motor unit activity and isokinetic dynamometry with torque measurement during externally induced flexion and extension of the knee.

Surface EMG signals were recorded from selected muscle groups with a 16-channel electroencephalograph (sensitivity 100 μV, bandwidth 800 Hz) with the patient supine.

The recordings began with 10 min of complete relaxation, following which the patient was asked to perform three times a standardized series of reinforcement maneuvers with nonparalyzed muscles to determine their influence on activity, and was also examined during passive stretch of individual muscle groups for information about muscle tone and abnormal irradiation of activity to nonstretched muscles. Phasic stretch reflex evaluation was done with tendon jerks and ankle and patellar clonus. Properties of the tonic stretch reflex were explored through the application of vibration to tendons of the quadriceps and triceps surae muscles. Evaluation of the segmental organization of the withdrawal reflex was carried out by mechanical stimulation of the plantar surface, both during relaxation and during attempts by the patient to suppress the withdrawal movement.

Isokinetic Dynamometry

Recordings of torque measurements of passive knee motion were performed with a Cybex isokinetic dynamometer with the patient supine while the leg was extended and flexed at a rate of stretch at 30, 60 and 100° with 3 repetitive measurements for each rate of stretch during which the EMG was recorded from the quadriceps and hamstring muscles.

Results

PEMG recordings in the 5 patients who sustained spinal cord injury revealed that 3 had absent volitional but partial postural motor control, and 2 had partial postural motor control and residual volitional motor control. All revealed severely increased muscle hypertonia during passive flexion and extension on isokinetic dynamometry with excessive motor unit activity in quadriceps more than in hamstrings.

In all 5 head-injured patients PEMG revealed upper motor neuron dysfunction with excessive motor unit activity during postural and gait activities and simple volitional motor acts. However, at the same time isokinetic dynamometry revealed nothing more than normal muscle tone during passive stretch.

Thus, in the presence of clinical neurological findings of upper motor neuron dysfunction in both categories of patients, there was physiologic evidence of impaired volitional activity, remote muscle contraction on attempted contraction of paretic or paralyzed muscles and characteristic features for released phasic stretch reflex functions. Additionally, isometric dynamometry definitely divided these two groups of patients into hypertonic and normotonic groups, with spinal cord-injured patients demonstrating release and head-injured patients showing suppression of tonic stretch reflex functions.

Discussion

This preliminary observation suggests that upper motor neuron dysfunction can be present without abnormal tone during passive stretch when caused by the spinal cord. Poor motor control, paresis and distrubances of volitional, postural and gait motor control with signs of released phasic stretch reflex phenomena in chronic head-injured patients is not necessarily accompanied by muscle hypertonia of tonic stretch reflex origin.

P.L. Gildenberg, MD, PhD, 6560 Fannin, Suite 1530, Houston, TX 77030 (USA)

Proc. 9th Meeting World Soc. Stereotactic and Functional
Neurosurgery, Toronto 1985
Appl. Neurophysiol. *48:* 111-116 (1985)

Bioengineering Changes in Spastic Cerebral Palsy Groups following Cerebellar Stimulation

Ross Davis[a], *Edward Gray*[a], *Thomas Ryan*[a], *Joseph Schulman*[b]

[a] Department of Neurological Surgery, Mount Sinai Medical Center, Miami Beach, Fla., and [b] Neurodyne Corporation, Sylmar, Calif., USA

Key Words. Spastic cerebral palsy · Performance testing · Cerebellar stimulation · Respiratory function

Abstract. Quantitative bioengineering tests were performed on 30 spastic cerebral palsy (CP) patients who underwent chronic cerebellar stimulation (CCS) using the fully implantable pulse generator (Neurolith 601, 1.1-1.8 $\mu C/cm^2$/phase). Using respiratory inductive plethysmography to measure 8 patients with paroxysmal and/or ataxic breathing patterns, 5 were shown to revert to normal with 3 others markedly improved within 5 months of CCS. Compliance testing of the ankle was performed on 4 patients who showed improvement in 9 of the 16 tests performed. Motor performance ability was evaluated with 9 comprehensive tests in 17 patients. Following 1-2 weeks of CCS, 52% showed performance increases greater than 10%, increasing to 62% during the first year.

Introduction

Bioengineering studies have been published relating to quantitative changes in spasticity, athetosis and motor performance in humans as a result of CCS. Results have shown an increase in respiratory muscle coordination [8], improvement in developmental reflexes [9], and a shift of muscle compliance towards normal [5, 9, 10]. In support of this, reduction of spasticity and co-contraction in primates has been shown [4, 6]. Improvement in neurological function of fine hand control has been shown [1, 2]. Gait analysis has shown changes with CCS that include a smoothing of angle-angle diagram [7] and increases in coordination and knee flexion [2]. Quantitative measurements have been carried out in 30 spastic CP patients and presented here.

Method

Clinical Series and Equipment

Of the 314 spastic patients undergoing CCS since February 1974 through March 1982, 160 spastic patients (146 with CP - 91%) were studied as a separate group from May 1979 onwards [3]. This latter group comprised only those given the fully implanted lithium battery stimulator (Neurolith 601, Neurodyne Corp., Sylmar, Calif.). This unit was preset in the factory to produce pulses of 1.0–1.4 mA, 0.5 ms, 150 pulses/s intermittently 4 min on and 4 min off. The Neurolith stimulator was used in conjunction with the two 4-button electrode arrays (Avery Lab., Inc., Farmingdale, N.Y.), which were situated bilaterally on the cerebellar superior paramedian surface. The charge density so produced was 1.1–1.8 $\mu C/cm^2$/phase. The 146 spastic CP patients were grouped according to A (1 to 3) - bedridden or strapped in a wheelchair, possessing little or no independence; B (4 and 5) - wheelchair bound, with upper extremity usage in varying degrees; C (6) - walking with walker/braces; C (7) - walking with a cane/crutches; D (8 and 9) - mildly affected, walking without aid(s).

Respiratory Testing

Ten very spastic CP patients were tested (A, n = 3; B, n = 6; C, n = 1). Because the patients could not be tested with oral connection to the pulmonary pathways, an inductive plethysmograph (Respitrace, Ambulatory Monitoring, Inc., Ardsley, N.Y.) was used to monitor respiratory function. One band was positioned around the rib cage and the other around the abdomen.

Compliance Testing

Four very spastic patients were studied (A, n = 1; B, n = 3). The ankle compliance measurement was accomplished by placing the foot on a rotating foot plate or cradle which was connected by a mechanical chain drive to a torque-producing motor. The resistance was measured through a bridge circuit and provided an output proportional to the motor position. The torque and position were recorded simultaneously on a polygraph. The frequency of the sinusoidal movement was increased from 1 to 10 Hz.

Motor Performance Testing

17 spastic CP patients were selected because their intellectual and motor performances could be tested quantitatively; 9 were wheelchair bound (5-B4, 4-B5) and 8 were ambulatory (2-C6, 4-C7, 2-D8). No patient increased medication during these trials. One patient had his system removed 3 months postoperatively because of infection; he underwent total recovery but a return of his spasticity. Another patient died 11½ months after the implantation; this was 3 days postoperatively following the removal of a Harrington rod and thoracic fusion.

The testing covered (1) range of motion encompassing speed, coordination, fatigue, strength and capacity for movement and (2) response time. A battery of 9 tests could provide up to 27 measurements per patient depending upon their ability. Of the 17 who were studied during the first and second week with CCS, 10 were followed 1.5–13.5 (6.3) months with CCS. Statistical methods were used to allow each value to be individually weighed. By comparing a patient's value with himself, compensation is made for the range of severity of the patients which may exceed two orders of magnitude. Standard error of the mean was used when no normal population existed for comparison.

Results

Respiratory Function

Of the 10 severely spastic CP patients, 2 showed normal patterns prior to CCS and remained so in follow-up testing. Eight patients showed abnormal patterns, including 'ataxic' and/or paroxysmal respiration between the intercostal and diaphragmatic movements. Following 1 week of CCS, 3 progressed to normal and 3 showed marked improvement, 1 showed a moderate improvement and 1 was unchanged. Two patients were retested following 5 months of CCS. One had previously showed marked improvement while the other was unchanged following the first week of CCS: both patients had improved to normal. Thus of 8 patients with abnormal patterns prior to CCS, 5 had normal breathing patterns and 3 showed marked improvement with CCS. Respiration rates showed no significant changes overall.

Compliance Testing

Four spastic patients were tested by recording the compliance at frequencies varying between 1 and 10 Hz. The patient was asked to voluntarily rotate the foot cradle, if possible. Of the 16 tests (4 per patient: left/right ankles, above/below 4 Hz), 9 (56%) showed signs of improvement following CCS. *Penn and Etzel* [9] using similar compliance testing showed that 5 of the 9 patients (55%) showed improvements with CCS.

Performance Testing

The 17 moderately and less affected CP patients chosen were tested 2–4 days prior to implantation and again with 1–2 weeks of CCS; 10 patients were tested again in the follow-up period of 1.5–13.5 (mean 6.3) months of CCS. Each patient was compared with himself, practice was given with each test until the patient was proficient. (A) *Complex visual-motor coordination:* a maze board (No. 2706E, Lafayette Instrument Co. (LIC), Lafayette, Ind.) was placed before the seated patient to gauge speed and coordination. Eight patients performed this test (table I). (B) *Static strength:* Grip strength was measured using a hand

Table I. Results of battery of tests

Test	% change (post-op)	Patients, n	p	% change follow-up	Patients, n	p
Complex visual-motor coordination	+20.4	8	<0.001	+31.2	3	NS
Static strength	+32.2	13	<0.001	+46.7	7	0.001
Finger dexterity	+11.7	8	<0.05	− 7.0	4	0.025
Gross arm movement	+ 8.3	15	<0.001	+26.8	9	0.001
Gross leg movement	+18.6	7	<0.001	+12.3	2	NS
Reaction time (push)	+ 4.4	13	<0.001	+21.5	9	0.001
Reaction time (pull-off)	− 3.9	12	<0.001	+10.6	9	0.01
Tracking error	+13.1	6	<0.01	+ 6.8	2	NS
Tracking velocity	+ 1.3	6	NS	+22.3	2	NS
Tracking reaction time	+ 7.4	5	<0.005	+23.5	2	NS

Note: Values denote performance increase. NS = not significant.

dynomometer (No. 76502, LIC) that registered kilograms of force. Thirteen patients were tested (table I). (C) *Finger dexterity:* A peg board with T-shaped slots for 25 pegs (No. 32025, LIC) was used to gauge finger dexterity in 8 patients (table I). (D) *Gross upper and lower extremity movement:* The patient's speed of gross movements was measured by alternately tapping two plates during a 10-second period (No. 32012, LIC). A probe was positioned either in the hand or foot. The distance between the conducting plates was 28 cm. Fifteen patients were tested for upper extremity movement and 7 for lower extremity movements (table I). (E) *Reaction time:* A device was built to measure the lag time between light stimulus presentation and the patient's reaction in the pressing push mode or release pull-off mode. Thirteen patients undertook this test (table I). (F) *Visual pursuit tracking:* Five patients' ability to follow a moving display on an oscilloscope by hand controlling a joystick by use of a 4-channel signal averager (No. 5480B, Hewlett-Packard) was tested. Reaction time, velocity and integrated absolute error were calculated (table I). (G) *Gait analysis:* Gait was analyzed in 5 patients by recording hip and knee movements and walking speed (cadence). Polarized light source sensors were affixed to the waist, thigh and leg; all knee or hip motions in the sagittal plane cause sensor-induced voltages in a TECA (PN22) electrogoniometer. Dia-

Table II. Patient distribution according to the percentage of their tests showing performance increases greater than 10%

Performance increased	Postoperative status		Follow-up status (1.5–13.5 months)	
	n	%	n	%
60–100% (marked improvement)	4	24	6	60
50–59% (moderate improvement)	7	41	2	20
30–49% (mild improvement)	6	35	2	20
Total patients	17		10	

grams of hip versus knee angles are an indicator of general walking ability. A coordination index (CI) was obtained by dividing the perimeter of the closed loop-angle diagram by the square root of the area. The range in normals was found to be 4.5–6.0 [7]. In the 5 patients tested, 3 showed bilateral increases towards normal and 2 showed unilateral increases. Cadence showed a 4.1% decrease, and has been shown not to affect CI [7]. A better synchrony between the hip and knee was seen in the curves.

Discussion

Although quantitative performance improvements were seen after 1–2 weeks of CCS, further improvements are measured in the follow-up period (1.5–13.5 months) with the 10 patients, indicating ongoing and increasing benefits. Table II shows patient distribution when placed according to percentage of their tests that showed performance increases greater than 10%. When comparing results of each of the above patients clinically graded into marked, moderate and mild improvements in our clinical paper [3], 6 of the 10 patients followed showed a direct correlation; 3 others were within 1 grade, while 1 patient was given a marked improvement by the bioengineering tests and only graded mild for clinical improvements. It is assumed that CCS induces muscle tone relaxation and lessening of cocontraction which allows the increases in range of motion, speed, coordination, accuracy, and strength, as well as improvements in respiratory patterns.

References

1 Allen, M.; Malik, A.; Flanigin, H.: Performance evaluation of four spastic patients using chronic cerebellar stimulation; in Davis, Bloedel, Cerebellar stimulation for spasticity and seizures, pp. 189–194 (CRC Press, Boca Raton 1984).

2 Davis, R.; Engle, H.; Kudzma, J.; Gray, E.; Ryan, T.; Dusnak, A.: Update of chronic cerebellar stimulation for spasticity and epilepsy. Appl. Neurophysiol. *45:* 44–50 (1982).

3 Davis, R. Kudzma, J.; Gray, E.; Engle, H.; Ryan, T.: Graded clinical effects in spastic cerebral palsy groups following chronic cerebellar stimulation; in Davis, Bloedel, Cerebellar stimulation for spasticity and seizures, pp. 223–240 (CRC Press, Boca Raton 1984).

4 Ebner, T.J.; Vitek, J.L.; Schwartz, A.B.; Bloedel, J.R.: Effects of cerebellar stimulation on abnormal proprioceptive reflexes in spastic primates. Expl. Neurol. *70:* 721–725 (1980).

5 Gottlieb, G.L.; Agarwal, G.C.; Penn, R.: Sinusoidal oscillation of the ankle as a means of evaluating the spastic patient. J. Neurol. Neurosurg. Psychiat. *41:* 32–39 (1978).

6 Hemmy, D.C.; Larson, S.J.; Sances, A., Jr.; Millar, E.A.: The effect of cerebellar stimulation of focal seizure activity and spasticity in monkeys. J. Neurosurg. *46:* 648–653 (1979).

7 Milner, M.; Hershler, C.; Bruin, H. de; Baker, R.S.; Upton, A.R.M.; Cooper, I.S.: Preliminary investigation of influence of cerebellar stimulation on gait analysing angle-angle diagrams; in Cooper, Cerebellar stimulation in man, pp. 123–144 (Raven Press, New York 1978).

8 Miyasaka, K.; Hoffman, H.J.; Froese, A.B.: The influence of chronic cerebellar stimulation on respiratory muscle coordination in a patient with cerebral palsy. Neurosurgery *2:* 262–265 (1978).

9 Penn, R.D.; Etzel, M.L.: Chronic cerebellar stimulation and developmental reflexes. J. Neurosurg. *46:* 506–511 (1977).

10 Upton, A.R.; Cooper, I.S.: Some neurophysiological effects of cerebellar stimulation in man. Can. J. neurol. Sci. *3:* 237–254 (1976).

Dr. Ross Davis, 150 Dresden Avenue, Gardiner, ME 04345 (USA)

Session III: CT-Guided Stereotaxis for Radiation Therapy

Proc. 9th Meeting World Soc. Stereotactic and Functional
Neurosurgery, Toronto 1985
Appl. Neurophysiol. *48:* 117–120 (1985)

Stereotactic Interstitial Brachytherapy – Current Concepts and Concerns in Twenty Patients

L. Dade Lunsford, Melvin Deutsch, Virgil Yoder

Departments of Neurological Surgery, Radiology (Radiation Therapy) and Radiation Physics, University of Pittsburgh School of Medicine, and Presbyterian-University Hospital, Pittsburgh, Pa., USA

Key Words. Stereotactic surgery · Brain tumor · Brachytherapy

Abstract. Recent advances in imaging and stereotactic techniques have resulted in wider application of interstitial brachytherapy (IBT) for brain tumors. The advantages of brachytherapy alone or in combination with teletherapy have been detailed, and may be responsible for increasing survival time. We report the preliminary results of 20 patients who underwent CT stereotactic IBT for malignant brain tumors. Despite both old and recent evidence about the efficacy of IBT, concerns remain about the proper grade neoplasm, the target, the dose, and the timing for treatment. Current usage of IBT should be limited to centers with both stereotactic and radiotherapeutic expertise, and where the risks and benefits are being investigated.

The advantages of removable radiation isotopes (interstitial brachytherapy, IBT) for treatment of both benign and malignant brain tumors have been detailed [1]. Spurred by the availability of precise stereotactic devices coupled with advanced imaging tools, numerous centers recently have embarked on clinical treatment programs using IBT. A retrospective review of our initial experience with stereotactic IBT revealed both encouraging preliminary results and raised serious questions about further widespread development of stereotactic interstitial radiation.

Methods and Materials

Twenty patients (12 males, 8 females, age range 27–67 years) underwent stereotactic IBT using ^{125}I after-loaded in removable catheters. The Leksell stereotactic coordinate

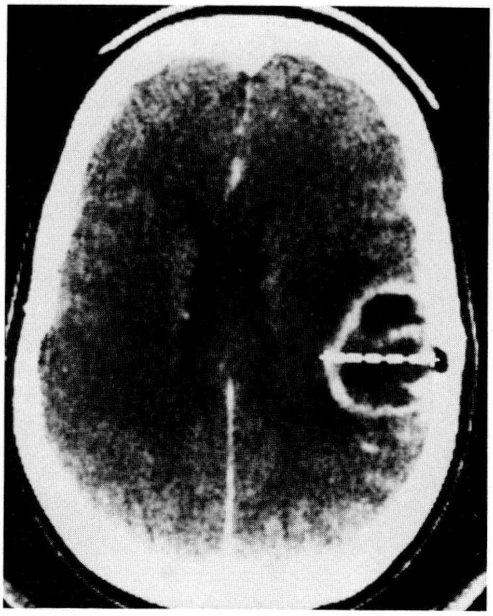

A

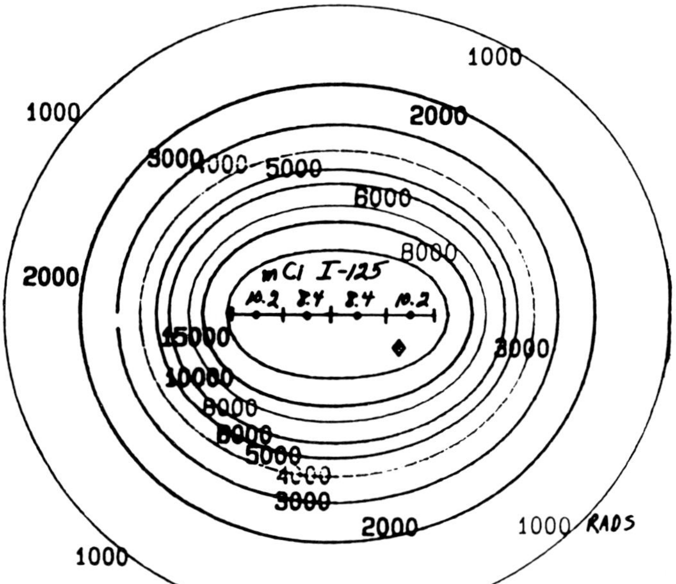

B

Fig. 1. A Contrast enhanced CT scan disclosed a mass lesion in the left frontal parietal region. The projected pathway of the ^{125}I catheter is shown. **B** Computer isodose planning for brachytherapy of the lesion.

Table I. Factors in treatment and survival of patients with malignant brain tumors treated by IBT

1.	Method to determine lesion size (CT versus magnetic resonance imaging?)
2.	Appropriate and tolerable dose to tumor and brain
3.	Histological grade of neoplasm (cell cycle time?)
4.	Timing of IBT (prospective versus recurrent?)
5.	Adjunctive therapy (cytoreductive debulking, teletherapy, chemotherapy?)
6.	Length of follow-up
7.	Choice of isotope
8.	Length of total survival; quality of survival

frame (AB Elekta Instruments, Decatur, Ga.) was used. Preoperative dosimetry was done with computer technique using CT scan derived measurements of the tumor volume (fig. 1A,B). A primary (prospective) group of 10 patients (7 had glioblastomas, 3 had anaplastic astrocytomas) were treated after diagnosis to a total dose to the enhancing tumor margin of 11,000–13,000 rad, including 6,000 rad by external beam and 5,000–7,000 rad by IBT. Ten patients (8 anaplastic astrocytomas, 1 glioblastoma, 1 metastasis) were treated as secondary (recurrent) cases after being declared failures of prior treatment regimes. Follow-up range was from 12 to 92 weeks (median was 44 weeks) for these 20 patients.

Results

In the primary (prospective) trial (n = 10), 2 patients died of disease progression at 44 and 58 weeks respectively. At the time of review, median life survival for glioblastoma patients (n = 7) was 40 weeks, but 6 patients were still living 40–60 weeks after diagnosis. In our secondary (recurrent) trial, median life survival after treatment for anaplastic astrocytoma (n = 8) was 50 weeks, but 5 were still living, and 2 had died 92 and 52 weeks after IBT. Median total survival for anaplastic astrocytoma patients after diagnosis was 141 weeks with 5 patients still living. No mortality or neurological morbidity occurred from surgery; 1 patient developed a delayed catheter site infection. Before or after IBT, 10 patients underwent craniotomy for tumor debulking and 8 patients had chemotherapy.

Discussion

Spurred by the encouraging results of *Mundinger* [3] and *Gutin* et al. [2], among others, many investigators have pursued IBT as both a primary and an adjunctive treatment for malignant brain tumors. Our own preliminary results are encouraging and provide further evidence that IBT is potentially equal to or superior to conventional treatment of malignant gliomas. In the assessment of results of IBT, many factors must be analyzed in a larger group of patients with prolonged follow-up (table I). Each factor must be separately analyzed, since results seem quite different when lesion size, histological grade, dosage, timing of treatment, and the role of adjunctive therapies are considered. At present, stereotactic IBT must be regarded as a potentially promising treatment of malignant tumors. Widespread application of IBT should be reserved for those centers with both stereotactic and radiotherapeutic expertise, and where active investigation as to its applicability is being pursued. Controlled clinical trials will be necessary before IBT can be confirmed as a definitive therapy in patients with lesions of suitable size and histology.

References

1 Bernstein, M.; Gutin, P.H.: Interstitial irradiation of brain tumors: a review. Neurosurgery *9:* 741–750 (1981).

2 Gutin, P.H.; Phillips, T.L.; Wara, W.M.; Leibel, S.A.; Hosobuchi, Y.; Levin, V.A.; Weaver, K.A.; Lamb, S.: Brachytherapy of recurrent malignant brain tumors with removable high-activity iodine-125 sources. J. Neurosurg. *60:* 61–68 (1984).

3 Mundinger, G.: Implantation of radioisotopes (curietherapy); in Schaltenbrand, Walker, Stereotaxy of the human brain, pp. 410–435 (Thieme/Stratton, New York 1982).

L. Dade Lunsford, MD, Room 9402, Presbyterian-University Hospital,
230 Lothrop Street, Pittsburgh, PA 15213 (USA)

Proc. 9th Meeting World Soc. Stereotactic and Functional
Neurosurgery, Toronto 1985
Appl. Neurophysiol. *48:* 121–126 (1985)

Treatment of Low Malignancy Brain Neoplasms by Means of Stereotactic Interstitial Radiotherapy

F. Frank[a], *A.P. Fabrizi*[a], *R. Frank-Ricci*[b], *C. Sturiale*[a], *G. Nuzzo*[c]

[a] Division of Neurosurgery, [b] Neuropathology Service, and [c] Division of Neuroradiology, Bellaria Hospital, Bologna, Italy

Key Words. Biopsy · Iodine-125 · Brain tumor · Interstitial radiotherapy · Social reentry · Stereotactic interstitial radiotherapy

Abstract. The authors report their results of 37 patients with low malignancy brain tumors seated in deep or highly functional areas not amenable to traditional surgery, nor to conventional radiochemotherapy. In the past 5 years these patients were treated by means of stereotactic interstitial radiotherapy. The isotope employed in all cases was ^{125}I. Stereotactic radioisotope implants were always preceded by multiple stereotactic biopsies affording precise histological diagnoses. A 6-month to 5-year follow-up shows a survival rate of 72.6% (29 patients), and of these patients, 80.9% (26 out of 29) had complete social reentry.

Radioisotope implantation in the treatment of cerebral neoplasms is part of the realm of the brachytherapeutic intercavitary approach to tumors. With the success of interstitial therapy in the late 1960s for various neoplasms, *Talairach* et. al. [5] and *Szikla and Peragut* [4] performed the first isotope implants in brain tumors.

The uncertain results obtained with these first studies led to the abandonment of this procedure. The related problems were numerous: difficulty in obtained true volumetric and topographic reconstruction of the lesions, and difficulty in obtaining radioisotopes that gave a useful dose distribution in the tumor. With the advent of the CT scanner in the 1970s, the problem of precise volumetric and topographic calculations were for the most part resolved [1, 2]. During these years new isotopes were developed [3] (i.e., ^{125}I), with characteristics of easier handling and more uniform dose distribution, favoring the return to this surgical procedure in the treatment of neoplasms that were considered inoperable.

Inoperable cerebral neoplasms that correspond to the criteria for radioisotope implants must be: small to medium sized (max. 4.5 cm in diameter); in deep-seated areas, that present either difficult approaches, or highly functional areas, that would cause grave neurological disorders. These tumors must also be low malignancy types, that would scarcely respond to conventional radiochemotherapy [3].

We based our study employing interstitial radiotherapy on the work of the Freiburg group [2, 3], using the same therapeutic protocol.

Materials and Method

From 1981 to date, 37 patients with small- to medium-sized low grade neoplasms were treated with stereotactically implanted radioisotopes.

^{125}I was the isotope chosen for the following 3 reasons: (1) dose distribution is homogeneous; (2) radius of maximum activity is 2.5 cm from the source to the periphery of the tumor, therefore theoretically limiting damage to the surrounding normal brain tissue, and also does not require special radiation protection for the patient and relatives; (3) half-life of 60.2 days, therefore in a relatively short period it is possible to evaluate the first effects of the treatment and the eventual successive therapeutic possibilities.

In all the patients treated with brachytherapy, the implants were performed stereotactically and preceded by serial biopsies. The Riechert stereotactic frame (Fischer Inc., Freiburg im Breisgau, FRG) was employed and the biopsy specimens were obtained with special biopsy forceps, (Fischer Inc.), that allow for 1 mm^3 tissue samples. The neoplasms were reconstructed directly from CT images into radiograms taken during the stereotactic procedure. The implants were performed under local anesthesia with the exception of children. No mortality or morbidity was reported during the intervention.

Results

The tumor site and the histopathological diagnoses are presented in tables I and II respectively. Table III presents the follow-up that ranges from 6 months to 5 years. At the follow-up, 29 patients (72.6%) are still alive, and 8 patients (27.4%) died. The authors stress that in 75% of the deceased patients, there was a histological grading error and the tumor was a grade III astrocytoma and the mean survival rate of these patients was 20 months (8–36 months).

From an analysis of the quality of life of the survivors, 84% (25 patients) recovered their normal life-style or their clinical course remained stable, while 16% (4 patients) showed progressive clinical deterioration.

Table I. Site of the tumoral lesions (n = 37) treated with ^{125}I

Frontal lobe	9	suprasellar region	6
Parietal lobe	2	basal ganglia	5
Temporal lobe	2	third ventricle	3
Pineal region	7	brainstem	3

Table II. Histopathological type of neoplasms (n= 37) treated with ^{125}I

Subependymomas	2	craniopharyngiomas	3
Pineocytomas[1]	2	oligodendrogliomas	1
Pituitary adenomas	1	ependymomas	1
Astrocytomas[2] (grade II)	27		

[1] Patients responded poorly to interstitial radiotherapy, at rebiopsy the tumor was a germinoma.
[2] Three of the 27 grade II astrocytomas, after a second biopsy, proved to be grade III astrocytoma; these responded poorly to ^{125}I implant.

Table III. Clinical follow-up of 29 cases (6 months – 5 years)

Improved	20 patients	social reentry
Unchanged	5 patients	25 patients (84%)
Worsened	4 patients	permanent handicap
Total	29 patients	4 patients (16%)

Discussion

Interstitial radiotherapy in brain tumors is a direct development from previous experience with neoplasms of other organs (particularly intracavitary tumors). To date there are few specific publications that allow for a precise long-term evaluation of this therapy. It is certain that even if the survival rate is not augmented compared to other similar untreated slow-growing neoplasms, the quality of life of these patients is improved. Our 5-year study clearly indicates partial or complete social reentry in 80.9% of the treated patients, who are still alive

(26 out of 29 patients). On the basis of this high percentage of good results on the quality of life of the survivors, we believe that in slow-growing neoplasms radioisotope implant is the correct therapeutic procedure.

Numerous problems exist that are not easily resolved, such as diagnostic (radiological or histopathological), radiobiological (dosimetry), and the stereotactic procedure. The neuroradiological diagnostic difficulties are not of the order of the late 60s when fractionated gas encephalography localized tumoral site poorly, and could not define the volume of the cerebral neoplasms. With CT these topographical problems have disappeared, but the exact tumor volume may still be uncertain, especially certain subcortical astrocytomas, with no precise boundaries between tumor, perifocal edema and normal brain tissue. Even nuclear magnetic resonance (NMR) has done little to the volumetric quantification of the neoplasm. Often NMR tumor images may be confused with perifocal edema, and small neoplasms may appear larger than their true dimensions and lead to erroneous radioisotopic treatment.

In these neoplasms, usually grade I and II astrocytomas, the histopathological diagnoses may be difficult to obtain on the basis of these minute tissue fragments. Furthermore, there are dosimetric problems due to the uncertain tumoral volume. If the dosage is radiobiologically insufficient, little therapeutic value ensues; and if it is excessive, the dosage may cause damage to surrounding tissue, and cause possible neurological deficits.

Lastly, there are technical problems (strictly surgical) that may cause irregular dose distributions. The stereotactic procedure is a fine and rigorous technique; however, when placing a radioisotope, the proceeding biopsy may cause an irregular lacuna, and the seed could fall into a deeper position than what was calculated as the target point, altering the spatial dose distribution.

Despite these problems and the need for further refinement of the procedure, our experience is positive and leads us to affirm that, at the present moment, interstitial brachytherapy is the treatment of choice in low malignant inoperable neoplasms (fig. 1).

In subcortical tumors,with poorly defined borders, massive demyelinization of the surrounding white matter may occur, possibly due to excessive dose, that, however, does not impinge on either the quality or the quantity of life. In deep-seated tumors that show spectacular CT

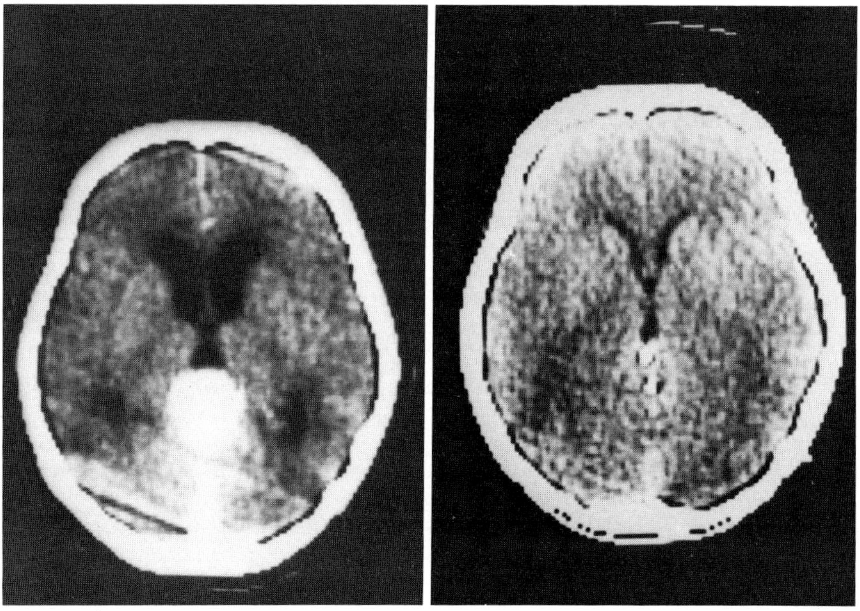

a b

Fig. 1. CT image low grade pineal astrocytoma in young female. **a** Tumor image prior to treatment. **b** Disappearance of the neoplasm 2 years after the implant with ^{125}I.

resolution, the prognosis is also unclear, due to the possible disorders caused by the necrosis of surrounding vital areas. Only 18 months after the implant (when the radiobiological effect subsides) in the absence of massive necrosis, can one be optimistic in these types of tumors. Our study also shows that neoplasms with high calcium content are difficult to treat, because the radiodosimetric calculations are seldom sufficient, since the calcium forms a radiation barrier. Chiasmatic gliomas responded poorly to brachytherapy. In two previously blind patients treated with ^{125}I, the lesion showed no modification at follow-up.

Conclusions

Although limited to only 5 years, our experience in the treatment of slow-growing cerebral neoplasms by means of brachytherapy using ^{125}I appears positive.

The advantages of this procedure are absence of postoperative mortality and morbidity; relative ease of execution of the intervention; and highly manageable isotope (^{125}I), with no special protective measures and relatively short half-life (60.2 days).

This procedure may be repeated, if necessary, and also allows for good social recovery in cases with tumors located in deep-seated and/or highly functional areas.

References

1 Birg, W.; Mundinger, F.; Klar, M.: Computer assistance for stereotactic brain operations. Adv. Neurosurg. *4:* 287–291 (1977).

2 Mundinger, F.; Ostertag, C.: Computerized tomography in stereotactic interstitial curietherapy of midline tumors; in Lanksch, Kazner, Cranial computerized tomography, pp. 110–113 (Springer, Berlin 1976).

3 Mundinger, F.: Rationale and methods of interstitial iridium-192 brachycurietherapy and iridium-192 or iodine-125 protracted long term irradiation; in Szikla, Stereotactic cerebral irradiation. Inserm Symp. No. 12, pp. 101–116 (Elsevier/North-Holland Biochemical, Amsterdam, 1979).

4 Szikla, G.; Peragut, J.C.: Irradiation interstitielle des gliomes; in Schlienger, Radiothérapie des tumeurs du système nerveux central de l'adulte. Neurochirurgie *21:* suppl. 2, pp. 187–228 (1975).

5 Talairach, J.; Bonis, G.; Szikla, G.; Schaub, G.; Boucaud, J.; Covello, L.; Bordas-Ferrer, F.: Stereotaxic implantation of radioactive isotopes in functional pituitary surgery. Techniques and results; in Wang, Paoletti, Radionuclide applications in neurology and neurosurgery, pp. 267–325 (Thomas, Springfield 1970).

Dr. F. Frank, Division of Neurosurgery, Bellaria Hospital, I-40139 Bologna (Italy)

Proc. 9th Meeting World Soc. Stereotactic and Functional
Neurosurgery, Toronto 1985
Appl. Neurophysiol. *48:* 127–132 (1985)

Epileptogenic Cerebral Low-Grade Tumors: Effect of Interstitial Stereotactic Irradiation on Seizures

G.F. Rossi, M. Scerrati, R. Roselli

Institute of Neurosurgery, Catholic University, Rome, Italy

Key Words. Epilepsy · Stereotactic brachycurietherapy · Stereotactic surgery · Tumor epilepsy

Abstract. 15 patients with various types of surgically inaccessible epileptogenic cerebral neuroepithelial tumors were treated with stereotactic interstitial irradiation. Epilepsy was improved in all cases, being abolished in 6 and markedly reduced in another 7. The effects which became apparent soon after the radioisotope implant persisted. Possible mechanisms of the phenomenon are discussed.

Epilepsy is a common symptom of supratentorial cerebral tumors [1]. In slowly developing gliomas it may be the only symptom for several years. In surgically macroscopically accessible tumors (frontopolar, temporopolar, occipitopolar), complete removal is possible and there is thus a good chance of cure of epilepsy. On the other hand, when the tumor is not amenable to surgery, pharmacological treatment fails to completely control the seizures in a relevant number of case. We report an experience treating this second type of patient with stereotactic interstitial curietherapy.

Material and Method

15 patients of both sexes, with epileptogenic surgically nonresectable cerebral tumors (2 recurrences), from 17 to 51 years of age, are considered. All had repeated seizures for a minimum of 6 months to a maximum of 18 years (fig. 1). In all cases pharmacological treatment was maintained for at least 4 months. The study of the electroclinical seizure pattern (repeated long-lasting EEG accompanied by TV monitoring) revealed a partial origin in all patients with a secondary generalization in 8 (fig. 2). The frequency

Table I. Histology and location of the tumors

	Dienceph.	Deep frontal	Rolandic	Temporal	Temporo parietal	Temporo parieto occipital
Pilocytic astrocytoma (I)		1				
Astrocytoma (II)		1	4	1	2	1
Oligodendro-glioma (II)	1		1			
Oligoastrocytoma (II)			2			
Anaplastic astrocytoma (III)			1			

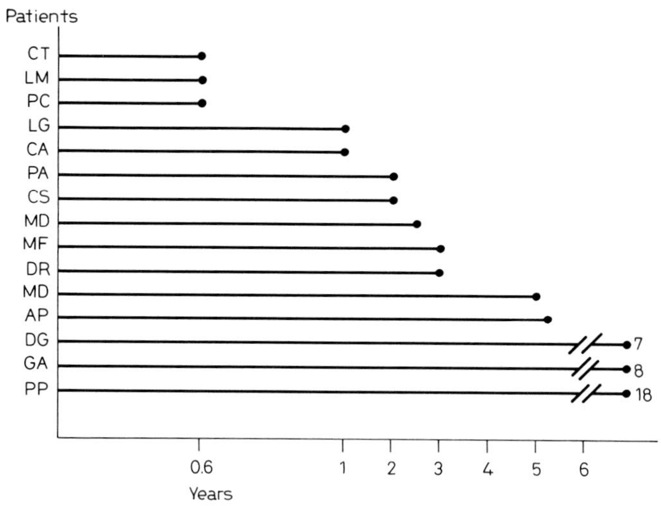

Fig. 1. Duration of epilepsy before treatment.

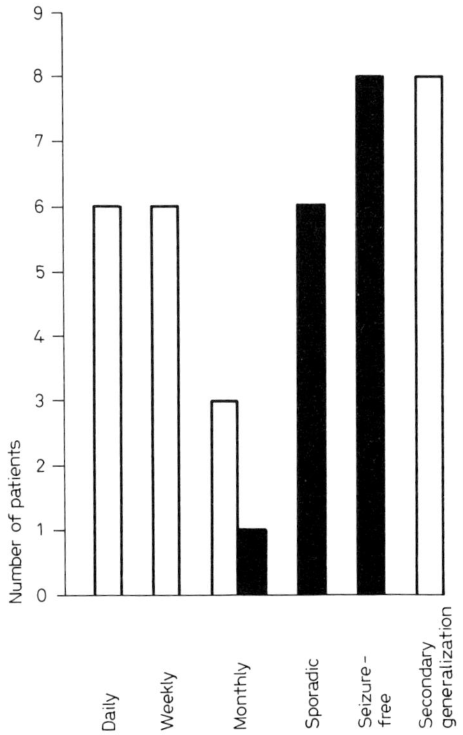

Fig. 2. Frequency and character of seizures before (□) and after (■) interstitial stereotactic irradiation.

of the seizures was of at least one per day in 6 patients, weekly in 6 and monthly in the remaining 3 despite pharmacological treatment (fig. 2). The Karnovsky evaluation of performance status ranged from 0.40 to 0.80.

Stereotactic biopsy (Talairach apparatus integrated with the polar accessorium designed in our laboratory [7]) was always performed. Multiple stereotactic tracks permitted definition of the nature of the tumor as well as its volume and spatial configuration [2, 3, 8, 9]; the results are synthetized in tables 1 and 3. The location of the tumor is also indicated in table 1.

Stereotactic brachycurietherapy was performed with permanently implanted ^{125}I in 11 cases. The modalities of the treatment were planned by integrating neuroradiological data and morphovolumetric information provided by the stereobiopsy (fig. 3). The isotope implant was performed in such a way as to reach (165–205 days, according to the isotope) a dose of 100–120 Gy: (i) at the periphery of relatively compact and circumscribed tumors, showing very scarce tumor cell infiltration (4 patients; maximum volume 17 cm^3) (ii) at the periphery of the compact nucleus (maximum volume 56 cm^3) of tumors showing obvious scattered cell infiltration in the surrounding tissue, bringing the theoretical

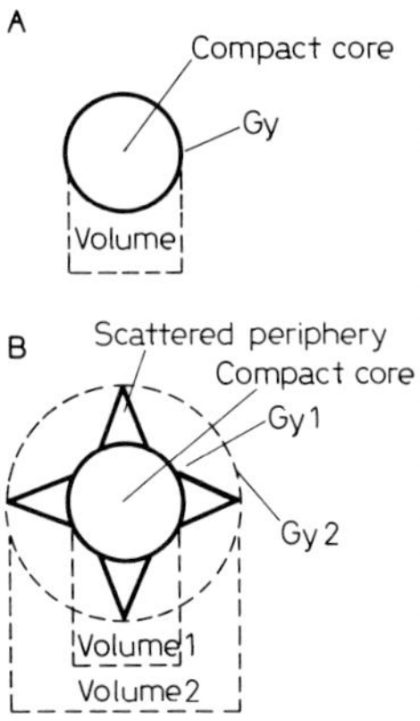

Pts n	Volume	Gy	External RxT
4	max 17 cm^3	100 - 130	no
11	1 max 56 cm^3 2 max 142 cm^3	1 100 - 130 2 30 - 80	yes (40-50 Gy in 4-6 weeks)

Fig. 3. Schematization of the modalities of treatment according to the volume and spatial configuration of the tumor.

'global' volume of the tumor to a maximum of 142 cm^3 [4-6, 10-12]; in this second group of patients (11 cases) in addition to the above dose, a dose of 30-80 Gy was delivered at the periphery of the 'global' volume and external radiotherapy was suggested [6, 10-12]. When accepted (9 cases), the latter was performed with fields exceeding the 'global' limits of the tumor by at least 2 cm, in fractioned (4-6 weeks) doses of 40-50 Gy; in this way the total dose (brachytherapy plus teletherapy) at the 'global' volume periphery reached at least 80 Gy.

Follow-up ranged from 5 to 57 months (mean 24 months). The pharmacological antiepileptic treatment was maintained, though reduced with respect to the preradiation treatment in some cases.

Results

Seizure Occurrence and Frequency (fig. 2). In 8 patients, seizures were completely suppressed; in 6, only sporadic seizures occurred; 1 patient reported monthly seizures. Daily and weekly frequencies were abolished.

Characteristics of the Seizures. When persisting, the seizures were of partial type only. Secondary generalization disappeared (fig. 2).

Time of Appearance and Duration of the Effect. The effect of brachycurietherapy on the seizures became evident very early. Actually, in the patients with daily seizures, in whom such an evaluation was easier, seizure disappearance could appear on the day of treatment. The effect persisted (maximum follow-up 57 months) in 13 patients. Two patients showed a return of the seizures 9 and 11 months after the treatment. Neuroradiological studies showed that this seizure recurrence was coincident with the development of radionecrosis. The seizures disappeared again along with the spontaneous reduction of radionecrosis.

Comments

Our findings clearly indicate that the stereotactic insertion of radioactive sources within epileptogenic cerebral gliomas is quite effective in reducing and even suppressing epilepsy. The previous data by *Szikla* et al. [11, 12] are thus confirmed.

The nature of the phenomenon is not known. At least two mechanisms can be suggested: (1) The epileptogenic action of the tumor is lowered because of the reduction of the tumor mass. This hypothesis seems supported by (i) the evidence of progressive mass reduction shown by serial CT scans (all of our cases); (ii) the progressive neurological improvement (all of our cases); (iii) the seizure recurrence with development of radionecrosis and subsequent improvement with radionecrosis reduction (2 of our cases), and (iv) the seizure reappearance following tumor recurrence (as shown by *Szikla* [11]). (2) The epileptogenicity of the cerebral neurons in the vicinity of the tumor or mixed with the neoplastic cells [1], which is responsible for the seizures, is directly affected by the radiation. This second hypothesis is justified by the early appearance of the full effect almost immediately after implantation of the radioactive sources and certainly before they could affect the tumoral mass.

Both the above-mentioned mechanisms are likely to be involved. Further investigation into this matter seems worthwhile.

References

1 Bancaud, J.; Talairach, J.; Geier, S.; Scarabin, J.M.: EEG et SEEG dans les tumeurs cérébrales et l'épilepsie (Edifor, Paris 1973).
2 Daumas-Duport, C.; Monsaingeon, V.; Szenthe, L.; Szikla, G.: Serial stereotactic biopsies: a double histological code of gliomas according to malignancy and 3D

configuration, as an aid to therapeutic decision and assessment of results. Appl. Neurophysiol. *45:* 431–437 (1982).
3 Daumas-Duport, C.; Vedrenne, C.; Szikla, G.: Contribution of stereotactic biopsies to the 3D localization of brain tumors, gliomas in particular; in Szikla, Stereotactic cerebral irradiation, pp. 33–41 (Elsevier/North-Holland, Amsterdam 1979).
4 Mundinger, F.: The treatment of brain tumors with interstitially applied radioactive isotopes; in Wang, Paoletti, Radionuclide applications in neurology and neurosurgery, pp. 199–265 (Thomas, Springfield 1970).
5 Mundinger, F.: Rationale and methods of interstitial iridium-192 brachycurietherapy and iridium-192 or iodine-125 protracted long-term irradiation; in Szikla, Stereotactic cerebral irradiation, pp. 101–115 (Elsevier, Amsterdam 1979).
6 Scerrati, M.; Arcovito, G.; D'Abramo, G.; Montemaggi, P.; Pastore, G.; Piermatei, A.; Romanini, A.; Rossi, G.F.: Stereotactic interstitial irradiation of brain tumors: preliminary reports. Rays *7:* 93–99 (1982).
7 Scerrati, M.; Fiorentino, A.; Fiorentino, M.; Pola, P.: Stereotaxic device for polar approaches in orthogonal systems. Tech. note. J. Neurosurg. *61:* 1146–1147 (1984).
8 Scerrati, M.; Pizzolato, G.P.: The role of stereotactic biopsy in the 3-dimensional localization of cerebral tumor. Acta neurochir. *57:* 305–306 (1981).
9 Scerrati, M.; Rossi, G.F.: The reliability of stereotactic biopsy. Acta neurochir. *33:* suppl., pp. 201–205 (1984).
10 Schlienger, M.; Bouhnik, H.; Missir, O.; Constans, J.P.; Szikla, G.: Association of the temporary interstitial ^{192}Ir implantation and external radiotherapy in the management of supratentorial tumors. Technique and dosimetry; in Szikla, Stereotactic cerebral irradiation, pp. 117–121 (Elsevier, Amsterdam 1979).
11 Szikla, G.: Combined interstitial and external irradiation of gliomas. A progress report (cooperative study); in Szikla, Stereotactic cerebral irradiation, pp. 329–338 (Elsevier, Amsterdam 1979).
12 Szikla, G.; Schlienger, M.; Blond, S.; Daumas-Duport, C.; Missir, O.; Miyahara, S.; Musolino, A.; Schaub, C.: Interstitial and combined interstitial external irradiation of supratentorial gliomas. Results in 61 cases treated 1973–1981. Acta neurochir. *33:* suppl., pp. 355–362 (1984).

Dr. G.F. Rossi, Institute of Neurosurgery, Catholic University,
Largo A. Gemelli 8, I-00168 Rome (Italy)

Proc. 9th Meeting World Soc. Stereotactic and Functional
Neurosurgery, Toronto 1985
Appl. Neurophysiol. *48:* 133–145 (1985)

Stereotactic Radiosurgery Utilizing a Linear Accelerator

F. Colombo[a], *A. Benedetti*[a], *F. Pozza*[b], *A. Zanardo*[c], *R.C. Avanzo*[d], *G. Chierego*[d], *C. Marchetti*[d]

Departments of [a] Neurosurgery and [b] Radiotherapy, City Hospital, Vicenza; [c] Institute of Applied Mechanics, University of Padova, and [d] Service of Medical Physics, City Hospital, Vicenza, Italy

Key Words. Radiotherapy · Radiosurgery · Brain tumor · Stereotactic surgery

Abstract. The authors have developed a radiosurgical technique based on multiple arc irradiations. The target is fixed to the rotational isocenter of a Varian 4 MV linear accelerator. The first irradiation is carried out while the radiating source is rotating on a 100–140° arc. The patient is then rotated around a vertical axis passing through the target, and arc irradiations are repeated in different angular positions. By this technique it is possible to obtain very steep dose gradients at the borders of the target volume. High doses are usually delivered in two shots.

47 patients have been treated so far in a clinical trial that started in November 1982. The paper deals with the preliminary results (more than 6 months' follow-up) obtained in patients affected by nonresectable brain tumors and AVMs.

Introduction

Since the early sixties, at the Karolinska Institute of Stockholm, single dose, multiple beam stereotactic irradiation (radiosurgery) has been employed as a therapeutic tool [11]. The main advantages of this 'closed surgical technique' are the steep dose gradient and the high spatial accuracy obtainable with the Gamma Unit. Since the beginning of radiosurgical activity, a large series of selected intracranial tumors and AVMs has been treated [1, 12, 15, 16] and the procedure has been proven safe and reliable. The single and very important drawback is the high cost of the equipment. Meanwhile other radiosurgical techniques have been developed and tested. *Kjellberg* et al. [9] utilize the Bragg peak of the proton beam. *Barcia Salorio* et al. [2] use a special collimator coupled with a telecobalt unit. *Betti and Derechinski* [3] and

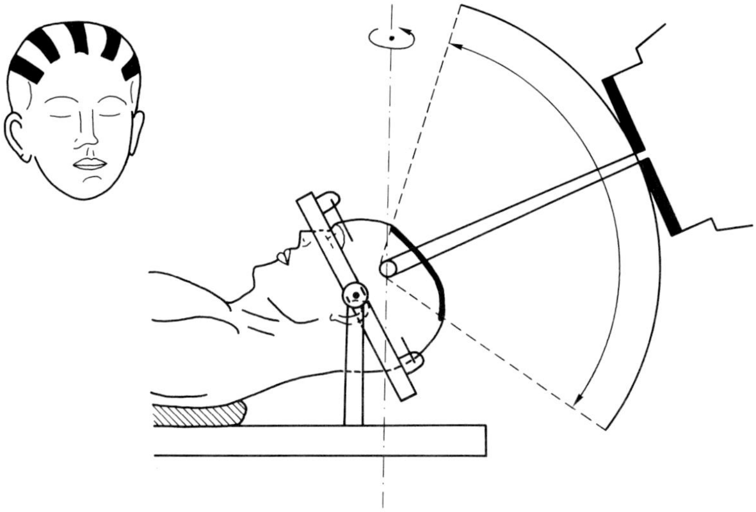

Fig. 1. Patient fixed to the treatment couch; target coincides with the isocenter. Arc irradiations are multiplied by rotating the patient around a vertical axis.

Hartmann et al. [7] have selected the highly collimated beam of the linear accelerator, but both of them require complicated and expensive machinery.

We have developed an original radiosurgical technique which employs a common isocentric linear accelerator coupled with our stereotactic apparatus, and have employed it in clinical practice since 1982. By this straightforward technique any isocentric linear accelerator can be converted into an efficient radiosurgical machine. The extra equipment needed is neither complicated nor expensive [5, 6].

The aim of this communication is to present the preliminary results obtained in a series of patients affected by deep-seated, nonresectable intracranial lesions.

Materials and Method

The technique and the set-up have been extensively described elsewhere [6]. The principle (fig. 1) is as follows: the target is fixed to the rotational isocenter of the linear accelerator. The first irradiation is undertaken through a 100–140° arc. The patient is then rotated around a vertical axis passing through the target and the arc irradiations are

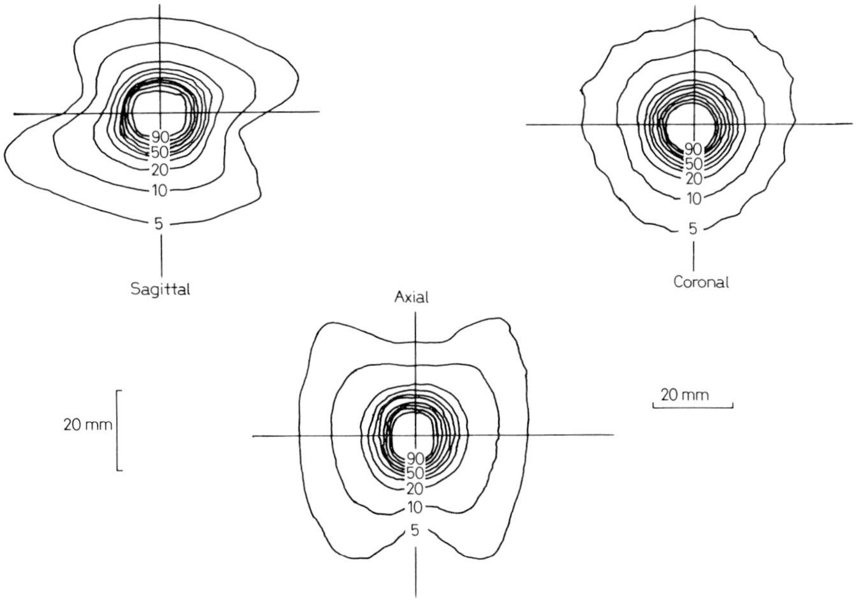

Fig. 2. Isodoses obtained by film dosimetry on paraffin phantoms. 9 arcs, field 15 × 15 mm.

repeated at different angular approaches spread over the hemisphere and overlying convexity of the skull.

Before undertaking a clinical trial, the performances of our technique in terms of dose concentration and dose gradient have been evaluated by film dosimetry employing anthropomorphic and paraffin phantoms. Isodoses read by the photodensitometer are shown in figure 2. To enhance the sparing of irradiation of healthy tissues, the collimator openings can be adapted to the variable cross section of the lesion.

The procedure is started by fixing the patient to our stereotactic apparatus [4]. After the localization procedures, either CT or angiography, a stereotactic biopsy is performed. Intraoperative cytological sampling is necessary to ascertain the pathology of the lesion and to verify the three-dimensional shape of the tumor [13]. Once the biopsy is completed, the multiple arc irradiation procedure is simulated.

A millimetric ruler is fixed to the tool holder. By moving this ruler the appropriate plans of arc irradiations are selected to avoid radiosensitive structures. The depth of the tissues that must be passed through by the beam before reaching the target are recorded and transmitted to the dose-planning computer system. The computer then provides the parameters of irradiation.

A head frame adaptor has been built for the treatment couch of our Varian Clinac 4 MV linear accelerator. Preliminary tests have demonstrated that the 4–6 MV energy range is the most suitable for radiosurgery of intracranial targets. The accelerator has

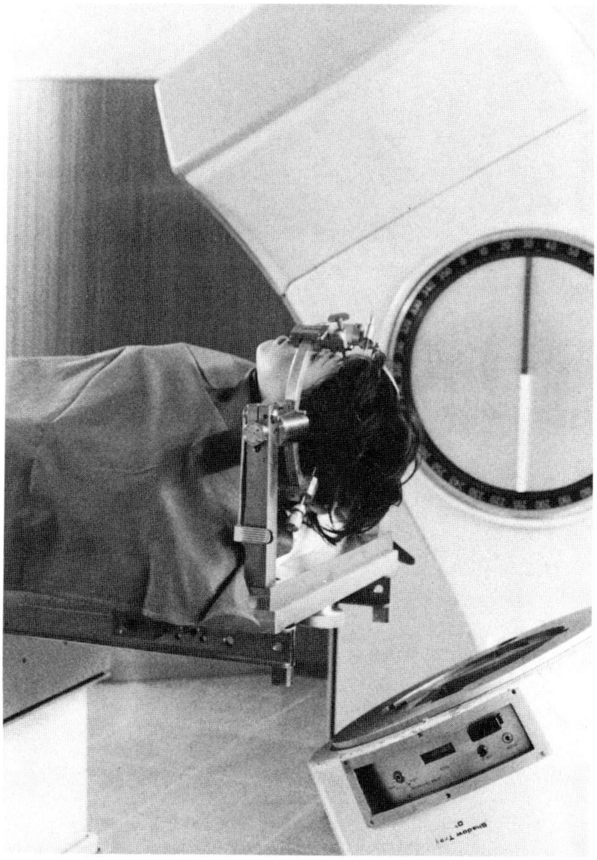

Fig. 3. The patient positioned ready for treatment.

two main features that are indispensable for performing radiosurgical operations. The first is the high mechanical accuracy in the movement of the couch. The second is the possibility to obtain without any adjunctive collimators very small fields free of penumbra.

The target point (the center of the target volume) is made to coincide with the linear accelerator isocenter marked by the front-pointer by controlled movements of the couch and the aid of a base ring phantom. The patient is substituted for the phantom and the irradiation is undertaken (fig. 3).

The radiosurgical technique has been employed in clinical practice since November 1982. Our series presently consists of 47 patients, of which 36 have been followed up for more than 6 months (table I). All patients were deemed not suitable for open craniotomy, since most of the lesions were deep-seated or located in highly functional cortical areas.

Table I. Radiosurgery with linear accelerator (Nov. 82–Dec. 84)

Glial tumors		22
Low grade astrocytoma	9	
Anaplastic astrocytoma	7	
Glioblastoma	1	
Oligodendroglioma	2	
Ependymoma	2	
Choroid plexus papilloma	1	
Pinealomas		4
Pineocytoma	1	
Pineoblastoma	1	
Germinoma	2	
Medulloblastoma		1
Meningioma		1
Metastasis		2
Craniopharyngioma		2
Pituitary adenoma		1
Arteriovenous malformation		3
Total		36

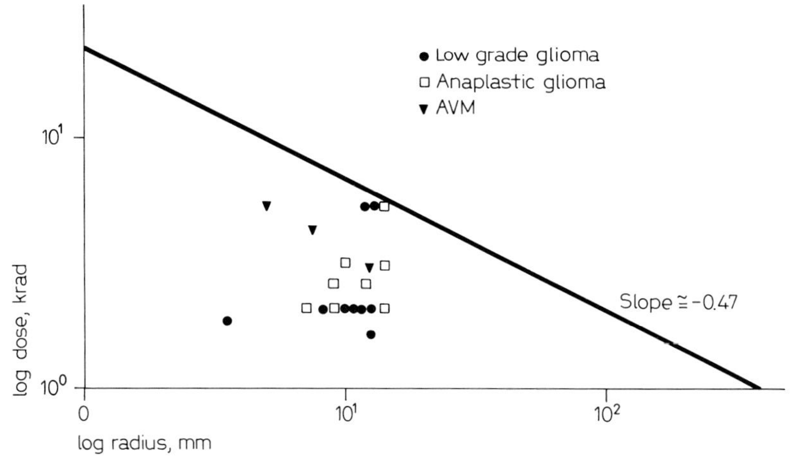

Fig. 4. Kjellberg's diagram log dose/log radius of three most important groups of patients.

Table II. Low grade astrocytoma

Case	Sex	Age years	Symptoms	Lesion	Radiation	Follow-up
1	M	14	raised ICP hemiparesis	lt. thalamic ∅ 24 mm	2 × 2,500 rad 5 arcs 28 × 28 mm	31 months - CT: shrinkage of the lesion normalized clinical picture
2	F	25	mental deterioration	corpus callosum ∅ 25 mm	2 × 2,500 rad 9 arcs 30 × 30 mm	25 months - CT: shrinkage of the lesion unchanged clinical picture
3	M	11	hydrocephalus	lt. thalamic ∅ 25 mm	2 × 800 rad 9 arcs 30 × 30 mm	18 months - CT: shrinkage of the lesion normal ventricular size
4	M	16	Parinaud's syndrome	pineal region ∅ 7 mm	2 × 900 rad 9 arcs 10 × 10 mm	18 months - CT: shrinkage of the lesion normal ocular motility
5	M	12	amaurosis	optic chiasm ∅ 23 mm	2 × 1,000 rad 9 arcs 25 × 25 mm	15 months - CT: shrinkage of the lesion unchanged clinical picture
6	F	21	hemiparesis	rt. thalamic ∅ 20 mm	2 × 1,000 rad 17 arcs 25 × 25 mm	13 months - CT: unchanged unchanged clinical picture
7	F	12	Parinaud's syndrome	pineal region ∅ 17 mm	2 × 1,000 rad 17 arcs 22 × 22 mm	13 months - CT: unchanged unchanged clinical picture
8	M	25	hemiparesis	lt. parietal ∅ 25 mm	2 × 1,000 rad 17 arcs 30 × 30 mm	8 months - CT: unchanged unchanged clinical picture
9	F	30	hydrocephalus	rt. thalamic ∅ 21 mm	2 × 1,000 rad 17 arcs 25 × 25 mm	6 months - CT: shrinkage of the lesion normal ventricular size

Target volumes displayed clear-cut borders and usually had a spherical three-dimensional shape. Collimator openings were selected to have the 80% isodose (where the dose gradient is steepest) coinciding with the borders of the target volume.

The total dose to be applied (usually in two sessions) was determined taking into account the volume of the lesion, the age of the patient, and the spatial relationship with

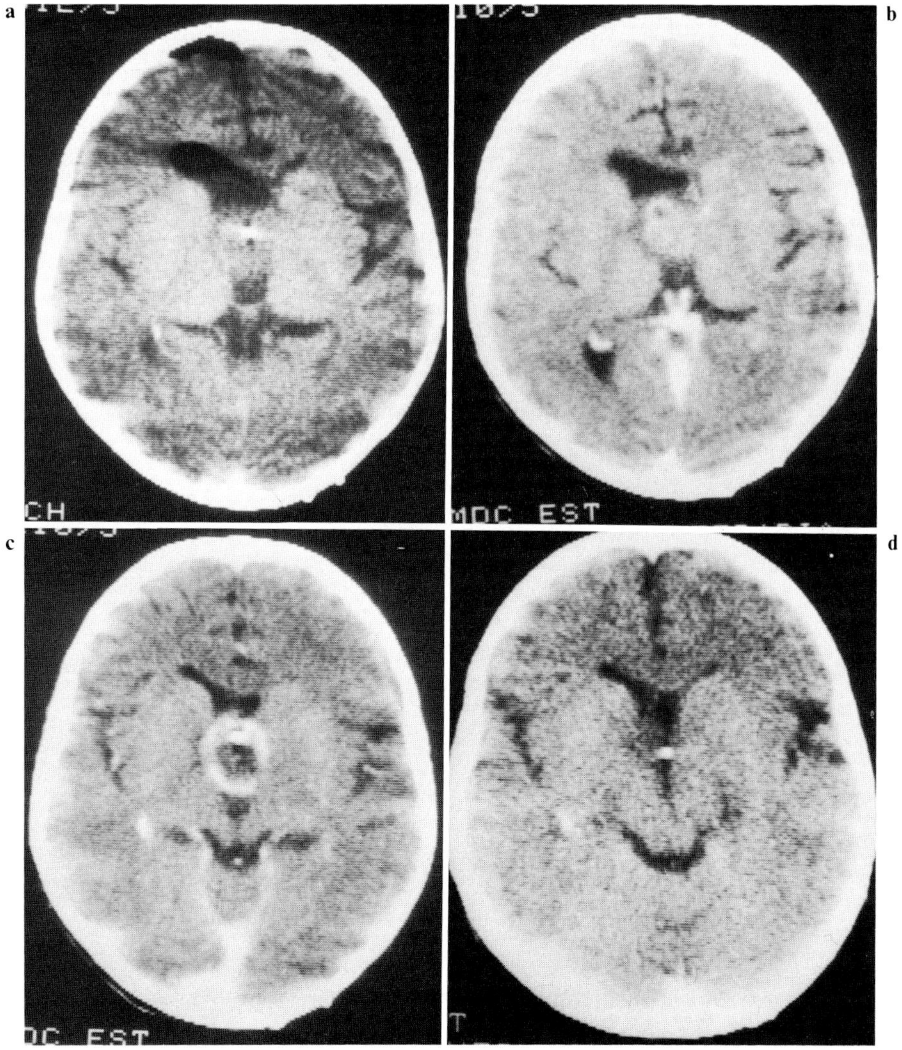

Fig. 5. Patient No. 3 (low grade astrocytoma): **(a)** before treatment, metallic marker on the biopsy site, **(b)** 1 month, **(c)** 3 months, and **(d)** 12 months after radiosurgery.

nearby radiosensitive structures. In figure 4 the dose applied to our most important groups of patients has been plotted in relation to the target volume radius. The upper limit represents the limit for a high risk of radionecrosis, according to *Kjellberg* [10]. In our experience a dose of 2,000–2,500 rad delivered in two sessions, 8 days apart, is both safe and well tolerated for lesions up to 30 mm in diameter.

Table III. Anaplastic astrocytoma

Case	Sex	Age years	Symptoms	Lesion	Radiation	Follow-up
1	F	34	diencephalic syndrome	hypothalamus ∅ 27 mm	2 × 2,500 rad 9 arcs 30 × 30 mm	27 months - CT: shrinkage unchanged clinical picture
2	F	14	hydrocephalus hemiparesis	rt. thalamic ∅ 18 mm	2 × 1,250 rad 17 arcs 23 × 23 mm	18 months - CT: shrinkage clinically improved
3	M	50	raised ICP hemiparesis	lt. temporal ∅ 27 mm	2 × 1,500 rad 9 arcs 35 × 35 mm	9 months - CT: worsened died
4	M	45	hemiparesis	rt. thalamic ∅ 28 mm	2 × 1,000 rad 9 arcs 35 × 35 mm	16 months - CT: unchanged unchanged clinical picture
5	M	21	hydrocephalus hemiparesis	lt. thalamic ∅ 25 mm	2 × 1,250 rad 17 arcs 30 × 30 mm	12 months - CT: unchanged clinically improved
6	F	12	hemiparesis	rt. thalamic ∅ 20 mm	2 × 1,500 rad 17 arcs 25 × 25 mm	6 months - CT: worsened died
7	M	11	raised ICP	mediofrontal ∅ 18 mm	2 × 1,000 rad 17 arcs 25 × 25 mm	4 months - worsened clinical picture operated on

Results

Low-Grade Astrocytomas

Nine patients were affected by low-grade astrocytomas (table II). In 7 patients we obtained good results from both the clinical and CT point of view. The therapeutic effect usually took 6–12 months to become evident. A typical evolution is displayed by patient 3. In this patient the CT picture before treatment showed a hypodense lesion without any contrast. One month after, the central core of the lesion was greatly enhanced by the contrast. Three months after, a typical ring feature was evident. At 12 months the tumor is almost completely gone (fig. 5a–d).

Table IV. Malignant radiosensitive tumors

Case	Sex	Age years	Symptoms	Lesion	Radiation	Follow-up
Pineo-blastoma	F	6	raised ICP Parinaud's syndrome cerebellar syndrome	pineal region ∅ 32 mm	3,000 rad refr. 2 × 1,000 rad 9 arcs 35 × 35 mm	31 months - CT: shrinkage of the lesion improved clinical picture
Medullo-blastoma	M	18	raised ICP cerebellar syndrome	mesencephalon ∅ 27 mm	1 × 1,500 rad 5 arcs 35 × 35- mm + 3,000 rad refr.	19 months - CT: shrinkage of the lesion normalized clinical picture
Germi-noma						
1	M	21	diencephalic syndrome tetraparesis	third ventricle ∅ 30 mm	1 × 1,000 rad 5 arcs 35 × 35 mm	28 days - CT: shrinkage died (unrelated) autopsy
2	M	14	hydrocephalus Parinaud's syndrome	pineal region ∅ 20 mm	1 × 1,000 rad 17 arcs 25 × 25 mm + 3,000 rad refr.	12 months - CT: shrinkage normalized clinical picture

Anaplastic Astrocytomas

Seven patients were affected by anaplastic astrocytomas (table III). Three patients showed a significant improvement of the clinical or CT picture. One patient is unchanged after 16 months. Two patients, both in poor clinical condition before radiosurgery, died presumably of their disease. One patient was operated on 4 months after radiosurgery for increasing intracranial pressure. Pathological examination of the specimen did not disclose any change attributable to radiosurgery.

Malignant Radiosensitive Tumors (table IV)

A heterogeneous group of radiosensitive tumors has been treated with stereotactically focalized dose. The aim of this radiosurgical in-

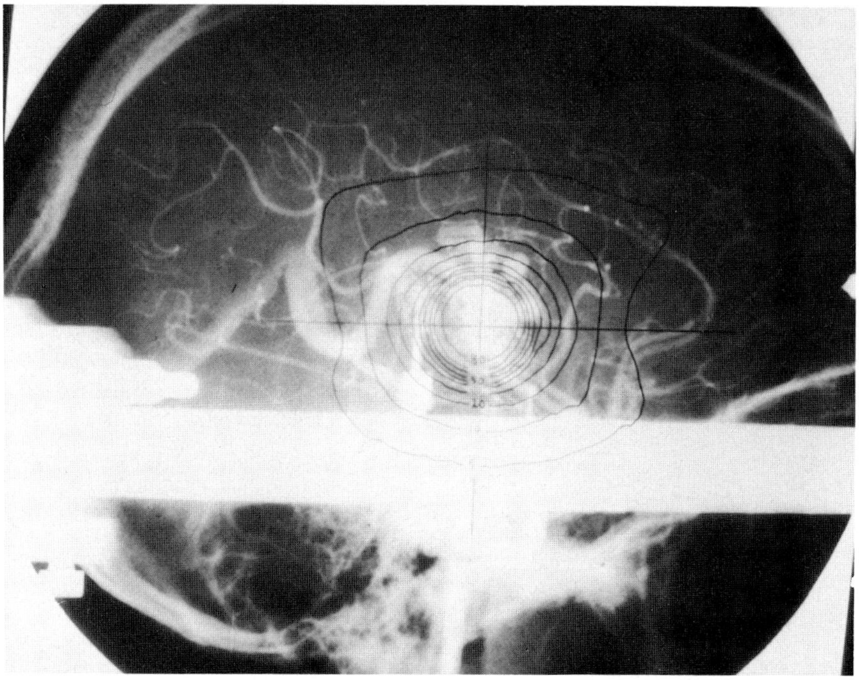

Fig. 6. Stereotactic angiography of a left thalamic arteriovenous malformation. Isodoses obtained with 9 arcs, 120° wide, field 20 × 20 mm. Two sessions of 2,000 rad, 8 days apart.

verse boost was to obtain a rapid debulking effect of the tumor mass following which the treatment was combined with extended field refracted dose radiotherapy to prevent cell seeding. The results were extremely good in 3 patients. One patient died of renal failure. Usually the debulking effect was strikingly evident 10–15 days after treatment, with complete shrinkage of the lesion.

Vascularized Tumors and AVMs

The unresectable part of an angioblastic meningioma infiltrating the cavernous sinus was left in place after a craniotomy operation on a 42-year-old female. This large (25 mm diameter) mass caused exophthalmos, chemosis, ophthalmoplegia and unbearable first division pain. Six months after surgery this patient was treated with two sessions of 1,250 rad. The lesion gradually shrunk (complete regression at 12 months) with clinical normalization.

Three patients affected by AVMs were treated with two shots of 1,500–3,000 rad. A minor hemorrhage recurred 1 month after treatment in 1 case. The clinical picture is unchanged in all patients. Follow-up angiography is planned 1 year after treatment (fig. 6).

Pathology

No low grade glioma underwent biopsy or autopsy examination after treatment. The specimen obtained in 1 patient, a 69-year-old male harboring a pineocytoma, may be of interest. In this patient, follow-up CT scans showed the development of a typical ring feature. The patient died 14 months after treatment of a chronic liver disease. At autopsy, the central core of the lesion was ischemic and necrotic. Blood vessels of the outermost shell of the tumor showed an intense endothelial proliferation with hyalinosis of the vessel wall.

The single patient affected by a glioblastoma was operated on 3 months after radiosurgery. Histological examination showed a largely necrotic tumor mass. Polynucleated giant cells were prominent in the still vital tumor tissue.

The autopsy specimen of the germinoma demonstrated a massive hemorrhagic necrosis of the entire tumor. No vital tumor tissue was still recognizable. There was no sign of radiation damage in the surrounding nervous tissue.

Conclusions

Radiosurgery with our technique has some theoretical and practical advantages. It is feasible on every isocentric linear accelerator. A large dose can be safely delivered to the target. Radiosensitivity of the lesion is not needed. An overkilling effect inside the target volume is obtained without risk of radiation damage outside it.

Although our follow-up is short, radiosurgery seems to be effective in low grade gliomas, where it can be considered a challenging alternative to radioisotope implantation. It can also be extremely useful to reduce rapidly the mass effect of radiosensitive malignant tumors. Moreover, it is the only stereotactic irradiation procedure that can be employed in vascularized tumors and AVMs.

With regard to the possible pathogenetic factors leading to the therapeutic effect, these seem to be more strictly related to the total amount of the radiation dose than to its time schedule of fractionation (two large doses 8 days apart). This fact is in agreement with a nonspecific damage induced by the radiosurgical focal dose. On the other hand, owing to the well-known low proliferating fraction in low grade gliomas [8], a cell cycle specific effect must be rejected, at least in these tumors.

The time lapse from the radiosurgical treatment to the actual shrinkage of slow growing tumors is more critical. In most of the patients the therapeutic effect took 9–12 months to be completed. In the first 6 months, a temporary increase of the mass effect, seldom requiring major therapeutic maneuvers, should be expected.

Our pathological evidence is too scanty to draw any definitive conclusions. However, we presume that the radiosurgery effect in slow growing tumors could be mediated by tumor vessels damage, which could be the intermediate step of the therapeutic effect. The same effect should be involved in cases of vascularized tumors and AVMs. The vessel damage, beginning in the central core, where a higher dose is delivered, could underlie also the appearance of the ring feature at CT follow-up [14].

The massive necrotization of highly malignant tumors induced by a single dose in a very short time (a constant feature of germinomas and 'small cell' tumors, still remains unexplained. But the main problem to be solved is the choice of the dose to be delivered. The radiosurgical experience of the Karolinska Institute (employing much higher doses) cannot directly be applied to ours. Our collimator openings are different (usually larger). The dose gradient for small fields seems to be steeper than that of the gamma unit, but for larger fields the trend is reversed. On the other hand, the Kjellberg diagram [9] radius/dose for radiosurgical procedures is based on few cases and has a large range of unreliability. The choice of the dose still remains a difficult one.

References

1 Backlund, O.: Stereotactic treatment of craniopharyngiomas. Acta neurochir. *21:* suppl., pp. 177–183 (1974).

2 Barcia Salorio, J.L.; Hernandez, G.; Broseta, J.; Gonzales Darder, J.; Ciudad, J.:

Radiosurgical treatment of carotid-cavernous fistulas. Appl. Neurophysiol. *45:* 520–522 (1982).
3 Betti, O.; Derechinski, V.: Irradiation stéréotaxique multifascieaux. Neurochirurgie *29:* 295–298 (1983).
4 Colombo, F.; Angrilli, F.; Zanardo, A.; Pinna, V.; Alexandre, A.; Benedetti, A.: A universal method to employ CT scanner spatial information in stereotactic surgery. Appl. Neurophysiol. *45:* 352–364 (1982).
5 Colombo, F.; Casentini, L.; Benedetti, A.; Pozza, F.: Biopsia e radioterapia stereotassica dei gliomi cerebrali. Minerva med. *75:* 1327–1331 (1984).
6 Colombo, F.; Benedetti, A.; Pozza, F.; Avanzo, R.C.; Marchetti, C.; Chierego, G.; Zanardo, A.: External stereotactic irradiation by a linear accelerator. Neurosurgery *16:* 154–160 (1985).
7 Hartmann, G.H.; Schlegel, W.; Sturm, V.; Kober, B.; Pastyr, O.; Lorenz, W.: Cerebral radiation surgery using moving field irradiation at a linear accelerator facility. J. radiat. Oncol. Biol. Phys. (in press, 1985).
8 Hoshino, T.: A commentary on the biology and growth kinetics of low grade and high grade gliomas. J. Neurosurg. *61:* 895–901 (1984).
9 Kjellberg, R.N.; Nguyen, N.C.; Kliman, B.: Le Bragg peak protonique en neurochirurgie stéréotaxique. Neurochirurgie *18:* 235–264 (1972).
10 Kjellberg, R.N.: Isoeffective dose parameters for brain necrosis in relation to radiosurgery dosimetry; in Szikla, Stereotactic cerebral irradiation, pp. 157–166 (Elsevier, Amsterdam 1979).
11 Leksell, L.: Stereotaxy and radiosurgery: an operative system (Thomas, Springfield 1971).
12 Noren, G.; Leksell, L.: Stereotactic radiosurgery of acoustic tumors; in Szikla, Stereotactic cerebral irradiation, pp. 241–244 (Elsevier, Amsterdam 1979).
13 Ostertag, C.; Mennel, H.D.; Kiessling, M.: Stereotactic biopsy of brain tumors. Surg. Neurol. *14:* 257–262 (1980).
14 Ostertag, C.; Weigel, K.; Birg, W.: CT changes after long-term interstitial iridium-192 irradiation of cerebral gliomas; in Szikla, Stereotactic cerebral irradiation, pp. 149–157 (Elsevier, Amsterdam 1979).
15 Rahn, T.; Amiko, M.; Arndt, J.: Stereotactic radiosurgery in the treatment of MB Cushing; in Szikla, Stereotactic cerebral irradiation, pp. 207–212 (Elsevier, Amsterdam 1979).
16 Steiner, L.; Leksell, L.; Forster, D.; Greitz, T.; Backlund, O.: Stereotactic radiosurgery of arteriovenous malformations. Acta neurochir. *21:* suppl., pp. 195–209 (1975).

Federico Colombo, Divisione di Neurochirurgia, Ospedale Civile,
Viale Rodolfi, I-36100 Vicenza (Italy)

Proc. 9th Meeting World Soc. Stereotactic and Functional Neurosurgery, Toronto 1985
Appl. Neurophysiol. *48:* 146–150 (1985)

Stereotactic Intracavitary Irradiation of Cystic Neoplasms of the Brain

L. Dade Lunsford[a], *L. Gumerman*[b], *G. Levine*[a]

Departments of [a] Neurological Surgery and [b] Nuclear Medicine, University of Pittsburgh School of Medicine, and Presbyterian-University Hospital, Pittsburgh, Pa., USA

Key Words. Cystic tumors · Computer tomography stereotaxis · Radiotherapy

Abstract. Ten patients with intracranial cystic tumors underwent stereotactic intracavitary irradiation using ^{32}P colloidal chromic phosphate. Accurate dosimetry (25,000–30,000 rad to the cast wall) was achieved by volume estimation using computed tomography. Between 1 and 15 months after surgery both craniopharyngioma and astrocytoma cysts regressed. Neurological, visual, and endocrinological deficits either stabilized or improved. Intracavitary irradiation should be the primary method of treating solitary cystic tumors of the brain.

Stereotactic intracavitary irradiation of cystic craniopharyngiomas has been performed sporadically in the United States since 1951. The superior results of intracavitary irradiation reported by *Backlund* and co-workers [1, 2], *Strauss* et al. [9], *Szikla* et al. [10], and others [3–5] have been neglected in favor of attempted radical resection by craniotomy. The long-term results of radical craniopharyngioma surgery have been discouraging, and increasingly radiation therapy has been advocated to improve postoperative longevity and intellectual and endocrinological function. For cystic tumors, implantation of beta-emitting isotopes such as ^{90}Y and ^{186}Re, with relatively short penetrance of the energy and short half-lives, has proven effective. These isotopes are not available in the United States due in part to the orphan drug phenomenon created by regulations of the Food and Drug Administration and supply and demand considerations. We report the results of stereotactic intracavitary irradiation using ^{32}P colloidal chromic phosphate in 8 patients with cystic craniopharyngiomas and 2 patients with cystic astrocytomas in the region of the third ventricle.

Methods and Materials

Ten patients (6 females, 4 males, age range 4–70 years) underwent surgery. Eight patients had solitary cystic craniopharyngiomas; 7 had no prior treatment. Two patients had cystic astrocytomas. The Leksell stereotactic coordinate frame (AB Elekta, Decatur, Ga.) was used in conjuction with a dedicated surgical GE 8800 CT scanner (GE Medical Systems, Milwaukee, Wisc.). All patients had visual, neurological or endocrinological deficits appropriate to the size and the location of the cyst. Radiation dosimetry of ^{32}P colloidal chromic phosphate (target dose of 25,000–30,000 rad to the cyst wall) was based upon volume calculation of the cyst. In 6 patients, CT estimated dosimetry was compared to that obtained by an isotope dilution technique using ^{99m}Tc sulfur colloid [7, 8]. Follow-up duration after treatment ranged from 6 to 36 months (mean 18.6 months).

Results

Cyst volumes ranged from 2.8 to 80 ml. Colloidal ^{32}P dosimetry using the CT technique alone proved accurate when compared to the isotope dilution technique [6], and 2 patients were treated by CT dosimetry alone. CT stereotactic puncture of the cyst was done with the fine needle technique to prevent isotope leakage [2]. Biopsies were not performed but the cyst fluid was examined. Three of 8 patients with craniopharyngiomas had cholesterol crystals seen by polarized light microscopy. Stereotactic repuncture of the cyst was performed in 6 patients from 14 to 70 days after implantation to reduce local mass effect. No significant amount of isotope was recovered from repuncture, since the isotope presumably adhered to the cyst wall. Subsequent biopsy of 1 patient with a large third ventricular cyst demonstrated an anaplastic astrocytoma of the septum pellucidum.

Follow-up CT, ophthalmological, and endocrinological evaluations were performed. All patients had CT evidence of gradual cyst regression from 2 to 8 months after surgery (fig. 1). All 8 patients with craniopharyngiomas had stabilization of endocrinological function. One patient subsequently required craniotomy for resection of a solid

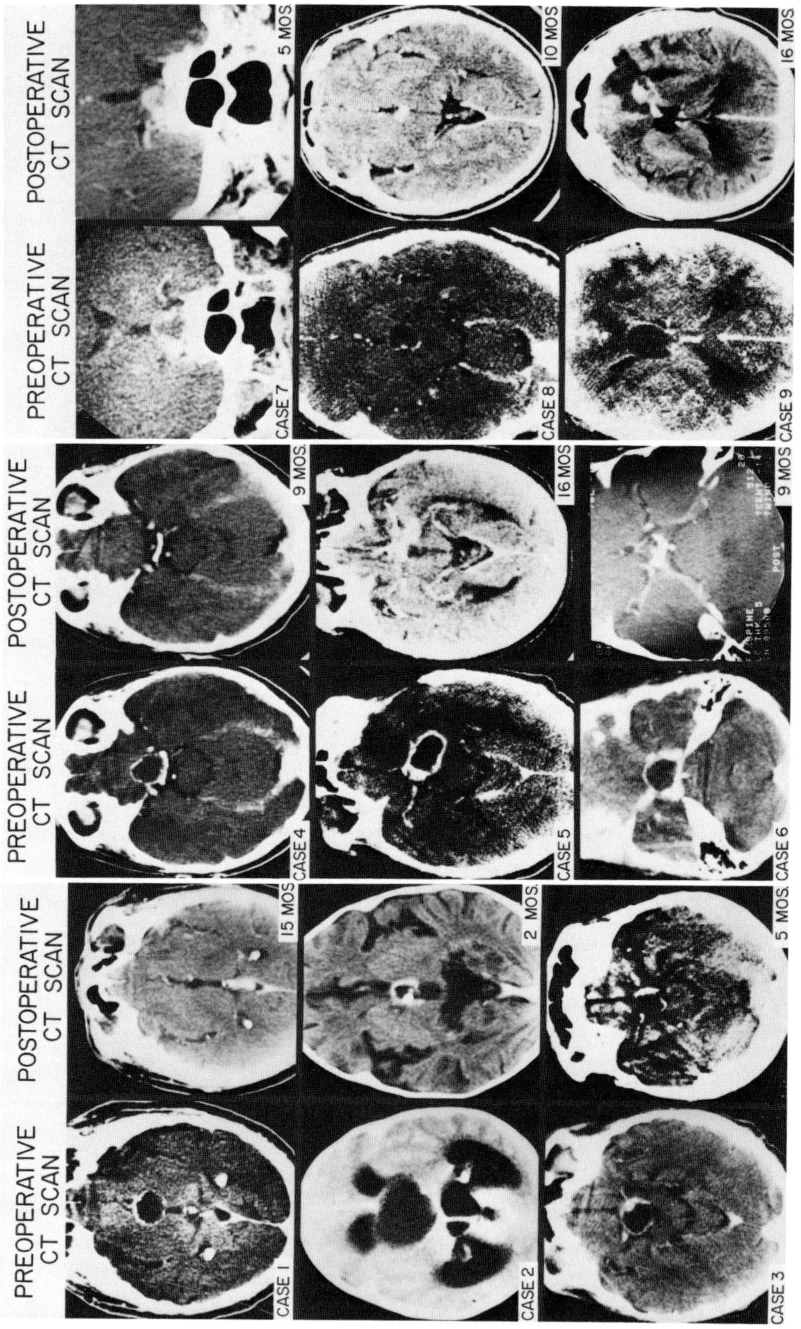
PREOPERATIVE CT SCAN
POSTOPERATIVE CT SCAN
CASE 1
15 MOS
CASE 2
2 MOS.
CASE 3
5 MOS.
PREOPERATIVE CT SCAN
POSTOPERATIVE CT SCAN
CASE 4
9 MOS.
CASE 5
16 MOS
CASE 6
9 MOS
PREOPERATIVE CT SCAN
POSTOPERATIVE CT SCAN
CASE 7
5 MOS
CASE 8
10 MOS
CASE 9
16 MOS

craniopharyngioma component resulting in progressive optic chiasm compression. Visual deficits improved in 8 of 10 patients.

Discussion

^{32}P colloidal chromic phosphate has certain attractive features as an agent to provide intracavitary beta-irradiation to thin-walled cystic tumors of the brain [5]. These include half value tissue penetrance of 0.8 mm and a half-life of 14.2 days. Surrounding structures are spared significant radiation, and radiation effects persist for up to 70 days (5 half-lives). Since no significant recovery of the isotope occurred with repuncture of the cyst, as may be necessary in cyst producing local mass effect, the extended half-life of this isotope in comparison to ^{90}Y may be beneficial.

Our experience in comparing CT dosimetry to that obtained by the isotope dilution technique as recommended by *Backlund* [2] confirmed that CT alone is adequate for defining cyst volumes [7]. Since minimal critical dose (i.e., 20,000 rad) seemed to be necessary, dose variations from 25,000 to 35,000 rad were satisfactory.

Eight patients with craniopharyngiomas all had cyst regression; 1 patient subsequently required craniotomy for removal of the solid tumor portion. One patient who had three prior operations and radiation therapy now has evidence of solid tumor growth and may require stereotactic radiosurgery using the gamma unit [1]. Preoperative endocrinological function was preserved in all patients, and visual function improved in 8. Both patients with cystic astrocytomas had regression of the cyst after intracavitary irradiation but both have subsequently deteriorated because of progressive growth of their neoplasms. Stereotactic intracavitary irradiation with ^{32}P colloid is a safe and effective method that resulted in cyst regression and preservation of endocrinological, visual and intellectual function. We believe that intracavitary irradiation should be the primary treatment for solitary cystic tumors of the brain.

Fig. 1. Treatment by stereotactic intracavitary ^{32}P. Preoperative and postoperative CT scans of 8 patients with solitary cystic craniopharyngiomas and 1 patient with a cystic anaplastic astrocytoma (case 9). Cyst regression occurred in each case, although case 9 deteriorated after 24 months because of solid tumor growth. Cyst volumes ranged from 2.8 to 80 ml.

Acknowledgments

Phyllis Shoemaker and *Mary Ann Vincenzini* aided in manuscript preparation.

References

1 Backlund, E.O.; Johansson, L.; Sarby, B.: Studies on craniopharyngiomas. II. Treatment by stereotaxis and radiosurgery. Acta chir. scand. *138:* 749–759 (1972).

2 Backlund, E.O.: Studies on craniopharyngiomas. III. Stereotaxic treatment with intracystic yttrium-90. Acta chir. scand. *139:* 237–247 (1972).

3 Gahbauer, H.; Sturm, V.; Schlegel, W., et al.: Combined use of stereotaxic CT and angiography for brain biopsies and stereotaxic irradiation. Am. J. nucl. Roentg. *4:* 715–718 (1983).

4 Huk, W.J.; Mahlstedt, J.: Intracystic radiotherapy (^{90}Y) of craniopharyngiomas: CT-guided stereotaxic implantation of indwelling drainage system. Am. J. Nuc. Roentg.: 803–806 (1983).

5 Kobayashi, T.; Kageyama, N.; Ohara, K.: Internal irradiation for cystic craniopharyngioma. J. Neurosurg. *5:* 896–903 (1981).

6 Levine, G.; Lunsford, L.D.; Shabason, L.B., et al.: Preparation and administration of ^{32}P colloidal chromic phosphate for stereotactic intracavitary irradiation of brain neoplasms (Abstract). 132nd Annual Meeting of the American Pharmaceutical Association, San Antonio, 1985.

7 Lunsford, L.D.; Levine, G.; Gumerman, L.W.: A comparison of computed tomographic and radionuclide methods to determine intracranial cystic tumor volumes. J. Neurosurg. (in press, 1985).

8 Lunsford, L.D.; Martinez, A.J.: Stereotactic exploration of the brain in the era of computed tomography. Surg. Neurol. *22:* 222–230 (1984).

9 Strauss, L.; Sturm, V.; Georgi, P., et al.: Radioisotope therapy of cystic craniopharyngiomas. Int. J. Radiat. Oncol. Biol. Phys. *8:* 1581–1585 (1982).

10 Szikla, G.; Musolino, A.; Schaub, C., et al.: Colloidal rhenium-786 endocavitary beta-irradiation of cystic craniopharyngiomas and active glioma cysts. Long-term results, side effects, and radiobiological data (Abstract). Sixth Meeting of the European Society for Stereotactic and Functional Neurosurgery, Rome 1983. Acta neurochir. Suppl. *33:* 331–340 (1984).

L. Dade Lunsford, Md, Department of Neurological Surgery, Room 9402,
Presbyterian-University Hospital, Pittsburgh, PA 15213 (USA)

Proc. 9th Meeting World Soc. Stereotactic and Functional
Neurosurgery, Toronto 1985
Appl. Neurophysiol. *48:* 151 (1985)

Somatosensory-Evoked Potentials in the Ventrolateral Thalamus

P. Birk, A. Struppler, H. Riescher, M. Keidel

Department of Neurology, University of Munich, FRG

Key Words. Evoked potentials · Movement disorders · Stereotactic surgery

Abstract. Electrical and physiological stimulation in the periphery evokes potentials which can be recorded in the target region during stereotactic surgery. This procedure, combined with intracerebral stimulation, is commonly used as a method to verify the localization of the tip of the probe. We recorded evoked potentials following electrical stimulation of a peripheral nerve during stereotactic operations of patients with parkinsonian tremor and spasmodic torticollis, in order to qualify the functional modalities of the fiber system which might be interrupted by a lesion in the target area. Therefore, mixed nerves (median nerve at the wrist, ulnar and median nerve in the brachial sulcus) were stimulated with a bipolar surface electrode contralateral to the operated side. In contrast, skin nerves were stimulated by a loop electrode around the tips of fingers 2–5 on the same side. The evoked potentials recorded in the target region were generally biphasic with an initially positive deflection at a latency of about 14 ms following median nerve stimulation at the wirst. No significant potential was recorded when the skin afferents were stimulated. The recording sites were plotted by computer with reference to the third ventricle and transferred to the stereotactic atlas using special software.

P. Birk, MD, Department of Neurology, University of Munich, Moehlstrasse 28,
D-8000 München 80 (FRG)

Proc. 9th Meeting World Soc. Stereotactic and Functional
Neurosurgery, Toronto 1985
Appl. Neurophysiol. *48:* 152 (1985)

Focus Irradiation in Epilepsy. Experimental Study in the Cat

J.L. Barcia Salorio, V. Vanaclocha, M. Cerda, P. Roldan

Department of Neurosurgery, University Hospital (Hospital Clinico),
Valencia, Spain

Key Words. Epilepsy · Radiosurgery

Abstract. An experimental model of chronic epilepsy has been developed in cats by means of placing cobalt oxide powder epidurally on the left frontal lobe. Radiosurgery of the epileptic focus with a total dose of 10 Gy was performed in a group of 6 animals, and behaviour and EEG observed.

The effect of focus irradiation of experimental epileptic focus in the cat is studied. Six cats with epilepsy caused by cobalt oxide powder placed epidurally on the left frontal lobe were used as a control group. All of them were clinically and electroencephalographically epileptic after a period of 1–3 weeks. None of the animals were free of the disease after 180 days, when they were sacrified for pathological examination. One animal died of intercurrent disease after a follow-up period of 540 days.

A second group of 6 cats underwent irradiation of their epileptic foci, 3 months after the placement of the epileptogenic material, when the epileptic phenomena could be considered chronic. They received a dose of 10 Gy. The colimeter had a diameter of 10 mm, with a 90% isodose of 9 mm. In 3 more cats the dose was of 20 Gy. All animals were cured of the disease 2–3 weeks after the procedure, and were sacrificed 3 months afterwards for pathological examination.

A third control group of 6 cats was submitted to the same surgical procedures, but without cobalt oxide implant. None of them underwent clinical or electroencephalographic changes at all.

Conclusion: the previous results suggest consideration of focus irradiation as a therapeutic measure in epilepsy.

J.L. Barcia Salorio, MD, Department of Neurosurgery, University Hospital (Hospital Clinico), Paseo Blasco Ibañez 17, Valencia (Spain)

Proc. 9th Meeting World Soc. Stereotactic and Functional
Neurosurgery, Toronto 1985
Appl. Neurophysiol. *48:* 153–165 (1985)

Central Nervous System Mechanisms for Pain Modulation

W.D. Willis, Jr.

Marine Biomedical Institute, Departments of Anatomy and of Physiology and Biophysics, University of Texas Medical Branch, Galveston, Tex., USA

Key Words. Spinothalamic tract · Analgesia · Brain stem · Thalamus

Abstract. Although a great deal has been learned about the neural basis for stimulation-produced analgesia, it is evident that the 'analgesia systems' are much more complex than was initially thought. Part of the complexity derives from the fact that a number of different pathways, using several different neurotransmitters, can affect nociceptive transmission. Further complexity stems from evidence that nociceptive transmission can be modulated both at a spinal cord level and at higher levels of the nociceptive projection system, such as the thalamus. Hopefully, a greater understanding of the 'analgesia systems' will lead to explanations for a number of puzzling aspects of pain and perhaps to improved therapy.

Introduction

The contemporary concept that pain can be modulated by electrical stimulation of the brain derives from efforts during the 1960s to develop the technique of electroanesthesia [31]. The paper by *Reynolds* [30] in 1969 showing the focal stimulation at the lateral margin of the periaqueductal gray (PAG) prevented nociceptive responses of rats during abdominal surgery without concomitant drug administration provoked a major and continuing effort in a number of laboratories to characterize neural structures capable of inducing what is known in the field of pain mechanisms as 'stimulation-produced analgesia' [see 26 for introduction of this term; much of the work in this field has been reviewed in 4, 8, 27, 33]. Of particular interest has been the association of neural systems utilizing certain neurotransmitters, including monoamines (serotonin, norepinephrine) and the endogenous opioids with antinociceptive pathways [e.g., 37, 38], since this provides a rationale for the clinical effectiveness of many drugs known to be helpful in pain control, including the narcotics.

The analysis of neural systems that modulate pain can be accomplished most efficiently through the use of animal models. Evidence summarized in the reviews cited above has led to the concept that antinociceptive actions can be mediated by pathways descending from the brain, where they exert an inhibitory action on the circuits that process nociceptive information arriving in the spinal cord by way of nociceptive afferent fibers. A substantial effort has been made to characterize nociceptive circuits in the dorsal horn of the spinal cord. Some of this work has been summarized recently [34]. The ways in which descending control systems interact with dorsal horn circuits are then taken as an indication of how analgesia is produced when structures in the brain are stimulated.

However, evidence is now accumulating suggesting that there may well be important mechanisms for modulation of pain that depend upon interactions at other levels of the pain transmission system. For example, some of the brain structures that are involved in 'stimulation-produced analgesia' have connections not only downstream with the spinal cord but also upstream with the thalamus.

In this review, findings that are consistent with the notion that there are descending inhibitory pathways from the brain that may contribute to analgesia will be described first. Then, some of the evidence for ascending pathways that may modulate pain transmission at the thalamic level will be discussed.

Descending Antinociceptive Pathways

In 1978, *Basbaum and Fields* [4] proposed a neural circuit model for some of the descending pathways believed to modulate pain transmission. This model is shown in figure 1. While details could be added to or subtracted from the model, the basic idea is still reasonably current. The components shown include neurons in the PAG and in the nucleus raphe magnus (NRM) that form a pathway from the midbrain to the dorsal horn of the spinal cord whose role is to inhibit nociceptive neurons, thus preventing the signalling of pain. Parallel projections from the locus coeruleus (LC), the subcoeruleus-parabrachial complex

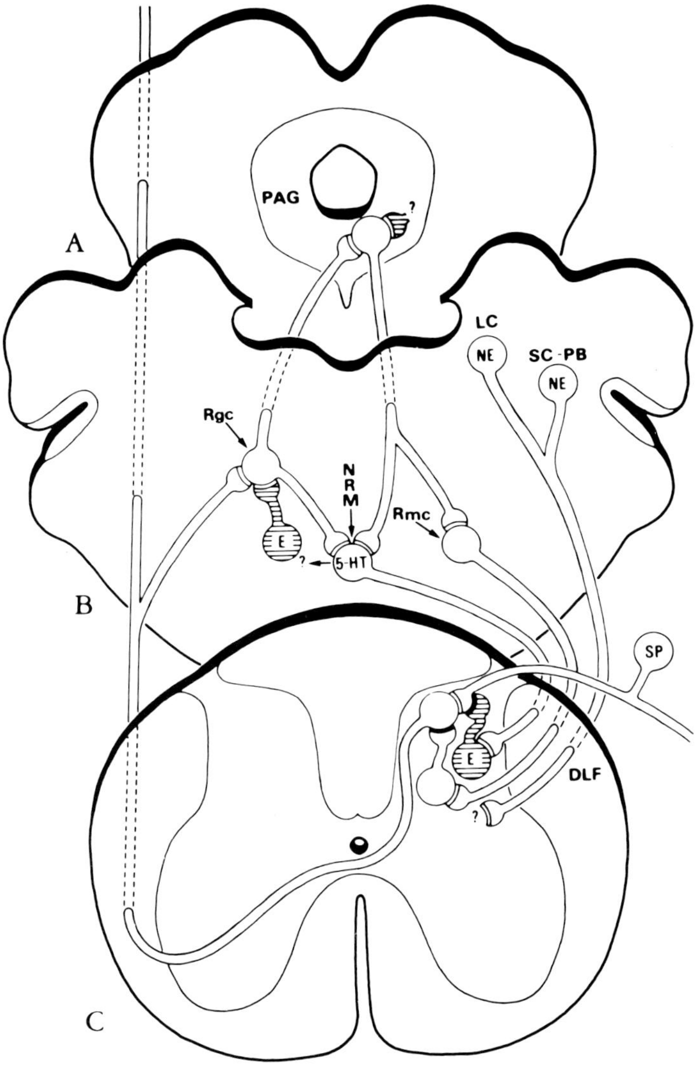

Fig. 1. Neural circuits thought to be involved in the endogenous analgesia system. From *Basbaum and Fields* [4].

(SC-PB) and the magnocellular part of the nucleus reticularis gigantocellularis (Rmc) are included in the model, but these will not be discussed here. The ascending tract cell shown in the spinal cord to send a crossed projection toward the brain would presumably belong to the spinothalamic tract (STT), a pathway believed to be crucial for pain transmission, at least in primates, including humans [34]. It is shown to receive a synaptic input from a dorsal root ganglion cell that contains a neuropeptide transmitter, substance P (SP). The cross-hatched elements represent neurons that contain endogenous opioid substances, such as enkephalin (E). The STT cell sends a collateral into the reticular formation, where it synapses on a neuron in the nucleus reticularis gigantocellularis (Rgc). The latter projects to the PAG and NRM. This component of the model would help account for the activation of the descending antinociceptive pathways.

The next section reviews evidence that the responses of primate STT cells to noxious stimuli can be inhibited when the PAG or NRM are stimulated electrically, that raphe-spinal neurons are excited by PAG stimulation, and that the conduction time in this descending system is consistent with that required to account for inhibition of STT cells by PAG stimulation.

Stimulation in PAG or NRM Inhibits STT Cells

Several studies have shown that electrical stimulation in either the PAG or the NRM can produce a powerful inhibition of primate STT cells [5, 14, 17, 20, 36, 39]. An example of such inhibition is illustrated in figure 2. In this instance, the STT neuron belonged to the high threshold (or nociceptive-specific) class [11], as shown by its preferential response just to very intense mechanical stimulation (squeezing the skin with serrated forceps, fig. 2A). The cell was located near lamina I of the dorsal horn (fig. 2C), and it had a restricted receptive field on the glabrous skin of the foot (fig. 2B). Stimulation in the NRM (fig. 2D) or in the PAG (fig. 2E) produced an inhibition of the activity of the cell that was evoked by squeezing the skin with forceps (fig. 2F, G).

The activity of both wide dynamic range (multiconvergent) and high threshold STT cells is inhibited by NRM [14, 36] or PAG [17] stimulation. Usually the responses to both tactile and noxious stimuli are inhibited, but sometimes there is a selective inhibition of nocicep-

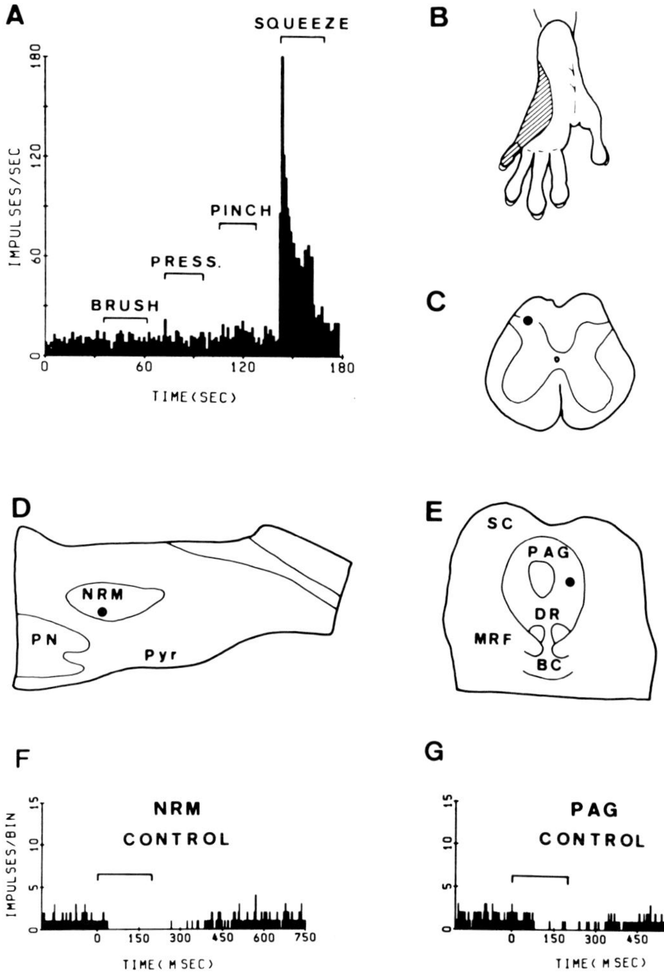

Fig. 2. Inhibition of a high threshold spinothalamic tract cell by stimulation in either the nucleus raphe magnus (NRM) or in the periaqueductal gray (PAG). The peristimulus time histogram in **A** shows the background discharge of the cell and the responses to graded intensities of mechanical stimulation (brushing the skin, pressure applied by an arterial clip, pinch produced by a different arterial clip with a stronger bite, and squeezing the skin forceps). The histograms in **F** and **G** resulted from 10 summed sweeps, during which the skin of the receptive field was squeezed with forceps. Stimulus trains were applied to the NRM or PAG during the times indicated by the brackets (200 ms trains, 0.1 ms, 200 μA pulses at 333 Hz). From *Yezierski* et al. [39].

tive responses. The latency of inhibition of STT cells following the onset of stimulation in the midbrain was 24.9 ± 7.2 ms (n = 35) [17].

In a study of raphe neurons, it was found that stimulation in the PAG at a site that inhibited an STT cell would typically excite raphe-spinal neurons (identified by antidromic activation from the upper lumbar spinal cord). Such a finding is shown in figure 3. In this experiment, the graded responses of an STT cell that were produced by a graded series of mechanical stimuli are shown in figure 3D. The cell was classified as a wide dynamic range (multiconvergent) neuron. Stimulation in the PAG at the site indicated in figure 3A resulted in the inhibition of the STT cell (fig. 3C). The same stimulation excited a raphe-spinal neuron (fig. 3B). The mean latency for excitation of raphe-spinal and reticulospinal neurons was 11.6 ± 11.1 ms [35].

In a series of recordings from antidromically activated raphe-spinal (and medial reticulospinal) neurons, the mean conduction time from the upper lumbar level to the medulla was 8.2 ± 7.1 ms (n = 132) [35].

Adding the latency for excitation of raphe- and reticulospinal neurons by PAG stimulation to the conduction time for propagation of activity to the lumbar spinal cord yields a period of 19.8 ms for activity in descending pathways to reach a level near the STT cells from which we recorded. Since the mean latency of inhibition of STT cells following PAG stimulation was longer, 24.9 ms, it could be concluded that the inhibitory pathway from the PAG could include a relay in the NRM or adjacent medullary reticular formation, as postulated by *Basbaum and Fields* [4].

While recordings were being made from raphe- and reticulospinal neurons, it was often possible to demonstrate their excitatory receptive fields by applying stimuli to the body surface. The neurons were generally of the high threshold class, being excited just by noxious intensities of mechanical or thermal stimuli [35]. The excitatory receptive fields were often very large, including the entire surface of the body and face. An example of such a receptive field is shown for a neuron in the magnocellular reticular formation in figure 4A. Similar fields were observed also for neurons in the NRM. Presumably, the excitatory input to such neurons would be conveyed by spinoreticular neurons or by collaterals of STT cells to the reticular formation [22, 23].

It is interesting to note that STT cells often have both excitatory and inhibitory receptive fields [16]. For example, the receptive fields of

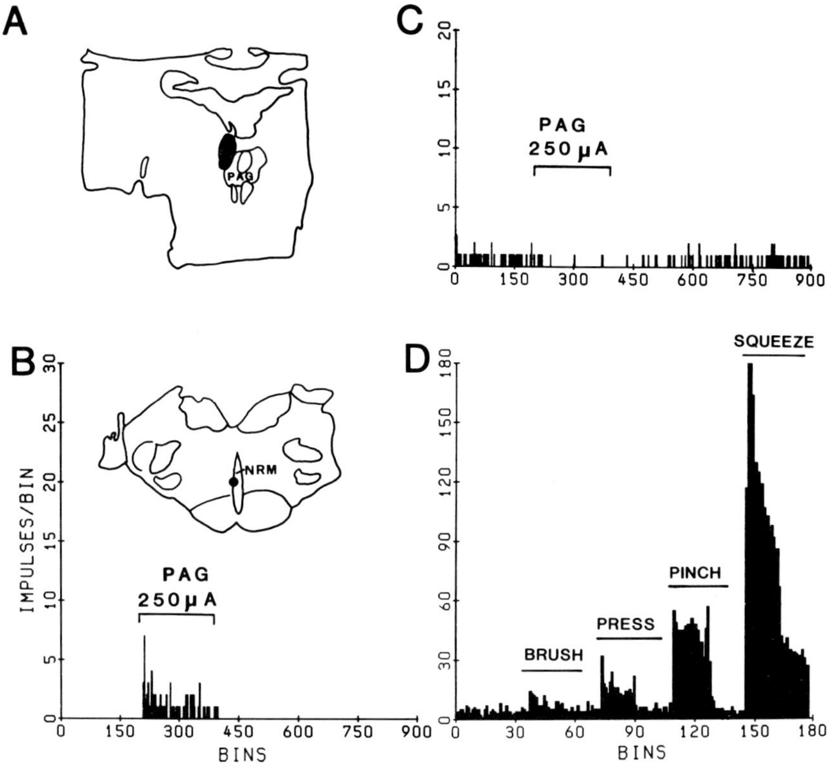

Fig. 3. Excitation of a raphe-spinal neuron and inhibition of a spinothalamic tract cell following stimulation at the location in the PAG shown in **A**. The single pass peri-stimulus time histogram in **D** shows the responses of the STT cell to graded intensities of mechanical stimulation. The histograms in **B** and **C** show the summed responses during 10 repetitions of PAG stimulation. In **B** is the excitatory response of a raphe-spinal cell recorded at the site shown in the inset, while in **C** is the inhibition of the STT cell. From *Willis* et al. [35].

an STT cell are shown in figure 4B. Squeezing the skin produced an excitation from one foot but comparable stimulation over the remainder of the surface of the body and face resulted in an inhibition [35]. Part of the neural mechanism of this inhibition depends upon spinal cord circuits, but part appears to depend upon a loop through the brain stem, perhaps through the NRM and adjacent reticular formation [16, 24, 25].

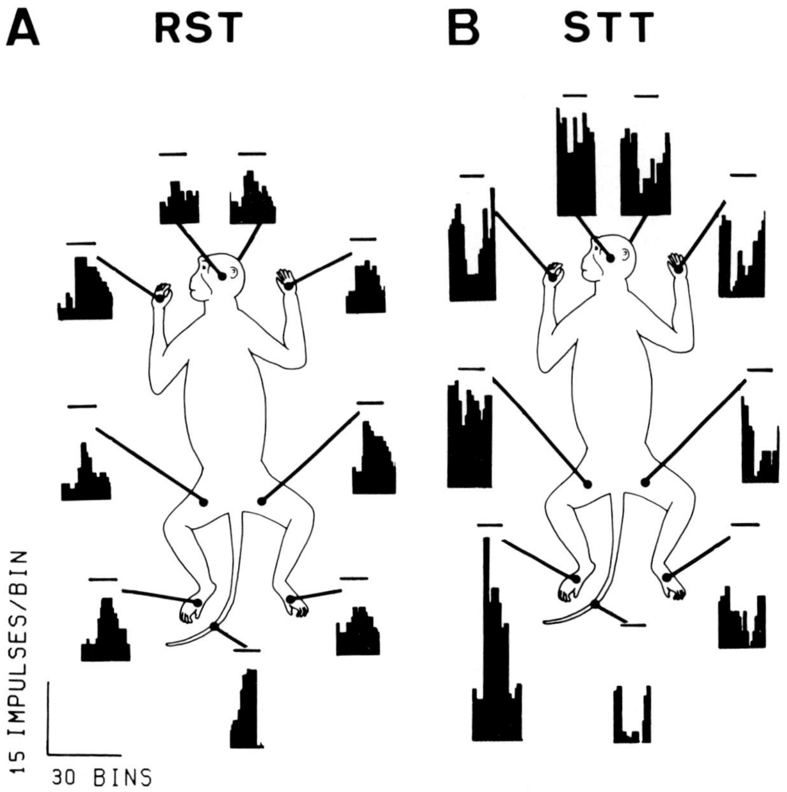

Fig. 4. Excitatory receptive field of a reticulospinal neuron and inhibitory receptive field of a spinothalamic tract cell in the same experiment. The reticulospinal neuron was in the magnocellular part of the nucleus reticularis gigantocellularis. The responses were to squeezing the skin with serrated forceps. From *Willis* et al. [35].

These results by no means prove that the raphe- and reticulospinal neurons from which we recorded in fact inhibited STT cells or that this system in fact operates as an antinociceptive pathway. Nevertheless, the results are consistent with the model proposed by *Basbaum and Fields* [4] for the descending 'analgesia system' shown in figure 1.

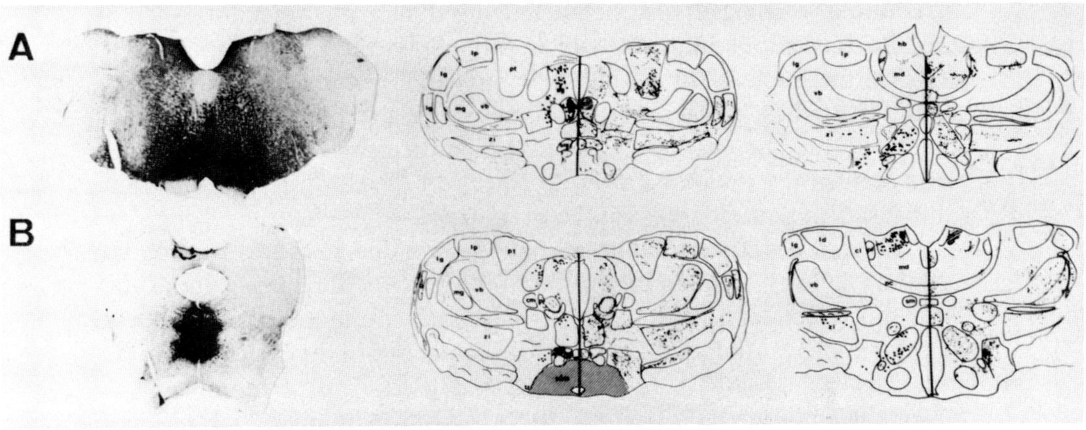

Fig. 5. The pattern of anterograde and retrograde labelling in the thalamus of the rat is shown following injections of wheat germ agglutinin-conjugated horseradish peroxidase into the region of the nucleus raphe magnus **(A)** and the median raphe nucleus **(B)**. Injection sites are shown at the left. Anterograde labelling is indicated by stippling; retrogradely labelled neurons are shown by dots. Dense label was seen in the hatched area. cl = nucleus centre median; hb = habenula; ld = nucleus lateralis dorsalis; lg = lateral geniculate; lp = nucleus lateralis posterior; md = mediodorsal nucleus; mg = medial geniculate; pc = nucleus paracentralis; sm = nucleus submedius; vb = ventrobasal complex; vl = ventrolateral nucleus; zi = zona incerta. From *Peschanski and Besson* [29].

Brain Stem Control of Thalamus

In addition to centrifugal control of the ascending flow of nociceptive information near its point of origin in the spinal cord, there is likely also to be control of the processing of that information at higher levels of the nervous system [19], for example in the thalamus. There are brain stem connections to both the ventrobasal and intralaminar complexes, and there is some evidence for modulation of nociceptive transmission in the thalamus.

It is well known that the brain stem reticular formation projects to the thalamus [9, 28]. Most of the reticular projections have been found to terminate medially in the intralaminar nuclei and to the ventrobasal complex [3, 10, 18]. Finally, there is a substantial serotonergic projection to the thalamus, with endings in the posterior complex and the intralaminar nuclei [12]. Raphe nuclei with thalamic connections include the nucleus raphe magnus, which projects to the intralaminar nuclei and to the nucleus submedius (areas receiving spinothalamic inputs), and the median raphe nucleus, which projects to the ventrobasal complex and the nucleus submedius [29]. The pattern of anterograde labeling seen in the thalamus after an injection of wheat germ agglutinin-horseradish peroxidase is shown in figure 5.

Electrophysiological studies have shown that electrical stimulation in the PAG results in an inhibition of the activity of neurons in the ventral posterior lateral nucleus [32] and that stimulation in the dorsal raphe nucleus inhibits the responses of neurons in the nucleus parafascicularis to noxious stimuli [2]. After depletion of serotonin, dorsal raphe stimulation no longer produces inhibition but rather causes facilitation of the discharges of Pf neurons [2]. Furthermore, iontophoretically released serotonin inhibits the nociceptive discharges of neurons of Pf [1]. These observations suggest that the inhibition of Pf neurons by stimulation in dorsal raphe nucleus is due to the release of serotonin. It is argued that these effects are caused by an action at the level of the thalamus.

Another line of evidence favoring the idea of analgesia mechanisms that involve interconnections of the brain stem and thalamus are recent observations on the action of morphine. Microinjection of morphine into the PAG causes a naloxone-reversible reduction in the responses of neurons in the ventrobasal complex to noxious stimuli, even when the dose of morphine used is less than that which produces a clear-cut reduction in activity of nociceptive dorsal horn neurons [21]. Similarly, systemic administration of morphine causes a reduction in the nociceptive responses of ventrobasal thalamic neurons at doses much lower than are required to depress the firing of spinal cord neurons [7].

A third line of evidence supporting the concept of supraspinal analgesia mechanisms is the recent report that stimulation in the VPL nucleus of the rat can produce inhibition of the nociceptive responses of neurons in the Pf nucleus through a mechanism that is not affected by naloxone [6], and the inhibition did not appear to involve dorsal horn neurons of the spinal cord, since stimuli that inhibited Pf neurons did not affect the responses of a limited sample of dorsal horn interneurons. One mechanism that was suggested was that stimulation in the VPL nucleus may have activated an inhibitory projection from the thalamic reticular nucleus. However, the possibility that part of the inhibitory action was secondary to a spinal cord action should not be ruled out, since stimulation in the VPL nucleus in other species (cat, monkey) can result in the inhibition of dorsal horn interneurons, including spinothalamic tract cells [13, 15].

Acknowledgements

The author thanks his colleagues who participated in the experiments done in his laboratory and mentioned here. He also thanks *Phyllis Waldrop* for typing the manuscript. The work in the author's laboratory was supported by NIH grants NS 09743 and NS 11255.

References

1 Andersen, E.; Dafny, N.: Microiontophoretically applied 5-HT reduces responses to noxious stimulation in the thalamus. Brain Res. *241:* 176–178 (1982).
2 Andersen, E.; Dafny, N.: An ascending serotonergic pain modulation pathway from the dorsal raphe nucleus to the parafascicularis nucleus of the thalamus. Brain Res. *269:* 57–67 (1983).
3 Barbaresi, P.; Conti, F.; Manzoni, T.: Periaqueductal grey projection to the ventrobasal complex in the cat: a horseradish peroxidase study. Neurosci. Lett. *30:* 205–209 (1982).
4 Basbaum, A.I.; Fields, H.L.: Endogenous pain control mechanisms: review and hypothesis. Ann. Neurol. *4:* 451–462 (1978).
5 Beall, J.E.; Martin, R.F.; Applebaum, A.E.; Willis, W.D.: Inhibition of primate spinothalamic tract neurons by stimulation in the region of the nucleus raphe magnus. Brain Res. *114:* 328–333 (1976).
6 Benabid, A.L.; Henriksen, S.J.; McGinty, J.F.; Bloom, F.E.: Thalamic nucleus ventro-postero-lateralis inhibits nucleus parafascicularis response to noxious stimuli through a non-opioid pathway. Brain Res. *280:* 217–231 (1983).
7 Benoist, J.M.; Kayser, V.; Gautron, M.; Guilbaud, G.: Low dose of morphine strongly depresses responses of specific nociceptive neurones in the ventrobasal complex of the rat. Pain *15:* 333–344 (1983).
8 Besson, J.M.; Guilbaud, G.; Abdelmoumene, M.; Chaouch, A.: Physiologie de la nociception. J. Physiol., Paris *78:* 7–107 (1982).
9 Bowsher, D.: Diencephalic projections from the midbrain reticular formation. Brain Res. *95:* 211–220 (1975).
10 Chi, C.C.: An experimental silver study of the ascending projections of the central gray substance and adjacent tegmentum in the rat with observation in the cat. J. comp. Neurol. *139:* 259–272 (1970).

11 Chung, J.M.; Kenshalo, D.R., Jr.; Gerhart, K.D.; Willis, W.D.: Excitation of primate spinothalamic neurons by cutaneous C-fiber volleys. J. Neurophysiol. *42:* 1354–1369 (1979).

12 Cropper, E.C.; Eisenman, J.S.; Azmitia, E.C.: An immunocytochemical study of the serotonergic innervation of the thalamus of the rat. J. comp. Neurol. *224:* 38–50 (1984).

13 Fraunhoffer, M.; MacKinnon, J.D.; Carstens, E.: Map of diencephalic sites at which stimulation inhibits spinal nociceptive transmission. Soc. Neurosci. Abstr. *8:* 767 (1982).

14 Gerhart, K.D.; Wilcox, T.K.; Chung, J.M.; Willis, W.D.: Inhibition of nociceptive and nonnociceptive responses of primate spinothalamic cells by stimulation in medial brain stem. J. Neurophysiol. *45:* 121–136 (1981).

15 Gerhart, K.D.; Yezierski, R.P.; Fang, Z.R.; Willis, W.D.: Inhibition of primate spinothalamic tract neurons by stimulation in ventral posterior lateral (VPL_c) thalamic nucleus: possible mechanisms. J. Neurophyisol. *49:* 406–423 (1983).

16 Gerhart, K.D.; Yezierski, R.P.; Giesler, G.J.; Willis, W.D.: Inhibitory receptive fields of primate spinothalamic tract cells. J. Neurophyisol. *46:* 1309–1325 (1981).

17 Gerhart, K.D.; Yezierski, R.P.; Wilcox, T.K.; Willis, W.D.: Inhibition of primate spinothalamic tract neurons by stimulation in periaqueductal gray or adjacent midbrain reticular formation. J. Neurophysiol. *51:* 450–466 (1984).

18 Hamilton, B.L.: Projections of the nuclei of the periaqueductal gray matter in the cat. J. comp. Neurol. *152:* 45–58 (1973).

19 Harvey, J.A.; Lints, C.E.: Lesions in the medial forebrain bundle: relationship between pain sensitivity and telencephalic content of serotonin. J. comp. physiol. Psychol. *74:* 28–36 (1971).

20 Hayes, R.L.; Price, D.D.; Ruda, M.; Dubner, R.: Suppression of nociceptive responses in the primate by electrical stimulation of the brain or morphine administration: behavioral and electrophysiological comparisons. Brain Res. *167:* 417–421 (1979).

21 Kayser, V.; Benoist, J.M.; Guilbaud, G.: Low dose of morphine microinjected in the ventral periaqueductal gray matter of the rat depresses responses of nociceptive ventrobasal thalamic neurons. Neurosci. Lett. *37:* 193–198 (1983).

22 Kevetter, G.A.; Haber, L.H.; Yezierski, R.P.; Chung, J.M.; Martin, R.F.; Willis, W.D.: Cells of origin of the spinoreticular tract in the monkey. J. comp. Neurol. *207:* 61–74 (1982).

23 Kevetter, G.A.; Willis, W.D.: Spinothalamic cells in the rat lumbar cord with collaterals to the medullary reticular formation. Brain Res. *238:* 181–185 (1982).

24 Le Bars, D.; Dickenson, A.H.; Besson, J.M.: Diffuse noxious inhibitory controls (DNIC). I. Effects on dorsal horn convergent neurones in the rat. Pain *6:* 283–304 (1979).

25 Le Bars, D.; Dickenson, A.H.; Besson, J.M.: Diffuse noxious inhibitory controls (DNIC). II. Lack of effect on non-convergent neurones, supraspinal involvement and theoretical implications. Pain *6:* 305–327 (1979).

26 Mayer, D.J.; Liebeskind, J.C.: Pain reduction by focal electrical stimulation of the brain: an antomical and behavioral analysis. Brain Res. *68:* 73–93 (1974).

27 Mayer, D.J.; Price, D.D.: Central nervous system mechanisms of analgesia. Pain *2:* 379–404 (1976).

28 Nauta, W.J.G.; Kuypers, H.G.J.M.: Some ascending pathways in the brain stem reticular formation; in Jasper et al., Reticular formation of the brain, pp. 3-30 (Little, Brown, Boston 1958).
29 Peschanski, M.; Besson, J.M.: Diencephalic connections of the raphe nuclei of the rat brainstem: an anatomical study with reference to the somatosensory system. J. comp. Neurol. *224:* 509-534 (1984).
30 Reynolds, D.V.: Surgery in the rat during electrical analgesia induced by focal brain stimulation. Science *164:* 444-445 (1969).
31 Reynolds, D.V.; Sjoberg, A.I.: Neuroelectric research (Thomas, Springfield 1971).
32 Schieppati, M.; Gritti, I.: Influences of locus ceruleus, raphe dorsalis, and periaqueductal gray matter on somatosensory-recipient thalamic nuclei. Expl Neurol. *82:* 698-705 (1983).
33 Willis, W.D.: Control of nociceptive transmission in the spinal cord; in Ottoson et al., Progress in sensory physiology, vol. 3, pp. 1-159 (Springer, Berlin 1982).
34 Willis, W.D.: The pain system. The neural basis of nociceptive transmission in the mammalian nervous system; in Gildenber, Pain and headache, vol. 8 (Karger, Basel 1985).
35 Willis, W.D.; Gerhart, K.D.; Willcockson, W.S.; Yezierski, R.P.; Wilcox, T.K.; Cargill, C.L.: Primate raphe- and reticulospinal neurons: effects of stimulation in periaqueductal gray or VPL_c thalamic nucleus. J. Neurophyisol. *51:* 467-480 (1984).
36 Willis, W.D.; Haber, L.H.; Martin, R.F.: Inhibition of spinothalamic tract cells and interneurons by brain stem stimulation in the monkey. J. Neurophysiol. *40:* 968-981 (1977).
37 Yaksh, T.L.: Direct evidence that spinal serotonin and noradrenaline terminals mediate the spinal antinociceptive effects of morphine in the periaqueductal gray. Brain Res. *160:* 180-185 (1979).
38 Yaksh, T.L.; Rudy, T.A.: Narcotic analgetics: CNS sites and mechanisms of action as revealed by intracerebral injection techniques. Pain *4:* 299-359 (1978).
39 Yezierski, R.P.; Wilcox, T.K.; Willis, W.D.: The effects of serotonin antagonists on the inhibition of primate spinothalamic tract cells produced by stimulation in nucleus raphe magnus or periaqueductal gray. J. Pharmac. exp. Ther. *220:* 266-277 (1982).

W.D. Willis, Jr., MD, Marine Biomedical Institute, University of Texas Medical Branch, 200 University Boulevard, Galveston, TX 77550 (USA)

Proc. 9th Meeting World Soc. Stereotactic and Functional Neurosurgery, Toronto 1985
Appl. Neurophysiol. *48:* 166–171 (1985)

Deafferentation Pain and Stimulation of the Thalamic Sensory Relay Nucleus: Clinical and Experimental Study[1]

Takashi Tsubokawa, Yoichi Katayama, Takamitsu Yamamoto, Teruyasu Hirayama

Department of Neurological Surgery, Nihon University School of Medicine, Tokyo, Japan

Key Words. Electrical stimulation · Thalamic sensory relay nucleus · Periaqueductal gray · Neurogenic pain · Deafferentation pain · Retrogasserian rhizotomy · Dorsal horn

Abstract. This report summarizes our clinical experience in which the effects of both thalamic sensory relay nucleus (TSRN) and periaqueductal gray (PAG) stimulation were tested in the same series of patients with various forms of pain. The clinical data indicated that neurogenic pain due to deafferentation at the level of the peripheral nerves or the spinal cord was often controlled by TSRN stimulation but not by PAG stimulation. We also review the results of our experimental investigations in cats which were undertaken in an attempt to clarify the neurophysiologic basis of such differential clinical effects of TSRN and PAG stimulation. It appeared that abnormal hyperactivity within the trigeminal medullary dorsal horn following retrogasserian rhizotomy was far more frequently inhibited by TSRN stimulation than by PAG stimulation.

Introduction

Pain caused by deafferentation of sensory neural pathways (neurogenic pain) and pain caused by excess noxious impulses originating from active diseases (somatogenic pain) can be distinguished. *Hosobuchi* et al. [4] reported that thalamic sensory relay nucleus (TSRN) stimulation is useful for treating facial anesthesia dolorosa occurring after retrogasserian rhizotomy. *Mazars* [7] indicated that TSRN stimulation

[1] This work was supported by the Japan Education Ministry, Grant 60480333.

can also relieve other forms of neurogenic pain. Subsequently, TSRN stimulation has usually been employed as a treatment for neurogenic pain [e.g., 10]. In contrast, in our experience, periaqueductal gray (PAG) stimulation is apparently ineffective in relieving neurogenic pain. In order to clarify the differential effects of these two procedures, we summarize our clinical experience in which both the effects of TSRN and PAG stimulation were tested in the same series of patients with various forms of pain, and also review the results of our experimental investigations which were undertaken to elucidate the neural mechanisms underlying the differential clinical effects of TSRN and PAG stimulation as revealed by clinical data.

Methods and Results

The results of deep brain stimulation in a total of 24 patients with various forms of pain who had undergone implantation of at least two electrode arrays (Medtronic DBS system), one for TSRN (nucleus ventralis posterolateralis or posteromedialis) stimulation and the other for PAG stimulation, were analyzed in the present study. Among these patients, 6 had suffered deafferentation of sensory neural pathways apparently due to benign pathology at the level of the peripheral nerves or the spinal cord (group I patients), 8 had suffered pain due to lesions within the central nervous system above the level of the brain stem (group II patients) and 10 had suffered pain caused by malignant neoplasms (group III patients).

Results

In all of the group I and II patients, the effects of PAG stimulation had been found to be unsatisfactory during a period of test stimulation, and electrodes for PAG stimulation were not internalized. In contrast, TSRN stimulation produced excellent effects in alleviating pain in 4 of the group I patients and 2 of the group II patients. TSRN stimulation also helped control the pain in the 2 group I patients and 3 group II patients. PAG stimulation proved helpful in controlling the pain in 3 of the group III patients. TSRN stimulation was helpful in controlling the pain in another 3 group III patients (table I). We gained the impression that the TSRN stimulation exerted only transient effects in reducing pain in many of the group III patients. However, 3 of the group III patients reported continuing effects for a long time beyond the initial pe-

Table I. Clinical results with TSRN stimulation

	n	Excellent	Good	Fair
Group I	6	4 (67%)	2 (33%)	0
Phantom limb pain		1		
Stump pain		1		
Myelopathy		1	1	
Postherpetic neuralgia		1	1	
Group II				
Central pain	8	2 (24%)	3 (38%)	3 (38%)
Group III				
Cancer pain	10	3(30%)	1 (10%)	6 (60%)

Excellent: $\geqq$ 80% reduction of pain score; good: 60–80% reduction of pain score; fair: < 60% reduction of pain score [cf. 8].

This series of patients underwent electrode placements in both TSRN and PAG. PAG stimulation was effective in none of group I and II patients and 3 of group III patients.

riod of treatment with deep brain stimulation. A detailed review of the medical records of these patients suggested that the pain in 2 of them had been due at least in part to deafferentation of peripheral nerves since these 2 had suffered sensory loss within the painful area.

These clinical data indicated that TSRN and PAG stimulation may be beneficial in different groups of pain patients. In particular, differential effects of TSRN and PAG stimulation on neurogenic pain due to deafferentation at the level of the peripheral nerves or the spinal cord were apparently clear. We therefore attempted to clarify the neurophysiological basis of such differential clinical effects using experimental animals. Full details of the experimental techniques and results will be reported separately. Only those observations relevant to the issues presently under consideration will be summarized here.

It was found in intact cats that TSRN (nucl. ventralis posteromedialis) stimulation, similarly to PAG stimulation, inhibited nociceptive trigeminal medullary dorsal horn neurons [1]. However, while single PAG stimulation produced inhibition for more than 500 ms, single

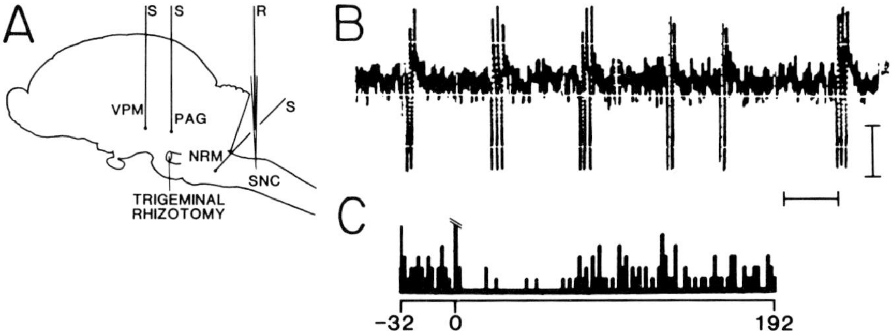

Fig. 1. A Stimulation and recording sites. NRM = nucleus raphe magnus; PAG = periaqueductal gray; R = recording; S = stimulation; SNC = trigeminal subnucleus caudalis; VPM = nucleus ventralis posteromedialis thalami. **B** An example of recordings from SNC 4 weeks after trigeminal rhizotomy. Calibration, 20 ms, 1 mV. **C** An example of poststimulus histogram. Bin width, 2 ms. A bar at time zero includes stimulus artefacts.

TSRN stimulation produced inhibition for only approximately 100 ms. Furthermore, the PAG-induced inhibition was antagonized by the opiate antagonist, naloxone, whereas the TSRN-induced inhibition was found to be resistant to naloxone. In cats in which retrogasserian trigeminal rhizotomy had been performed 4–6 weeks before the experiments, hyperactivity was observed in the trigeminal medullary dorsal horn (fig. 1), in agreement with previous studies [2, 5, 6]. We found that PAG stimulation often failed to inhibit such hyperactivity following rhizotomy. In contrast, TSRN stimulation was more frequently able to inhibit such hyperactivity.

Discussion

The clinical data in the present study suggested that neurogenic pain due to deafferentation at the level of the peripheral nerves or the spinal cord was often controlled by TSRN stimulation but not by PAG stimulation. The experimental data demonstrated that the physiological characteristics of dorsal horn neurons following peripheral deafferentation corresponded to such observed features of neurogenic pain. The experimental findings indicated that neural circuits within the dorsal horn may be reorganized following peripheral deafferentation in such a way that TSRN stimulation, but not PAG stimulation, can influence the resultant hyperactivity of dorsal horn neurons. Such neural reorganization within the dorsal horn may not be a cause of neurogenic pain by itself, but cases in which neurogenic pain occurred following peripheral deafferentation must have the same neural reorganization within the dorsal horn. Thus, differential effects of TSRN and PAG stimulation on abnormal hyperactivity of the peripherally deafferented dorsal horn may possibly underlie the differential effects of these two procedures on neurogenic pain due to peripheral deafferentation.

We previously reported clinical data indicating that TSRN stimulation can relieve morphine-resistant pain in humans [9] which has been thought not to be controlled by PAG stimulation [4]. Such data are consistent with the experimental observations in the present study indicating that TSRN-induced inhibition, unlike PAG-induced inhibition, of nociceptive dorsal horn neurons does not require opiate-mediated neural mechanisms. This represents another line of evidence to suggest that different mechanisms of inhibition of dorsal horn neurons following TSRN and PAG stimulation underlie the differential effects of these two procedures on various forms of human pain.

References

1 Gerhart, K.D.; Yezierski, R.P.; Fang, Z.R.: Inhibition of primate spinothalamic tract neurons by stimulation in ventral posterior lateral (VPL) thalamic nucleus: possible mechanisms. J. Neurophysiol. *49:* 406–423 (1983).

2 Hodge, C.J., Jr.; Apakarian, A.V.; Owen, M.P.: Changes in the effects of stimulation of locus coeruleus and nucleus raphe magnus following dorsal rhizotomy. Brain Res. *188:* 325–329 (1983).

3 Hosobuchi, Y.; Adams, J.E.; Rutkin, B.: Chronic thalamic stimulation for the control of facial anesthesia dolorosa. Archs Neurol. *19:* 158–161 (1973).

4 Hosobuchi, Y.; Rossier, J.; Bloom, F.E.; Guillemin, R.: Periaqueductal gray stimulation for pain suppression in humans; in Bonica, Liebeskind, Albe-Fessard, Advances in pain research and therapy, pp. 515–523 (Raven Press, New York 1979).

5 Loeser, J.E.; Ward, A.A., Jr.: Some effects of deafferentation on neurons of the cat spinal cord. Archs Neurol. *17:* 629–636 (1967).

6 Lombard, M.C.; Nashold, B.S., Jr.; Albe-Fessard, D.: Deafferentation hypersensitivity in the rat after dorsal rhizotomy: a possible animal model of chronic pain. Pain *6:* 163–174 (1979).

7 Mazars, G.L.: Intermittent stimulation of nucleus ventralis posterolateralis for intractable pain. Surg. Neurol. *4:* 93–95 (1975).
8 Tsubokawa, T.; Yamamoto, T.; Katayama, Y.; Hirayama, T.; Shibuya, H.: Thalamic relay nucleus stimulation for relief of intractable pain: clinical results and β-endorphin immunoreactivity in the cerebrospinal fluid. Pain *18:* 115–126 (1984).
9 Tsubokawa, T.; Yamamoto, T.; Katayama, Y.; Moriyasu, N.: Clinical results and experimental basis of thalamic relay nucleus stimulation for relief of intractable pain with morphine tolerance. Appl. Neurophysiol. *45:* 143–155 (1982).
10 Turnbull, I.M.; Shulman, R.; Woodhurst, B.: Thalamic stimulation for neuropathic pain. J. Neurosurg. *52:* 486–493 (1980).

Takashi Tsubokawa, MD, Department of Neurological Surgery, Nihon University School of Medicine, 30-1 Oyaguchikami-machi, Itabashi-ku, Tokyo 173 (Japan)

Proc. 9th Meeting World Soc. Stereotactic and Functional
Neurosurgery, Toronto 1985
Appl. Neurophysiol. *48:* 172–174 (1985)

Changes in Local Cerebral Glucose Utilization Induced by Electrical Stimulation of the Parafascicular and VPL Thalamic Nuclei in Rats

Yasutaka Aiko, Fumio Shima, Motohiro Kato,
Katsutoshi Kitamura

Department of Neurosurgery and Neurophysiology, Neurological Institute,
Kyushu University, Fukuoka, Japan

Key Words. Deep brain stimulation · Pf stimulation · VPL stimulation · Local cerebral glucose utilization

Abstract. A parallel bipolar stimulating electrode was stereotactically inserted in Pf and VPL. The parameter of Pf stimulating was adjusted so the withdrawal response of rats to tail-pinch was diminished. The stimulation started immediately before ^{14}C-deoxyglucose injection and lasted for 45 min, following which the rat was sacrificed. Coronal sections of the frozen brain were made and autoradiographs of these sections were prepared. LCGU was measured by Sokoloff's 2-deoxyglucose method.

In our clinical experience, electrical stimulation of Pf nucleus of the thalamus resulted in relief of bilateral intractable pain, while VPL stimulation relieved pain only on the contralateral side. In order to clarify the differences between the mechanisms of pain relief by Pf and VPL stimulation, we observed modification of local cerebral glucose utilization (LCGU) induced by electrical stimulation of either VPL or Pf in conscious rats. VPL stimulation induced increased LCGU in VPL and VPM of the thalamus, substantia nigra and sensory cortex on the stimulated side. Pf stimulation, on the other hand, increased LCGU in bilateral Pf and central median nuclei of the thalamus, sensory cortex, substantia nigra, ventral part of the striatum and ipsilateral PAG. A bilateral analgesic effect of Pf stimulation may result from the bilateral modification of activities in these diverse central structures.

Result

On Pf stimulation, rats clearly showed a reduction of the withdrawal response to tail-pinch. However, no reduction of the withdrawal response was observed during VPL stimulation, even if the stimulation parameter was carefully varied.

LCGU Changes [4]. VPL stimulation induced increase in LCGU in the VPL and VPM nuclei, substantia nigra pars reticulata and compacta and sensory cortex exclusively on the stimulated side. Pf stimulation, on the other hand, induced bilateral LCGU increase in the Pf and central medial nuclei of thalamus, ventral part of striatum, substantia nigra and sensory cortex, although the increase was greater on the stimulated side. The globus pallidus, subthalamic nucleus, VM, centrolateral and paracentral nuclei of thalamus, periaqueductal central gray, deep layers of superior colliculus and parabrachial pontine tegmental nucleus also showed increase in LCGU on the stimulated side. Although the dorsal raphe, raphe magnus, medullary reticular nuclei, or dorsal horn in the spinal cord are assumed to be the relevant structures to the pain suppression system, significant LCGU increases were not observed in these structures.

Discussion

Unilateral Pf nucleus has direct or indirect fiber connections to all structures that demonstrated increased LCGU [2, 3]. Among these, the majority of the structures, particularly the sensory cortex, striatum, substantia nigra, PAG and parabrachial pontine nucleus were assumed to be relevant to the pain suppression system [1].

The present study clearly indicates that unilateral stimulation of Pf nucleus activates the metabolic activities of some of these structures bilaterally. The present study suggests that the analgesia induced by unilateral Pf stimulation involves three systems, namely the thalamocortical pathway, the nigrostriatal system and the descending system mediated by the PAG on both sides. Unilateral VPL stimulation, on the other hand, activates the ipsilateral thalamocortical pathway and substantia nigra, but the relationship between the VPL and nigra and its role in pain suppression system could not be clarified. The bilateral analgesic effect of Pf stimulation may result from the bilateral modification of activities of these diverse central structures.

References

1 Barasi, S.: Responses of substantia nigra neurones to noxious stimulation. Brain Res. *171:* 121–130 (1979).

2 Gerfen, C.R.; Staines, W.A.; Arbuthnott, G.W.; Fibiger, H.C.: Crossed connections of the substantia nigra in the rat. J. comp. Neurol. *106:* 283–303 (1982).

3 Scheibel, M.E.; Scheibel, A.B.: Structural organization of nonspecific thalamic nuclei and their projections toward cortex. Brain Res. *6:* 60–94 (1967).

4 Sokoloff, L.; Reivich, M.; Kennedy, C.; Des Rosiers, M.H.; Patlak, C.S.; Pettigrew, K.D.; Sakurada, O.; Shinohara, M.: The ^{14}C-deoxy-glucose method for the measurement of local cerebral glucose utilization: theory, procedure, and normal values in the conscious and anesthetized albino rat. J. Neurochem. *28:* 897–916 (1977).

Yasutaka Aiko, MD, Department of Neurosurgery and Neurophysiology, Neurological Institute, Faculty of Medicine, Kyushu University, Fukuoka 812 (Japan)

Proc. 9th Meeting World Soc. Stereotactic and Functional Neurosurgery, Toronto 1985
Appl. Neurophysiol. *48:* 175–180 (1985)

Possible Neurohumoral Mechanisms in CNS Stimulation for Pain Suppression

B.A. Meyerson[a], *E. Brodin*[b], *B. Linderoth*[a]

Departments of [a] Neurosurgery, Karolinska Hospital, and [b] Pharmacology, Karolinska Institute, Stockholm, Sweden

Key Words. Pain · Neuropeptides · Analgesia · Central nervous system stimulation · Human cerebrospinal fluid

Abstract. Improved knowledge about biochemical mechanisms underlying pain suppression by CNS electric stimulation is one condition for the further advancement of this form of treatment. In 6 patients treated with PVG stimulation and in 14 with spinal cord stimulation the concentration of substance P-like immunoreactivity in lumbar CSF increased significantly following stimulation. However, these changes may be unspecific and not directly related to the suppression of pain. Measurements of somatostatin, cholecystokinin, vasoactive intestinal polypeptide, neurotensin and monoamine metabolites in CSF showed no changes related to stimulation and the ensuing pain relief. Possible reasons for these negative findings are discussed.

Introduction

One of the intriguing features of CNS stimulation for pain is the protracted poststimulatory relief which may last for several hours or even days. This phenomenon has been assumed to depend upon the involvement of neurohumoral mechanisms. However, these mechanisms are still poorly understood and, with regard to dorsal column stimulation (DCS) and stimulation of the thalamic sensory nuclei, virtually nothing is known. A large number of putative transmitters/modulators with possible relation to nociception as well as to antinociception have been described (e.g., somatostatin, cholecystokinin, vasoactive intestinal polypeptide, neurotensin, angiotensin II, calcitonin gene-related peptide, etc.) [2]. There is presently a marked discrepancy between the many novel transmitter candidates found and structurally defined and the paucity of data on their functional roles. In particular, information from human beings is scarce except with regard to endogenous opioids and substance P [5]. There are several approaches which can be employed to elucidate the transmitter-modulator physiology of CNS stimulation for pain. However, such studies are met with a number of problems and fallacies. The number of putative substances which may be linked to pain and pain-relieving procedures has increased to the extent that selection has become a major and crucial problem. For obvious reasons, a search for the relevant substances has to be based principally on data derived from animal experiments [for review, cf. 1], but these are often difficult to evaluate with regard to chronic pain.

Studies of the biochemical mechanisms underlying the clinical effect of stimulation for pain involve special problems. In principle, two different approaches can be employed: (a) measurements of different transmitter substances or their metabolites in lumbar or ventricular CSF in order to assess changes induced by stimulation, and (b) administration of drugs which have transmitter antagonistic or agonistic properties and therefore may reverse or enhance the effect of stimulation. When dealing with intracerebral stimulation it is likely that the concentration of substances released as a result of stimulation is higher in ventricular than in lumbar CSF. However, the collection of ventricular fluid via a catheter and a reservoir is questionable from an ethical point of view, in particular in patients with nonmalignant pain. Another difficult, though trivial, problem is the fact that there are very few laboratories which can screen CSF samples for large numbers of substances, and besides, normative values for many of the substances analyzed in healthy subjects are not available.

The urgent need of further exploring the problems outlined above is a reason for reporting our preliminary findings and trials in the search for endogenous substances which may be related to the pain-relieving effect of DCS and intracerebral stimulation.

Patient Material and Methods

Lumbar CSF has been collected from 20 patients undergoing stimulation treatment for chronic pain. Six of the patients had an electrode implanted in the PVG/PAG region and the remaining 14 underwent DCS. Only 1 patient suffered from pain associated with malignancy. The first tap was performed when the patient had been without any form of stimulation for at least 24 h and reported his usual pain. In the majority of the cases it was possible to withhold analgesics. A second tap was performed when the patient had used the stimulator freely for at least 24 h in order to obtain maximal pain relief. The puncture was performed 30–60 min after cessation of the stimulation and meanwhile the patient had been out of bed.

In all patients the CSF content of substance P was analyzed, in 9 neurotensin, in 10 cholecystokinin, in 10 monoamine metabolites, in 7 somatostatin, and in 10 cases VIP. The analyses have been performed in different laboratories (see Acknowledgements). The peptides were measured with RIA and the monoamines with high performance liquid chromatography.

Results

Substance P-like immunoreactivity (SPLI) was measured in 6 patients with PVG stimulation and in 14 with DCS. The changes of concentration of SPLI following stimulation are graphically illustrated in figure 1. In the majority of the patients both types of stimulation caused an increase of the SPLI content, but there were also cases in whom there was instead a decrease. There was no clear evidence of a consistent relationship between the pain-relieving effect of stimulation and the presence and amount of increase of SPLI. The mean values for SPLI before stimulation were 2.75 fmol/ml in patients with PVG electrodes and 4.67 fmol/ml in those subjected to DCS. After stimulation the corresponding mean values increased to 6.07 and 5.85 fmol/ml, respectively. The mean values for all the patients were 3.85 before and 6.0 fmol/ml after stimulation. All these changes were statistically significant ($p < 0.05$). All values fall well in the normal range, 1.0–16.7 fmol/ml, mean 5.0, as assessed in 8 healthy subjects.

Somatostatin was measured in CSF samples from 6 patients with DCS and 1 patient with PVG stimulation. Concentrations ranged from 18.1 to 43.8 pg/ml. Normal values obtained from 6 healthy subjects ranged between 22 and 47 pg/ml. No changes of the content of the substance following stimulation could be demonstrated, no matter whether pain relief was obtained or not.

Neurotensin was measured in 8 patients with DCS and 1 with PVG stimulation. Concentrations varied little and ranged from 2.7 to 3.8 fmol/l. No measurement with this RIA on healthy subjects have been done. No changes of the content of the substance following stimulation could be demonstrated, no matter whether pain relief was obtained or not.

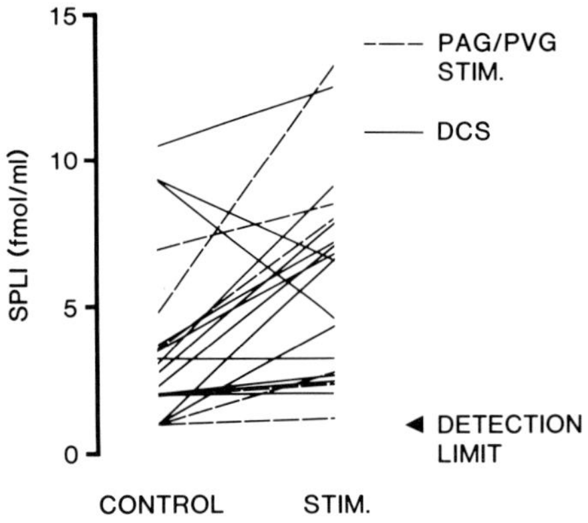

Fig. 1. Effect of PAG/PVG or dorsal stimulation on SPLI in lumbar CSF, sampled before and after stimulation, in patients with chronic pain.

Vasoactive intestinal polypeptide (VIP) was measured in 10 patients with DCS. Concentrations ranged from 2 to 24 p*M*, mean 13.6. No measurements with this RIA on healthy subjects have been done. No changes of the content of the substance following stimulation could be demonstrated, no matter whether pain relief was obtained or not.

Cholecystokinin (CCK) was measured in 8 patients with DCS and 2 with PVG stimulation. Concentrations ranged between values below 5, which was the detection limit, and 21.8 fmol/ml. Only 2 patients had values exceeding 10 fmol/ml. No measurements with this RIA on healthy subjects have been done. No changes of the content of the substance following stimulation could be demonstrated, no matter whether pain relief was obtained or not.

Metabolites from *monoamines* were measured in 8 patients with DCS, in 1 patient with PVG stimulation and 1 with sensory thalamic stimulation. Concentrations of HVA ranged between 10 and 500 pmol/ml with a mean value of 250. Two patients had values exceeding 300 pmol/ml. Normal range is 84–286 pmol/ml. Concentrations of MOPEG ranged between 35 and 52 pmol/ml, mean 42. Normal range is 29–51 pmol/ml. 5-HIAA ranged from 83 to 203 pmol/ml, mean 133. In 3 of the patients, concentrations exceeded 150 pmol/ml. Normal range is 46–154 pmol/ml. No changes of the content of these substances following stimulation could be demonstrated, no matter whether pain relief was obtained or not.

Discussion

The only transmitter/modulator substance found to be influenced by stimulation of the CNS was substance P. Before stimulation, the content of SPLI was found to be in the lower range of normal values. Considering the well-established notion that SP serves as a transmitter in the primary nociceptive neurons, one would expect comparatively high concentrations in the control samples when the patients reported pain. One possible explanation of the low concentrations of SPLI found at these occasions may be that the majority of the patients suffered from pain which may be classified as neurogenic [3]. It might be that such pain is less dependent on SP-mediated transmission than a nociceptive type of pain. No relationship could be demonstrated between pain relief and changes of concentration of SPLI. Substance P is contained in a number of other systems than those related to pain and it is likely that the effect of CNS stimulation reflects unspecific activation of descending spinal pathways and interneurons. At least one can assume that this unspecific release of SP completely neutralizes a moderate decrease which would otherwise have been expected to accompany pain relief.

There is much experimental evidence that the other endogenous substances analyzed in the present study are related to pain and pain suppression [2]. There are several possible reasons why we failed to demonstrate any changes of their concentrations following CNS stimulation and pain relief: (a) The generation and the inhibition of the types of pain represented by the patients in the present study may be independent of systems employing the substances selected for analyses. (b) It is conceivable that CNS stimulation activates a number of systems with no relation to pain and pain suppression, and that the pain-related substances are released in very small amounts. Besides, samples of CSF can rarely be collected close to the site of stimulation and substances released will hence become diluted. It might be that the methods of analysis are not sensitive enough to detect minute changes in concentration - and still we are left with the problem of the release of a particular substance from systems not related to pain. (c) It is known that many of the transmitter substances are rapidly metabolized and induced changes of their release would therefore not substantially influence the concentrations of the mother substances. (d) As long as analyses are performed on single samples of CSF subsequent to stimulation it might well be that the peak of the release is missed. Besides, little is known about the velocity of transport and concentration gradients of most transmitter substances in the subarachnoidal space [4].

The results obtained in the present study, performed with the aim to elucidate biochemical correlates to pain suppression with CNS stimulation, have indeed been discouraging. However, in view of the need to improve the efficacy of stimulation methods as treatment of pain the further exploration of the underlying mechanisms remains a challenge.

Acknowledgements

We are greatly indebted to those who performed the analyses: Prof. *Kerstin Uvnäs*, Department of Pharmacology (VIP); Prof. *Suad Efendic*, Department of Endocrinology (somatostatin); Prof. *Göran Sedvall* and Dr. *Alexandra Tylec*, Department of Psychiatry (monoamines); Dr. *Elvar Norheim*, Department of Clinical Chemistry (neurotensin), Karolinska Institutet, Stockholm.

Part of this study has been supported by grants from the Karolinska Institutet *(B.A.M., B.L.)* and from the Swedish Medical Research Council, No. 14X-6836 *(E.B.)*.

References

1 Abrams, G.M.; Recht, L.: Neuropeptides and their role in pain and analgesia. Acupunct. Electro-Ther. Res. *7:* 105–121 (1984).

2 Aronoff, G.; Sweet, W.H.: The future of pain management; in Aronoff, Evaluation and treatment of chronic pain, pp. 640–658 (Urban & Schwarzenberg, New York 1985).

3 Nutt, J.G.; Mroz, E.A.; Leeman, S.E.; Williams, A.C.; Engel, W.K.; Chase, T.W.: Substance P in human cerebrospinal fluid: reductions in peripheral neuropathy and autonomic dysfunction. Neurology *30:* 1280–1285 (1980).

4 Tamminga, C.A.; Le Witt, P.A.; Chase, T.W.: Cholecystokinin and neurotensin gradients in human CSF. Archs Neurol. *42:* 354–355 (1985).

5 Terenius, L.: The endogenous opioids and other central peptides; in Wall, Melzack, Textbook of pain, pp. 133–141 (Churchill Livingstone, Edinburgh 1984).

Björn Meyerson, MD, Department of Neurosurgery, Karolinska Sjukhuset, S-104 01 Stockholm (Sweden)

Proc. 9th Meeting World Soc. Stereotactic and Functional
Neurosurgery, Toronto 1985
Appl. Neurophysiol. *48:* 181–190 (1985)

Clinicoanatomical Study of Thalamic Stimulation for Pain Relief

R. Kuroda[a], *J. Nakatani*[a], *M. Ioku*[a], *K. Koshino*[b]

[a] Department of Neurosurgery, Kinki University, Osaka, and
[b] Department of Neurosurgery, Osaka University, Osaka, Japan

Key Words. Cordotomy · Corticofugal fibers from SI and SII · Deep brain stimulation · VPL stimulation · Pain · Spinothalamic tract

Abstract. Our small experiences with electrical stimulation in the VPL and VPM for dysesthetic pain show that it provoked only paresthesia and induced some relief of pain. It does not increase the beta-endorphin level in CSF. To clarify the anatomical substrata in VPL stimulation, neuroanatomical studies were done about the inputs to VPL in man, monkey and cat by the Fink-Heimer method. The spinothalamic tract terminates in VPL in a patchy fashion in the monkey. The corticothalamic fibers from SI and SII cortex project to VPL and VPM in somatotopical organization in the cat. SI and SII cortices have reciprocal connections, in addition to projections to area 5 or SIII cortex. The corticofugal fibers to the magnocellular and gigantocellular tegmental fields are suggested in addition to the dorsal column nuclei, spinal trigeminal nuclei and spinal posterior horn in cat. The medial lemniscus input to VPL and the above neural circuits are thought to be associated with VPL stimulation.

Introduction

To clarify the anatomical substrata of electrical stimulation of VPL and induced paresthesia, the terminal sites and pattern of the spinothalamic tract (STT) in man and monkey, and the corticofugal fibers from the somatosensory cortex (SI, SII) in cat were investigated by the Fink-Heimer method.

Materials and Methods

Two human cordotomy cases were investigated to study the STT fibers. The survival periods from each cordotomy were 3 weeks and 5 months, respectively. To eluci-

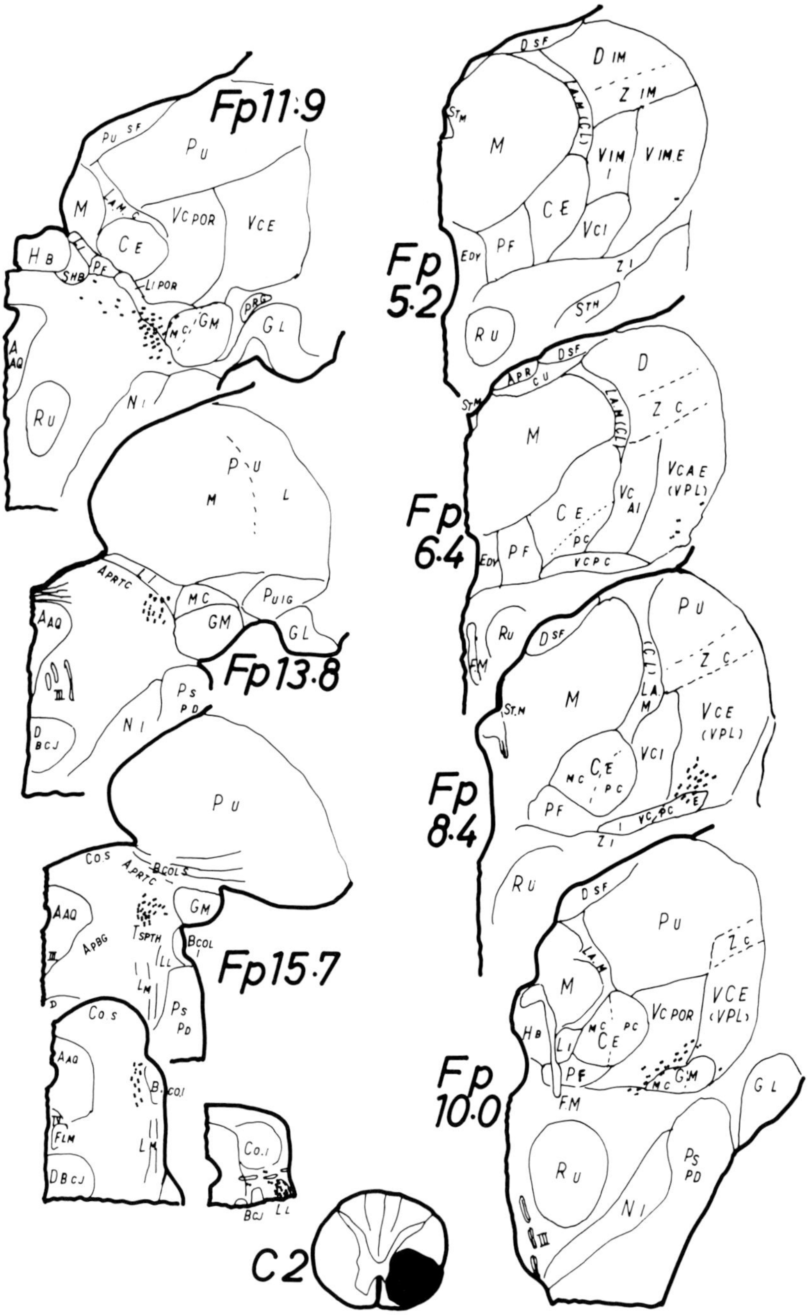
Fp11·9
Fp
5·2
Fp
6·4
Fp13·8
Fp
8·4
Fp15·7
Fp
10·0
C2

date some points, we also included monkeys in which experiments were made strictly on the anterolateral spinal column at the C3 level.

The corticofugal fibers from SI and SII were also investigated in 11 cats. A small electrolytic lesion was placed in the cortical gray matter. The survival periods of animal experiments were between 5 and 7 days.

Results

Terminal Sites and Pattern of the STT

In humans (fig. 1), degenerating STT fibers ascend just dorsal to the medial lemniscus and medial to the brachium inferior colliculus at the midbrain level. At the mesodiencephalic junction, the degenerating fibers pass medial to the medial geniculate nucleus and the main degenerating fiber stream ascends dorsolaterally to enter the thalamus, while a small amount of fibers turn medially just ventral to Li, Li. por and Pf. The termination of the latter group could not be traced into the intralaminar nuclei. The former group ascends into the thalamus and passes through Li, Li. por, Vc. por and Vc. pc. e, and terminates in Vce (VPL). Only a few fibers enter V. im. e. A small number of fibers seem to terminate in GMmc and Vc. pc. e. Probably due to the inadequate fixation and survival periods, any special terminal pattern in VPL and termination in CL could not be observed, although *Mehler* [9] has reported the archipelago-like pattern of termination in VPL and terminal degeneration in CL.

In monkeys (fig. 2), the degenerating fibers are divided into the lateral and medial groups entering the thalamus. The latter group passes mediodorsally through Li, CM, Pf, Pul. p and terminates in CL and the lateral part of MD. The lateral group ascends dorsolaterally into the

---

Fig. 1. Distribution of degenerating STT axons (dots) in human thalamus following percutaneous cordotomy at C2. The nomenclature and rough coordinates follow those of *Hassler* [4] and *Schaltenbrand and Wahren* [13]. Ce = nucleus centrum medianum; GMmc = nucleus geniculatus medialis magnocellularis; La m = lamella medialis; Li = nucleus limitans; Li por = nucleus limitans portae; Li = lamniscus lateralis; Lm = Lemniscus medialis; Pf = nucleus parafascicularis; Tspth = tractus spinothalamicus; Vcae = nucleus ventrocaudalis anterior externus; Vce = nucleus ventrocaudalis externus; Vc pc e = nucleus ventrocaudalis parvocellularis externus; Vc por = nucleus ventrocaudalis portae.

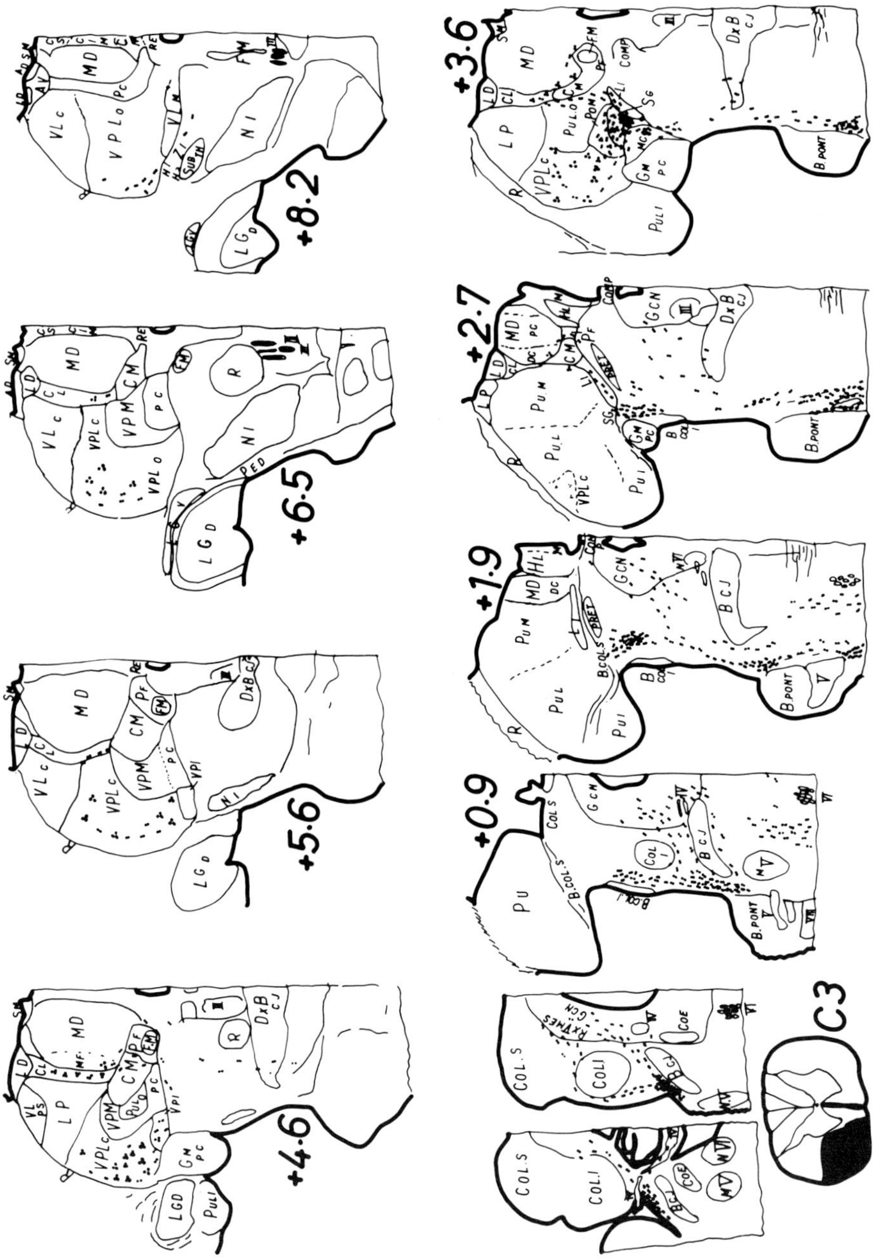
+8.2
+6.5
+5.6
+4.6
+3.6
+2.7
+1.9
+0.9
C3

thalamus, sending many terminal branches to GMmc, SG, posteromedial nucleus (POm), and terminates in VPLc and VPLo. In the VPL, dense terminal degenerations are distributed unevenly in a patchy pattern. Between each patchy termination there are sparse degenerating fibers. Using a magnifying-projecting apparatus, each patchy termination in VPL was magnified 100 times, projected and traced in drawings (fig. 3). Measurements show that there seems to be an average of seven patchy terminations in a section (24 μm thick) and the average diameter is about 200 μm. In a recent study using the WGA-HRP antegrade transport method, *Mantyh* [8] shows in monkey that this patchy termination in the coronal section extends in a rostrocaudal direction in three-dimensional reconstruction, thus forming a rod-like pattern.

Corticofugal Fibers from SI and SII Somatosensory Cortices

A small lesion in the gray matter of SI and SII cortices was observed in 4 and 6 cats, respectively. Ipsilateral cortical association fibers from SI and SII were studied. In general, both somatosensory cortices have reciprocal fiber connections between them and send fibers to MI (area 4) and area 5. The SII cortex, moreover, sends fibers to the insular cortex, suprasylvian fringe, vestibular representation and AI, AII. Although *Jones and Powell* [5] have reported that only SI cortex has fiber connection with area 5, this study shows that SII also sends fibers to area 5. It is interesting to note that a part of area 5 corresponds to the third somatosensory cortex (SII).

The corticothalamic connections from SI and SII seems essentially similar. Representative cases of each are shown in figure 3. In cat 721, which has a lesion in the face area of SI and small concomitant lesions in the posterior sigmoid gyrus, terminal degenerations were observed

---

Fig. 2. Distribution of degenerating STT axons (two dots) and terminations (three dots) in monkey thalamus following anterolateral cordotomy at C3. The nomenclature and rough coordinates mainly follow those of *Olszewski* [10]. B col i. = brachium colliculi inferioris; Cl = nucleus centralis lateralis; CM = nucleus centrum medianum; Gm mc = nucleus genicularis medialis, pars magnocellularis; Li = nucleus limitans; MD dc = nucleus medialis dorsalis, pars densocellularis; Pf = nucleus parafascicularis; Pom = nucleus posteromedialis; SG = nucleus suprageniculatus; VPI = nucleus ventralis posterior inferior; VPLc = nucleus ventralis posterior lateralis, pars caudalis; VPLo = nucleus ventralis posterior lateralis, pars oralis.

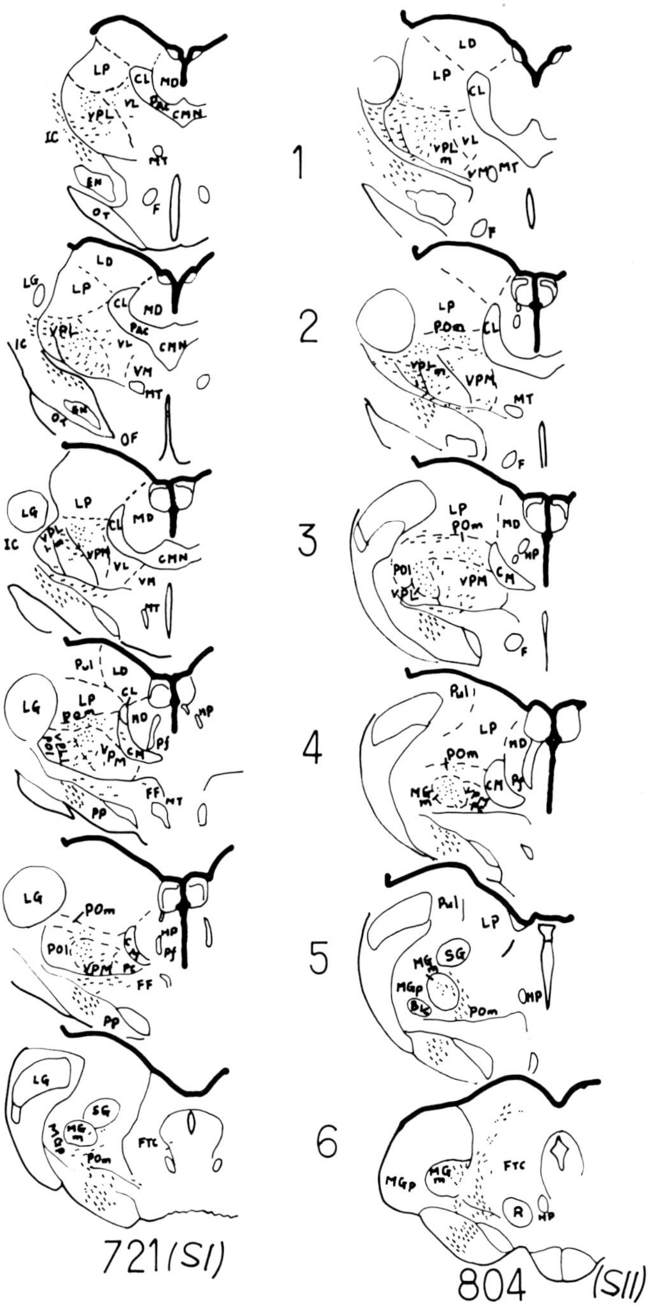
1
2
3
4
5
6
721(SI)
804(SII)
LD
LP
CL
MD
VL
VPL
CMN
IC
MT
OT
F
LG
VM
OF
VPM
Pul
POm
POl
CM
Pf
FF
PP
MP
SG
MGp
FTC
R

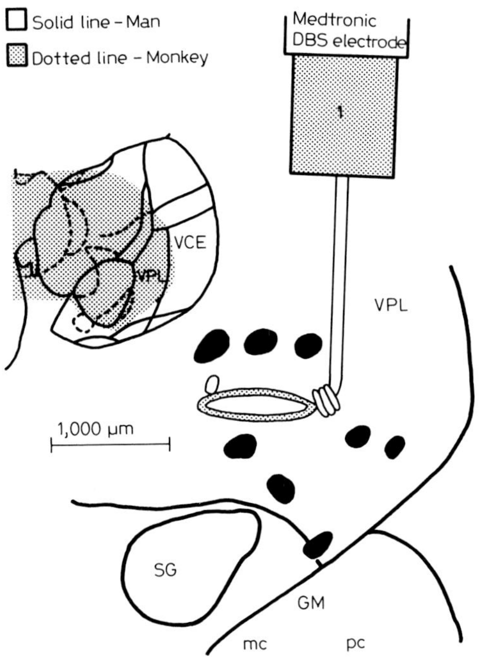

Fig. 4. Drawing of patchy terminal degenerations (solid circle) in VPL of monkey to compare the size of implantation electrode (Medtronic) with patches of STT termination. Number 0 and 1 of the electrode are designated to a distal loop electrode and the second contact point. In the left upper corner, a superimposed figure is shown to compare roughly the size of human thalamus with monkey's (stippled shadow).

Fig. 3. Distribution of degenerating axon (dots) and termination (single dot) of corticothalamic fibers from SI (cat 721) and SII cortex (cat 804). See text for explanation. The nomenclature used in this figure mainly follows that of *Berman and Jones* [2] and *Rinvik* [1]. CL = central lateral nucleus; CM = centre median nucleus; FF = nucleus of the field of Forel; FTC = central tegmental field; LP = lateral posterior complex; MGm = magnocellular medial geniculate nucleus; POm = posterior complex, medial region; SG = suprageniculate nucleus; VL = ventrolateral complex; VPLl = lateral part of nucleus ventralis posterior lateralis; VPLm = medial part of nucleus ventralis posterior lateralis; VPM = nucleus ventralis posterior medialis.

in VPLm, VPM, POm and MGm without a patchy pattern. In cat 804, in which the lesion was placed in the anterior part of anterior ectosylvian gyrus, terminal degenerations in VPLm, VPM, POm and MGm were observed. There appears to be essentially no differences in terminal site except in quantity. Somatotopic localization of the corticothalamic connections has been well documented in the literature [6, 7, 11], and we have made no attempt to consider this point because of concomitant lesions. It is interesting to note that there were no terminal degenerations in CL which receive direct fibers.

As has been well documented [7], SI cortex projects fibers mainly to the contralateral trigeminal nuclei complex and posterior column nuclei in a somatotopically organized manner in the brainstem. From SII cortex, projection to the brainstem appears to be much less intense than SI. Instead, it seems of interest to note that rather dense terminations in the ipsilateral superior colliculus and central tegmental field were observed in a cat with an SII lesion, in addition to a small amount of fibers which pass to the periaqueductal gray. Special attention was paid to the inferior central nucleus in the pons and medulla which corresponds to the nucleus raphe magnus. Small amounts of degenerating fibers were observed in inferior central nucleus, magnocellular, and gigantocellular tegmental fields bilaterally. The terminal degeneration, however, was not evident.

Only two sets of spinal cords were stained systematically. In cat 721 with lesions in SI cortex, degenerating fibers descend in the pyramidal tract in the dorsolateral funiculus after decussation in the medulla and were found to terminate in the IV, V, VI layers mainly and in the III, VII layers sparsely. The spinal cord of case 804 with a lesion in SII cortex has practically no degenerating fibers.

Discussion

The mechanisms of the modulation of pain by stimulation in the thalamic relay nucleus are still in debate. There is evidence that stimulation in VPL provokes inhibition of the STT neurons in the spinal posterior horn in the monkey [3] and excitation of the raphe-spinal neurons in NRM in the cat [14].

The size of an implantation electrode (Medtronic) is compared with the patches of STT termination in VPL (fig. 4). As our human VPL did not show the patches clearly, the electrode was drawn in one section of the monkey VPL, in which black circles show patchy terminations. Electric current passes between point 0 and 1, for example, during stimulation. It should be recognized that many STT terminations and other elements must be stimulated simultaneously by this macroelectrode.

Besides STT, VPL receives the medial lemniscus and somatosensory corticofugal fibers as well. According to *Berkley* [1], the medial lemniscus fibers terminate in the ventrobasal nucleus in dense terminal clusters like the STT terminations. The corticofugal and medial lemniscal fibers appear to fill the sparse area between the STT terminal patches. In this context, it will be clear that the macroelectrode will stimulate the STT, medial lemniscus, corticothalamic and thalamocortical fibers even in VPL. Thus, the stimulation may provoke paresthetic, not pure complex sensations and modulation of pain. The pathway and sites for the modulation of pain by VPL stimulation might be multiple.

References

1 Berkley, K.J.: Spatial relationships between the terminations of somatic sensory and motor pathways in the rostral brainstem of cats and monkeys. I. Ascending somatic sensory inputs to lateral diencephalon. J. comp. Neurol. *193:* 283–317 (1980).

2 Berman, A.L.; Jones, E.G.: The thalamus and basal telencephalon of the cat (University of Wisconsin Press, Madison 1982).

3 Gerhart, K.D.; Yezierski, R.P.; Fang, Z.R.; Willis, W.D.: Inhibition of primate spinothalamic tract neurons by stimulation in ventral posterior lateral (VPLc) thalamic nucleus: possible mechanisms. J. Neurophysiol. *49:* 406–423 (1983).

4 Hassler, R.: Anatomy of the thalamus; in Schaltenbrand, Bailey, Introduction to stereotaxis with an atlas of the human brain, vol. 1, pp. 230–290 (Thieme, Stuttgart 1977).

5 Jones, E.G.; Powell, T.P.S.: The ipsilateral cortical connections in somatic sensory areas in the cat. Brain Res. *9:* 71–94 (1968).

6 Jones, E.G.; Powell, T.P.S.: The projection of the somatic sensory cortex upon the thalamus in the cat. Brain Res. *10:* 369–391 (1968).

7 Kusama, T.; Otani, K.; Kawana, E.: Projections of the motor, somatic sensory research, vol. 21A, pp. 292–322 (Elsevier, Amsterdam 1966).

8 Mantyh, P.W.: The spinothalamic tract in the primate: a re-examination using wheatgerm agglutinin conjugated to horseradish peroxidase. Neuroscience: 847–862 (1983).

9 Mehler, W.R.: The anatomy of the so-called 'pain tract' in man: an analysis of the course and distribution of the ascending fibers of the fasciculus anterolateralis; in French, Porter, Basic research in paraplegia, pp. 26–55 (Thomas, Springfield 1962).

10 Olszewski, J.: The thalamus of the *Macaca mulatta*. An atlas for use with stereotaxic instruments (Karger, Basel 1952).

11 Rinvik, E.: The corticothalamic projection from the second somatosensory cortical area in the cat. An experimental study with silver impregnation methods. Exp. Brain Res. *5:* 153–172 (1968).

12 Rinvik, E.: A re-evaluation of the cytoarchitecture of the ventral nuclear complex of the cat's thalamus on the basis of corticothalamic connections. Brain Res. *8:* 254 (1968).

13 Schaltenbrand, G.; Wahren, W.: Atlas for the stereotaxy of the human brain (Thieme, Stuttgart 1977).

14 Tsubokawa, T.; Yamamoto, T.; Katayama, Y.; Moriyasu, U.: Clinical results and physiological basis of thalamic relay nucleus stimulation for relief of intractable pain with morphin tolerance. Appl. Neurophysiol. *45:* 143–155 (1982).

Dr. R. Kuroda, Department of Neurosurgery, Kinki University School of Medicine, Sayama-cho, Minamikawachi-gun, Osaka (Japan)

Proc. 9th Meeting World Soc. Stereotactic and Functional
Neurosurgery, Toronto 1985
Appl. Neurophysiol. *48:* 191–194 (1985)

Chronic Stimulation of the Septal Area for the Relief of Intractable Pain

Jorge R. Schvarcz

School of Medicine, University of Buenos Aires, Argentina

Key Words. Stereotactic surgery · Brain stimulation · Pain · Septal area

Abstract. Although brain stimulation techniques have changed the treatment of pain, their rationale has not yet been fully proved, and their clinical results are still frequently erratic or contradictory. In an attempt to provide alternate sites for stimulation, 10 patients were, in addition to conventional targets, chronically implanted at the septal area. Satisfactory relief of dysesthetic pain was induced by septal stimulation in 60% of the cases overall, without untoward effects. The follow-up ranged from 1 to 42 months. The available data conceivably suggest other mechanisms than the presumed exclusive activation of opiomimetic structures. They also seem to indicate that the septal area may be a suitable target for chronic stimulation.

The introduction of brain stimulation procedures has produced a dramatic change in the strategy to manage chronic intractable pain. Nevertheless, the pathophysiology of intracranial stimulation is only partially understood, and the results on pain obtained at the usual targets are often inconsistent or contradictory. Therefore, in an attempt to provide alternate sites for stimulation, 10 patients were, in addition to conventional targets, implanted at the septal area.

Material and Methods

Patients were operated under light sedation, with a modified Hitchcock stereotactic apparatus. The ventricular system was outlined by water-soluble positive contrast, and a standard DBS electrode was stereotactically placed at the PVG or at the VP. The patients, who had agreed to have an additional electrode implanted had then also a bipolar or a tetrapolar electrode stereotactically placed at the septal area (fig. 1). Its tip was aimed 5 mm in front and 2.5 mm below the anterior commissure in the coronal and horizontal planes, at 5.5 mm from the midsagittal plane. Both electrodes were externalized for a pe-

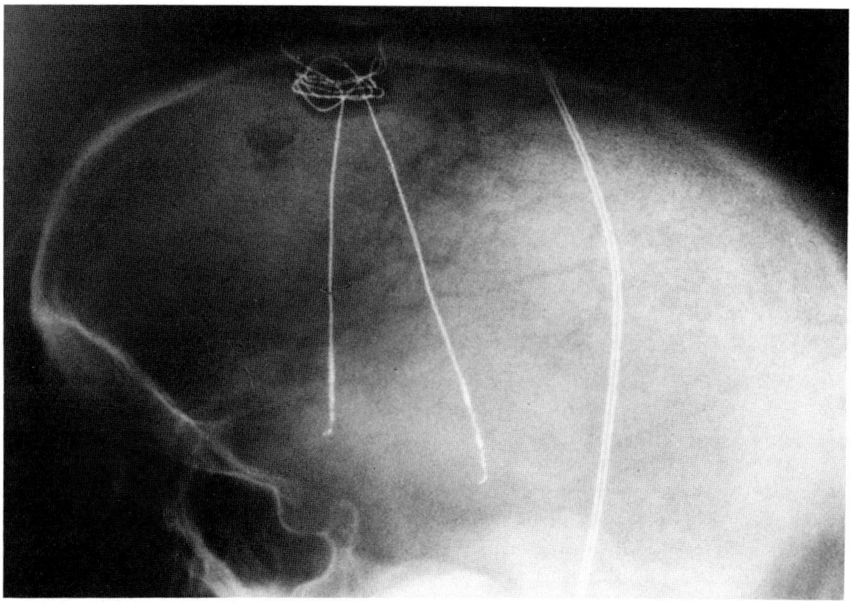

Fig. 1. Lateral radiograph showing chronic electrodes implanted in both the septal area and the periventricular gray region.

riod of percutaneous trial stimulation and, eventually, protracted stimulation or internalization.

The criteria for patient selection and the methods to assess the results on both clinical and acute pain have already been reported [9]. Ten patients underwent septal area stimulation. Five had pain of neoplastic origin, with gross deafferentation components related to plexus invasion, and 5 had neurogenic deafferentation pain. They all had severe pain, usually with both hyperpathia and deep background burning pain. They all have had extensive medical treatment, but none was presently on narcotic medication. Their pain history ranged from 1 to 4.5 years.

Results

Stimulation of the septal area usually produced clinical analgesia below the threshold to subjective sensations. However, just above threshold, a feeling of generalized warmth was often felt. Also a sensation of well-being and relaxation was frequently mentioned.

The clinical assessment of pain relief reflects the patient's own estimate of pain relief. Thus, 3 patients had significant pain relief, i.e., more than 75% reduction, although none of them achieved a complete abolition of pain; 3 had a moderate pain relief, i.e., from 50 to 75% reduction; and 4 of them failed to obtain any useful pain alleviation. The follow-up period ranged from 1 to 42 months.

There were no untoward side effects. There was no unequivocal reversal of pain relief by naloxone. Acute experimentally induced pain was not modified by stimulation.

Discussion

Although deep brain stimulation has produced significant advances in the elusive management of chronic intractable pain, knowledge about the mechanisms underlying pain relief is still fragmentary, and clinical results induced from current targets are rather unpredictable or even contradictory. Therefore, the protracted clinical evaluation of other areas presumably related to antinociceptive phenomena seems to be warranted.

Based on a neuropsychological rationale, very early attempts to correlate the positive rewarding effect of septal area stimulation in animals with human pain have been made by *Heath and Mickle* [3] and *Gol* [2], and more recently by *Obrador* et al. [5]. However, the presumably accepted rationale is presently based on the activation of opiomimetic structures. *Watson* et al. [10] have shown the anatomical distribution of immunoreactive β-lipotropin in the rat, which is located at the septal area, anterior hypothalamus, periventricular and periaqueductal gray. *Roldan* et al. [8] have demonstrated an increase in the plasma levels of immunoreactive β-endorphin after septal area stimulation in the rat. *Richardson* [6] has reported the results of acute stimulation of both the superior and inferior septal area in 5 cases with neurogenic pain, whereby a significant analgesic effect was obtained.

In the series herein reported, a satisfactory relief of pain was chronically induced in 60% of the cases overall. However, the effects on central pain, which theoretically should not be affected by such stimulation, or the rare reversal of pain relief by naloxone, strongly suggest nonopioid mechanisms. These clinical observations should then be accounted for if an exclusive morphiomimetic action is to be accepted. Stimulation can orthodromically or antidromically activate several neuronal circuits, and nonopioid mechanisms may well coexist with those related to endogenous opioids. This may be relevant when particular pain categories are considered vis-à-vis target selection. Similarly, stimulation of the periventricular gray has also been reported to influence deafferentation pain [1, 4, 7, 9]. These data seemingly indicate that the septal area is a suitable target for chronic stimulation, warranting further clinical evaluation.

References

1 Dieckmann, G.; Witzmann, A.: Initial and long-term results of deep brain stimulation for chronic intractable pain. Appl. Neurophysiol. *45:* 167–172 (1982).

2 Gol, A.: Relief of pain by electrical stimulation of the septal area. J. neurol. Sci. *5:* 115–120 (1967).

3 Heath, R.G.; Mickle, W.A.: Evaluation of seven years' experience with depth electrode studies in human patients; in Ramy, O'Doherty, Electrical studies on the unanesthetized brain, pp. 214–247 (Hoeber, New York 1960).

4 Martín-Rodriguez, J.G.; Obrador, S.: Therapeutic electrical stimulation of the brain. Biochemical changes induced in the ventricular cerebrospinal fluid with regard to opiate-like substances; in Hitchcock, Ballantine, Meyerson, Modern concepts in psychiatric surgery, pp. 47–56 (Elsevier, Amsterdam 1979).

5 Obrador, S.; Delgado, J.M.; Martín-Rodriguez, J.G.: The future of functional neurosurgery; in Sano, Ishii, Recent progress in neurological surgery, pp. 265–269 (Excerpta Medica, Amsterdam 1974).

6 Richardson, D.E.: Analgesia produced by stimulation of various sites in the human beta-endorphin system. Appl. Neurophyisol. *45:* 116–122 (1982).

7 Richardson, D.E.; Akil, H.: Pain reduction by electrical brain stimulation in man. Chronic self-administration in the periventricular gray matter. J. Neurosurg. *47:* 184–194 (1977).

8 Roldan, P.; Moreno, J.; Vincent, E.; Cerdá, M.; Ramos, S.; Barcia-Salorio, J.L.: Effect of electrical stimulation of periaqueductal gray and septal area on beta-endorphin plasma levels in a model of deafferentation pain. Experimental study in rats in Gybels, Hitchcock, Ostertag, Rossi, Siegfried, Szikla, Advances in stereotactic and functional neurosurgery 6. Acta neurochir. *33:* suppl., pp. 501–503 (1984).

9 Schvarcz, J.R.: Chronic self-stimulation of the medial posterior thalamus for the alleviation of deafferentation pain; in Gillingham, Gybels, Hitchcock, Rossi, Szikla, Advances in stereotactic and functional neurosurgery 4. Acta neurochir. *30:* suppl., pp. 295–301 (1980).

10 Watson, S.J.; Barchas, J.D.; Li, C.H.: Beta-lipotropin: localization of cells and axons in rat brain by immunocytochemistry. Proc. natn. Acad. Sci. USA *74:* 5155–5158 (1977).

Jorge R. Schvarcz, MD, Beruti 2926, Buenos Aires 1425 (Argentina)

Proc. 9th Meeting World Soc. Stereotactic and Functional
Neurosurgery, Toronto 1985
Appl. Neurophysiol. *48:* 195–200 (1985)

Pain Relief following Stimulation of the Pontomesencephalic Parabrachial Region in Humans: Brain Sites for Nonopiate-Mediated Pain Control[1]

Yoichi Katayama, Takashi Tsubokawa, Teruyasu Hirayama, Takamitsu Yamamoto

Department of Neurological Surgery, Nihon University School of Medicine, Tokyo, Japan

Key Words. Brain stimulation · Pain · Parabrachial nucleus · Locus coeruleus

Abstract. It has been demonstrated that stimulation of the pontomesencephalic parabrachial region (PBR) by microinjection of cholinergic drugs or electricity in the cat produces potent pain suppression which is not antagonized by the opiate antagonist, naloxone. We report the application of electrical PBR stimulation in 2 patients whose pain was resistant to conventional methods of treatment including morphine administration. Intermittent use of low-frequency PBR stimulation was found to relieve pain in these patients. The present results appear to suggest that PBR stimulation, unlike periaqueductal gray stimulation, may be useful for the control of morphine-resistant pain in humans.

Introduction

Chemical stimulation of the pontomesencephalic parabrachial region (PBR) by means of microinjection of cholinergic drugs [6–11] has been shown to produce potent behavioral pain suppression in cats. Unlike the pain suppression induced by periaqueductal gray (PAG) stimulation [4], the pain suppression induced by PBR stimulation has been found not to be antagonized by the morphine antagonist naloxone [13].

It has been reported that PAG stimulation does not relieve morphine-resistant pain [4]. However, among morphine-resistant types of pain, neurogenic forms of pain due to deafferentation are often relieved by thalamic sensory relay nucleus (TSRN) stimulation [e.g. 16],

[1] This work was supported by the Japan Education Ministry, Grant 60480333.

although TSRN stimulation is generally ineffective for the control of other forms of intractable pain. Thus, PBR stimulation could have unique advantages in the control of morphine-resistant pain which cannot be relieved by TSRN stimulation.

Although chemical stimulation more selectively influences restricted neural populations, clinical application of chemical stimulation is complicated by the possibility of accidental spread of the drug. Since it has recently been demonstrated in cats that certain parameters of electrical stimulation of the PBR can produce pain-suppressive effects similar to those induced by chemical stimulation and can dissociate pain suppression from effects on other neural functions [3, 7], it appears practical at this time to employ electrical stimulation for human use. We report the application of PBR stimulation in patients whose pain was morphine-resistant and was not sufficiently relieved by TSRN stimulation.

Methods

Two patients, 49- and 56-year-old males, both of whom suffered from severe chronic pain for several months due to lung cancer, underwent PBR stimulation. When they were referred to us, control of their pain by narcotics was entirely unsatisfactory even though a progressively larger dose was administered every day. It was suspected that these patients had become morphine tolerant due to long-term use of narcotics or their pain was neurogenic, rather than somatogenic, in nature. The latter possibility appeared less likely, since no peripheral skin region associated with sensory loss was noted. Electrodes for deep brain stimulation (Medtronic DBS system) were placed at the PBR in addition to the unilateral TSRN.

No single cytoarchitectural unit corresponds precisely to the PBR as identified physiologically. However, mapping of stimulation sites associated with pain suppression in the cat [6–11] has suggested that the dorsal and ventral nuclei of the brachium conjunctivum of *Winkler and Potter* [18], the nucleus parabrachialis (NPB) medialis et lateralis of *Taber* [15], the marginal nucleus of the brachium conjunctivum (MBC) of *Berman* [1], the caudal part of the nucleus tegmenti pedunculopontinus (NTPP) and the nucleus subcoeruleus (NSC) of *Taber* [15], as well as part of the paralemniscal tegmental field (FTP) and part of the Kölliker-Fuse (KF) nucleus of *Berman* [1] may be included. The NPB and MBC are both designated as medium-sized clusters and small neurons oriented parallel to the curved surface of the bundle of the brachium conjunctivum which extend from the level of the rostral pole of the nucleus nervi trigemini motorius [1, 15, 18]. The rostral limits of the cluster have not yet been clearly defined since these neurons disperse into rostral structures including the FTP [1, 15, 18] and meet the NTPP. It appears that the NPB and nuclei similarly named by others usually include areas more rostral than the MBC [12, 18]. The physiologically identified PBR may include these rostral areas as well. It has been indicated by *Kimura* et al. [12] that many cholinoceptive cells, as identified by choline acetyltransferase immunohistochemistry, are stained in the NPB including the MBC and the rostral areas, in agreement with the extent of the PBR identified by microinjection of cholinergic drugs. Rostrally, the cholinoceptive cells in the dorsal part of the NPB do not extend into the dorsally adjacent structures. The cells in the ventral part extend into the FTP. Caudally, the cholinoceptive cells are localized in the MBC and sparsely distributed in the NSC and KF.

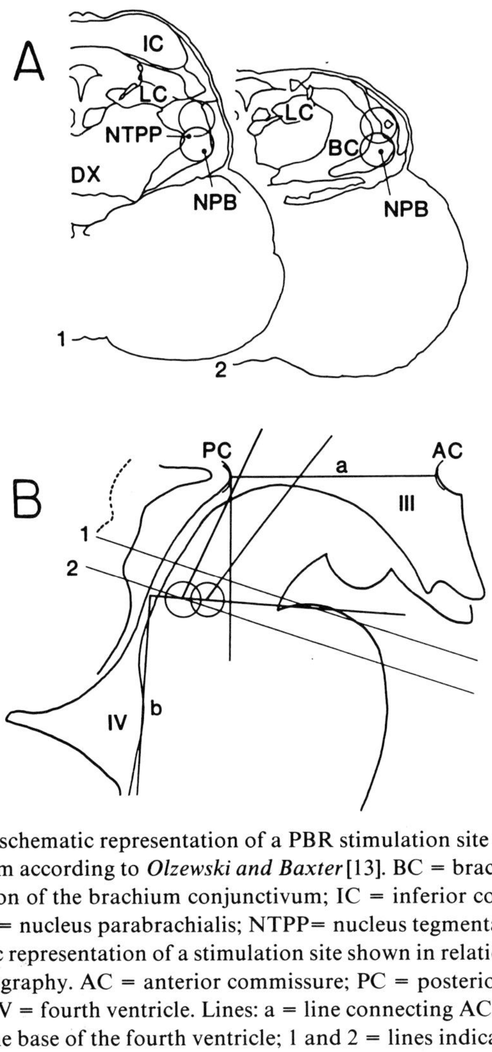

Fig. 1. A A schematic representation of a PBR stimulation site shown in sections of human brain stem according to *Olzewski and Baxter* [13]. BC = brachium conjunctivum; DX = decussation of the brachium conjunctivum; IC = inferior colliculus; LC = locus coeruleus; NPB = nucleus parabrachialis; NTPP= nucleus tegmentalis pedunculopontinus. **B** Schematic representation of a stimulation site shown in relation to the lateral view of the ventriculography. AC = anterior commissure; PC = posterior commissure; III = third ventricle; IV = fourth ventricle. Lines: a = line connecting AC and PC; b = line for the contour of the base of the fourth ventricle; 1 and 2 = lines indicating the levels of the sections of *Olzewski and Baxter* [13] shown in **A**.

Clusters of cells cytoarchitecturally similar to the cells of NPB or MBC in the cat can also be identified in primates including humans [5] as the MBC of *Crosby and Woodburne* [2]. Rostrally, these cells are intermingled with cells of the pars lateralis of the nucleus mesencephalicus profundus of Ziehen or the NTPP of Jacobsohn and *Olzewski and Baxter* [13] behind the level of the decussation of the brachium conjunctivum [2]. *Crosby and Woodburne* [2] suggested that the MBC described by Castaldi [2] in humans may correspond to the NTPP of Jacobsohn.

Based on these anatomical considerations, we placed electrodes for PBR stimulation within the rostral part of the MBC of *Olzewski and Baxter* [13] slightly caudal to the level of the decussation of the brachium conjunctivum (fig. 1A). Since experimental studies in cats have demonstrated that unilateral PBR stimulation produces bilateral effects, the electrodes for PBR stimulation in these patients were implanted unilaterally. According to the atlas of *Schaltenbrand and Wahren* [14], electrodes were introduced from a frontal burr hole to the brain stem 6.5–8.5 mm lateral to the midline, 1.0–5.0 mm posterior to the posterior commissure, 13–15.0 mm below the line connecting the anterior and posterior commissures and 2.0–4.0 mm anterior to the lateral contour of the base of the fourth ventricle (fig. 1B).

Results

During test stimulation periods, it was found that PBR stimulation with a frequency ranging from 10 to 30 Hz produced a reduction in pain in both of the patients. With this frequency of stimulation, no emotional/affective or autonomic effects, or cerebellar signs were induced, so the stimulation system was internalized. Although TSRN stimulation was also found to be moderately effective in these 2 patients, the pain control by TSRN stimulation alone was not satisfactory. We followed these 2 patients up for more than 2 months, respectively, until death due to cancer. During this period, the pain relief with intermittent use of PBR stimulation was satisfactory enough not to require the use of analgesics.

Discussion

The present finding that morphine-resistant pain in humans could be relieved by PBR stimulation is consistent with the data obtained in the cat indicating that pain suppression from PBR stimulation does not involve opiate-mediated neural pathways [8, 11]. No undesirable side effects were induced by low frequency PBR stimulation, in agreement with the results of experiments in the cat [3]. Although the present small number of cases does not permit us to draw any definite conclusions, the results do appear to suggest that PBR stimulation may be useful for the control of morphine-resistant pain.

References

1 Berman, A.L.: The brain stem of the cat: a cytoarchitectonic atlas with stereotaxic coordinates (University of Wisconsin Press, Madison 1968).
2 Crosby, E.C.; Woodburne, R.T.: The nuclear pattern of the non-tectal portions of the midbrain and isthmus in primates. J. comp. Neurol. *78:* 441-482 (1943).
3 DeSalles, A.A.F.; Katayama, Y.; Becker, D.P.; Hayes, R.L.: Pain suppression induced by electrical stimulation of the pontine parabrachial region: experimental study in cats. J. Neurosurg. *62:* 397-407 (1985).
4 Hosobuchi, Y.; Rossier, J.; Bloom, F.E.; Guillemin, R.: Periaqueductal gray stimulation for pain suppression in humans; in Bonica, Liebeskind, Albe-Fessard, Advances in pain research and therapy, pp. 515-523 (Raven Press, New York 1979).
5 Huber, G.C.; Crosby, E.C.; Woodburne, R.T.; Gillian, L.A.; Brown, J.O.; Tamthai, B.: The mammalian midbrain and isthmus regions. I. The nuclear pattern. J. comp. Neurol. *78:* 129-534 (1943).
6 Katayama, Y.; Becker, D.P.; Hayes, R.L.: New brain sites for pain control: selective activation of cholinoceptive cells in parabrachial region produces non-opiate analgesia. Proc. Am. Ass. Neurol. Surgeons, 1983, pp. 94-95.
7 Katayama, Y.; DeSalles, A.A.F.; Becker, D.P.; Hayes, R.L.: Nociceptive suppression induced by cholinergic and electrical stimulation of the pontine parabrachial region of the cat. Pain *2:* suppl., p. 325 (1984).
8 Katayama, Y.; DeWitt, D.S.; Becker, D.P.; Hayes, R.L.: Behavioral evidence for cholinoceptive pontine inhibitory area: descending control of spinal motor output and sensory input. Brain Res. *296:* 241-262 (1984).
9 Katayama, Y.; Tsubokawa, T.; Maejima, S.; Yamamoto, T.: Responses of raphe-spinal neurons to stimulation of the pontine parabrachial region which produces behavioral nociceptive suppression in the cat (submitted).
10 Katayama, Y.; Watkins, L.R.; Becker, D.P.; Hayes, R.L.: Evidence for involvement of cholinoceptive cells of the pontine parabrachial region in environmentally induced nociceptive suppression in the cat. Brain Res. *299:* 348-353 (1984).
11 Katayama, Y.; Watkins, L.R.; Becker, D.P.; Hayes, R.L.: Non-opiate analgesia induced by carbachol microinjection into the pontine parabrachial region of the cat. Brain Res. *296:* 263-283 (1984).
12 Kimura, H.; McGeer, P.L.; Peng, J.H.; McGeer, E.G.: The central cholinergic system studied by choline acetyltransferase immunohistochemistry in the cat. J. comp. Neurol. *200:* 151-201 (1981).
13 Olzewski, J.; Baxter, D.: Cytoarchitecture of the human brain stem; 2nd ed. (Karger, Basel 1982).
14 Schaltenbrand, G.; Wahren, W.: Atlas of stereotaxy of the human brain; 2nd rev. ed. (Thieme, Stuttgart 1977).

15 Taber, E.: The cytoarchitecture of the brain stem of the cat. I. Brain stem nuclei of cat. J. comp. Neurol. *116:* 27–70 (1961).
16 Tsubokawa, T.; Katayama, Y.; Yamamoto, T.; Hirayama, T.: Deafferentation pain and stimulation of the thalamic relay nucleus: clinical and experimental study. Appl. Neurophysiol. (in press, 1985).
17 Tsubokawa, T.; Yamamoto, T.; Katayama, Y.; Hirayama, T.; Shibuya, H.: Thalamic relay nucleus stimulation for relief of intractable pain: clinical results and β-endorphin immunoreactivity in the cerebrospinal fluid. Pain *18:* 115–126 (1984).
18 Winkler, C.; Potter, A.: An anatomical guide to the experimental researches on the cat's brain (Bersluys, Amsterdam 1914).

Yoichi Katayama, MD, PhD, Department of Neurological Surgery, Nihon University School of Medicine, 30-1 Oyaguchikami-machi, Itabashi-ku 173 (Japan)

Proc. 9th Meeting World Soc. Stereotactic and Functional Neurosurgery, Toronto 1985
Appl. Neurophysiol. *48:* 201–211 (1985)

An Experimental Model of Deafferented Pain in the Cat

Shimpei Namba, Yoji Shimizu, Takao Wani, Noriaki Fujiwara

Department of Neurological Surgery, Okayama University Medical School, Okayama, Japan

Key Words. Deafferented pain · Denervation hyperactivity · Experimental model · Pain

Abstract. Deafferentation hyperactivity, produced unilaterally in the neurons of the subnucleus caudalis of the spinal trigeminal nucleus (STNcd) in cats by left Gasserian ganglionectomy, was studied neurochemically and electrophysiologically. Analysis of neuronal activities on both sides of the STNcd was done 11–63 days after the denervation. On the denervated side, 37 (57%) of the 65 neurons identified showed deafferentation hyperactivity. Continuous and spontaneous firing of these hyperactive neurons were inhibited neither by the intraventricular administration of morphine or enkephalinamide nor by the electrical stimulation of periaqueductal gray. In contrast, the facilitation of the pain perceptive neuronal activities in the STNcd of the nondenervated side was remarkably inhibited, both by the administration of the same drugs and by periaqueductal gray stimulation. The deafferentation hyperactivity produced in this experiment in the STNcd of the denervated side might have a close physiological relationship to the deafferented pain of clinical patients.

Introduction

Intractable pain has been classified into two different types according to the etiology of the pain: peripheral and deafferented pain. A variety of pain models have been produced to study the pain evoking or suppressive mechanism. However, most are peripheral pain models based on the facilitation or excitation of peripheral pain-conducting fibers Aδ and C. It is important to design a model of deafferented pain, because deliberate study of this type of intractable pain is needed to approach the mechanism of pain in the patient with pain of central origin. In this report, a tentative model of deafferented pain is reported.

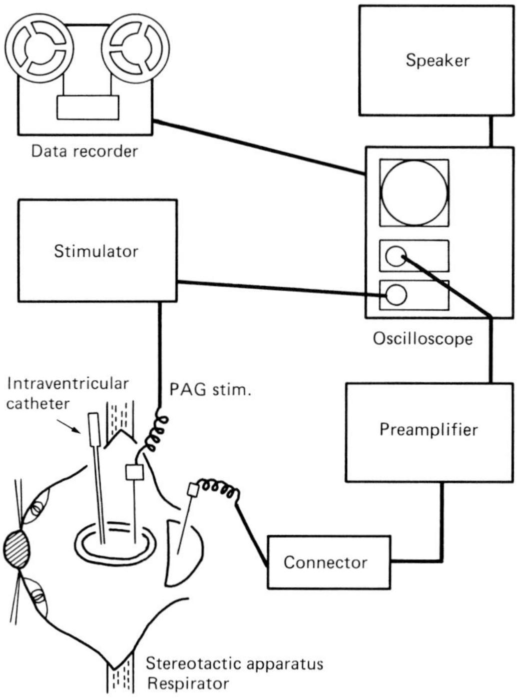

Fig. 1. Schematic drawing of the experimental set-up. A recording microelectrode was inserted in the STNcd, and a stimulating electrode stereotactically placed in the PAG. A small cannula was introduced into the lateral ventricle for the administration of drugs.

Method

Preliminary Experiment

Sixteen cats, weighing 2.5–4.0 kg, were used. They were anesthetized with ketamine (10 mg/kg i.m.), and intratracheal intubation was done. With 3 cats, an anatomical localization of subnucleus caudalis of the spinal trigeminal nucleus (STNcd) was first ascertained, according to Berman's atlas [2]. The heads of another 7 cats, immobilized with pancronium bromide (0.1 mg/kg/1–2 h), were fixed in the stereotactic apparatus. The distribution of STNcd neurons responsive to various modalities of stimuli on the face was determined. For this purpose, a suboccipital craniectomy including total removal of the posterior margin of the foramen magnum was performed, followed by the partial resection of the inferior portion of the cerebellum, thus exposing the obex and uppermost portion of the cervical spinal cord. A stainless steel electrode with tip diameter of 5 mm (500 K-1 Momega; Unique Medical Co., Japan) was inserted at various points from the level of the obex to 4 mm caudal to it, 2.5–4 mm lateral to the midline, where STNcd had been estimated to be located by the previous anatomical study. Extracellular neuronal activity responsive to various modalities of stimulation on the face was observed on the oscilloscope and recorded on tape for later analysis (fig. 1A, B). Thus, the distribution of the neurons responsive to facial stimuli was determined. In the remaining 6 cats, total Gasserian ganglionectomy of the left side was performed by electrocoagulation through the subtemporal extradural approach. The cats survived up to 51 days after the ganglionectomy. Neuronal activity in the STNcd of both denervated (left) and nondenervated (right) sides was examined at various intervals after the denervation operation, by inserting recording microelectrodes at various layers. Throughout these experiments, 0.5% lidocaine-HCl was periodically injected to the points on the face in touch with bars for the head fixation as well as to the skin incision. On finishing the experiments, the whole brain including the upper cervical spinal cord was removed and fixed with 10% formalin. Many serial preparations of 10 μm slices each were made for histological observation of the spinal trigeminal tract and determination of the exact electrode position by Nissl, Klüver-Barrera or HE stain.

Principal Experiment

Eighteen cats, weighing 2.3–4.0 kg, were used. Unilateral (left side) Gasserian ganglia (GG) of all cats were totally destroyed by the same procedure as in the preliminary experiments. The cats survived up to 63 days. Behavioral changes after the ganglionectomy were observed and recorded. Neuronal activity of STNcd of both denervated (left) and nondenervated (right) sides was examined 11–63 days after the ganglionectomy. The experimental design was the same as in the preliminary experiment, but the thorax was opened under artificial respiration to eliminate the movement of recording sites by respiration. In 6 of these 18 cats, 1 mg morphine-HCl in 2 ml solution (1 mg/2 ml) or enkephalinamide (0.55 mg/ml) was injected through a small cannula stereotactically introduced into the vicinity of the foramen of Monro (fig. 1). The influence of these substances on the neuronal activity in both sides of STNcd was observed, followed by intravenous naloxone (5 mg) injection. Electrical stimulation of the periaqueductal gray (PAG), the location of which was determined with Snider-Niemer's [8] or Jasper's [6] atlas (A: 6-7, L: 9-1, H: 0-1), was done in 4 cats using a stimulating electrode of 5 μm tip (Unique Medical Co.), with parameter of 2.0–3.0 V, 50 Hz, 20 ms train pulse. The effect of PAG stimulation on neuronal firing of both sides of STNcd was examined. On finishing the experiments, stimulating and recording sites were ascertained by the same procedure as in the preliminary experiment.

Result

Preliminary Experiment

The anatomical range of STNcd was found to be identical with Berman's atlas; 2.5–4.0 mm lateral to the midline, and 0.2–2.0 mm in depth from the dorsal surface of the uppermost cervical spinal cord. Accordingly, a recording microelectrode was inserted through that

2 A
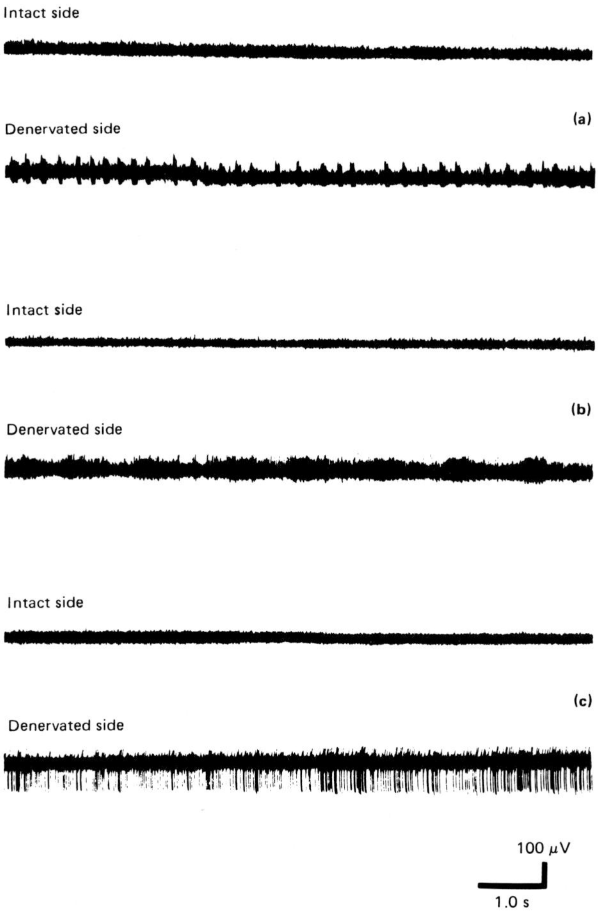

Fig. 2. **A** Spontaneous hyperactivity of the neuron in the STNcd of the denervated side became apparent from aobut 10 days after the ganglionectomy (denervation): (a) 11 days, (b) 25 days and (c) 50 days after the ganglionectomy. **B** The cat after the ganglionectomy; the upper photograph shows the broken vibrissae of the denervated (left) side with the palpebrae loosely sutured; the lower shows the ulcerations of coronea as well as facial skin on the denervated side.

range, the height being from the level of obex to 4 mm caudally. More extensive study elicited that the neuronal firing responsive to pin prick or pinch on the face was most frequently found from the height of the obex to caudal 2 mm and 3–4 mm lateral to the midline (fig. 3A). Denervation of the trigeminal nerve by ganglionectomy provoked the

2 B

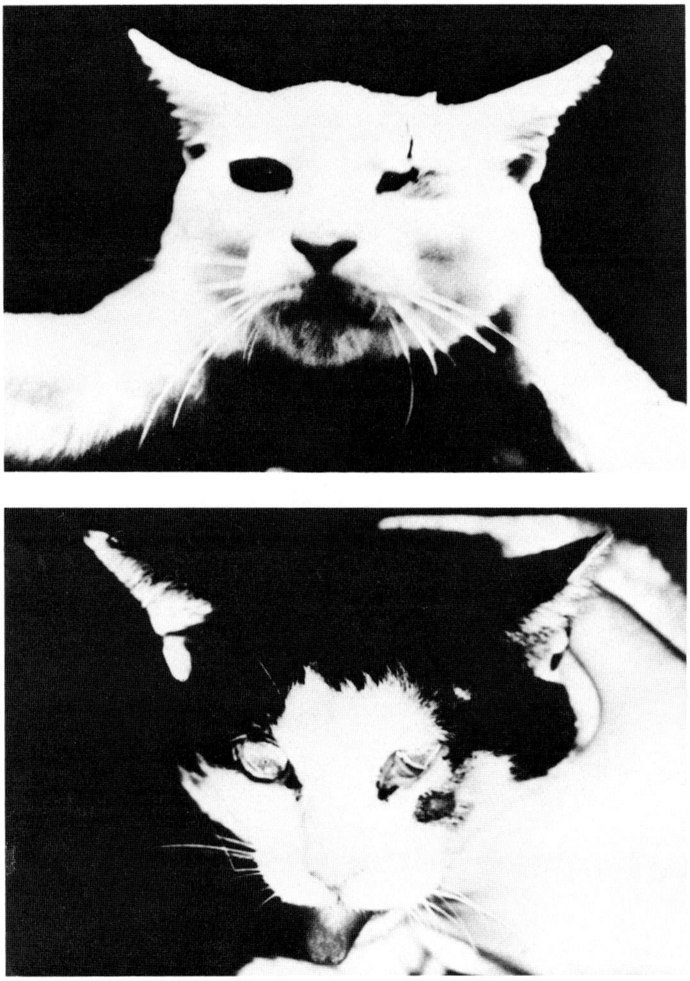

spontaneous neuronal hyperactivity in the STNcd of the denervated side, which continued throughout the period of observation without any stimulation on the face (fig. 2A). This neuronal hyperactivity became apparent by about 10 days after the denervation, and gradually grew to be so intensive as to show continuous high amplitude spontaneous firing so it was easily discriminated from the normal neuronal firing on the oscilloscope at sight. Histological examination of STNcds

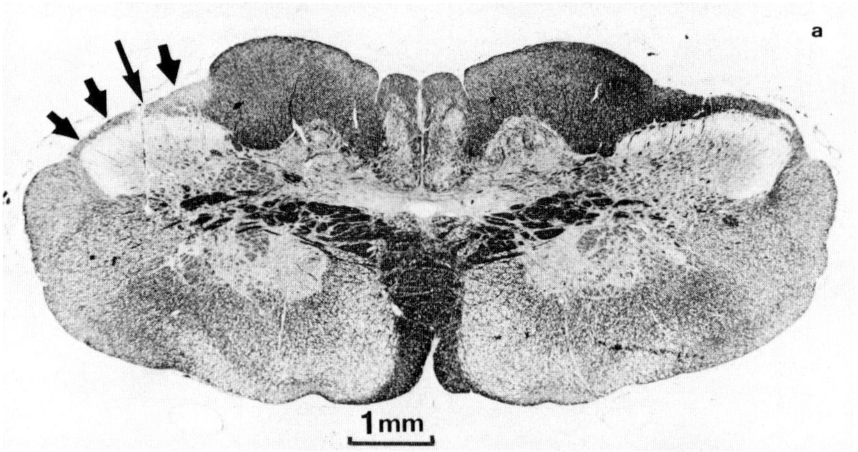
a
1mm

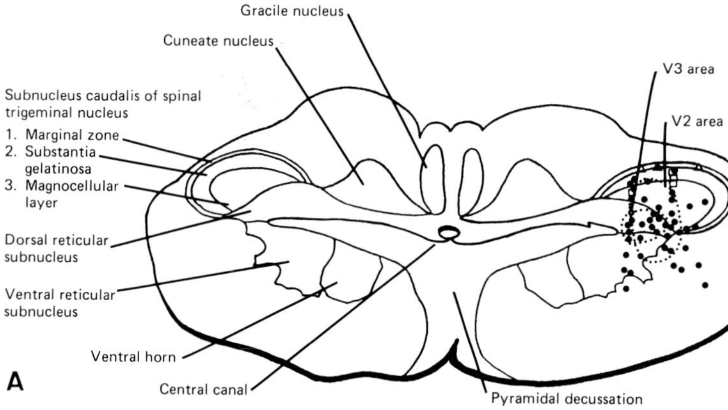
Gracile nucleus
Cuneate nucleus
Subnucleus caudalis of spinal trigeminal nucleus
1. Marginal zone
2. Substantia gelatinosa
3. Magnocellular layer
Dorsal reticular subnucleus
Ventral reticular subnucleus
Ventral horn
Central canal
Pyramidal decussation
V3 area
V2 area
A

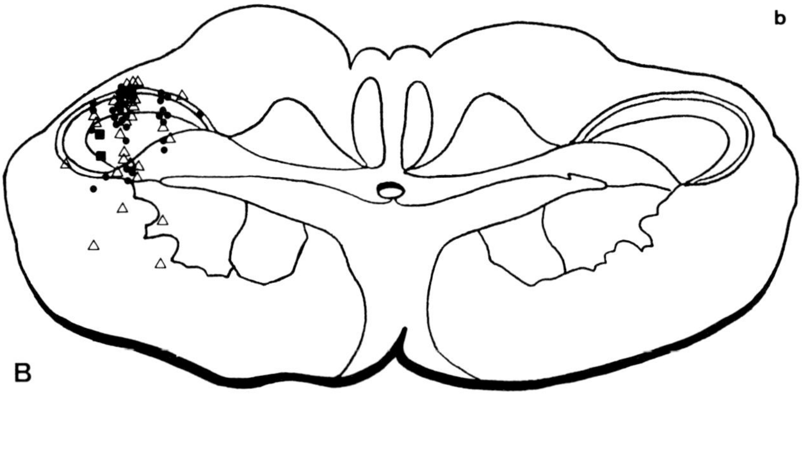
b
B

revealed a remarkable degeneration of the spinal trigeminal tract of the denervated side (fig. 3B).

Principal Experiment

The cats showed abnormal behavior starting from 7 to 10 days after the Gasserian ganglionectomy, which was never seen in those without ganglionectomy; incessant rubbing of the face on the denervated side (left side) against the cage caused the vibrissae to break and the skin to ulcerate. All cats without suture closure of the palpebrae showed corneal ulcer on the denervated side (fig. 2B). Figure 3 shows the distribution of the neurons in the STNcd of the right (nondenervated) side, which were responsive to various modalities of facial stimulation (fig. 3B). On the nondenervated side as many as 44 of the 51 neurons identified were wide dynamic range neurons (WDRN), which responded to pain as well as touch on the face. Only 3 of the 51 neurons were nociceptive specific neurons (NSN), which responded exceptionally to pain stimuli. The remaining 4 were low threshold mechanoreceptive neurons (LTMRN). WDRNs were predominantly distributed in the magnocellular layer of STNcd and more ventrally located dorsal or ventral reticular subnucleus. The ranges of the distribution of the neurons repsonsive to stimulation of the facial areas innervated by the second and third branches of the trigeminal nerve respectively, were overlapped and indistinct. On the denervated side, 37 (57%) of the 65 neurons identified showed spontaneous and continuous hyperactivity, which were easily discriminated from normal neuronal activity on the oscilloscope but was confirmed by spike frequency histogram analysis

---

Fig. 3. A Distribution of the neurons in the STNcd of the nondenervated (right) side, responsive to the various modalities of stimulation on the face. △ = Nociceptive specific neuron; □ = low threshold mechanoreceptive neuron; ● = wide dynamic range neuron. **B** (a) A Klüver-Barrera stain of the upper spinal cord 2 mm caudal to the obex of the cat after ganglionectomy. The short arrows indicate the degeneration of the spinal trigeminal tract and the long arrow indicates a tract of a recording microelectrode. (b) The distribution of the neurons with spontaneous hyperactivity after the denervation is shown. Thirty-seven (57%) of 65 neurons identified apparently showed denervation hyperactivity. ● = Neurons with denervation hyperactivity; △ = neurons without hyperactivity; ■ = hyperactive neurons in which the hyperactivity became more intensive in response to pain stimuli on the upper cervical skin (see fig. 5). Note, the neurons with denervation hyperactivity are predominantly distributed in the superficial layers of the STNcd.

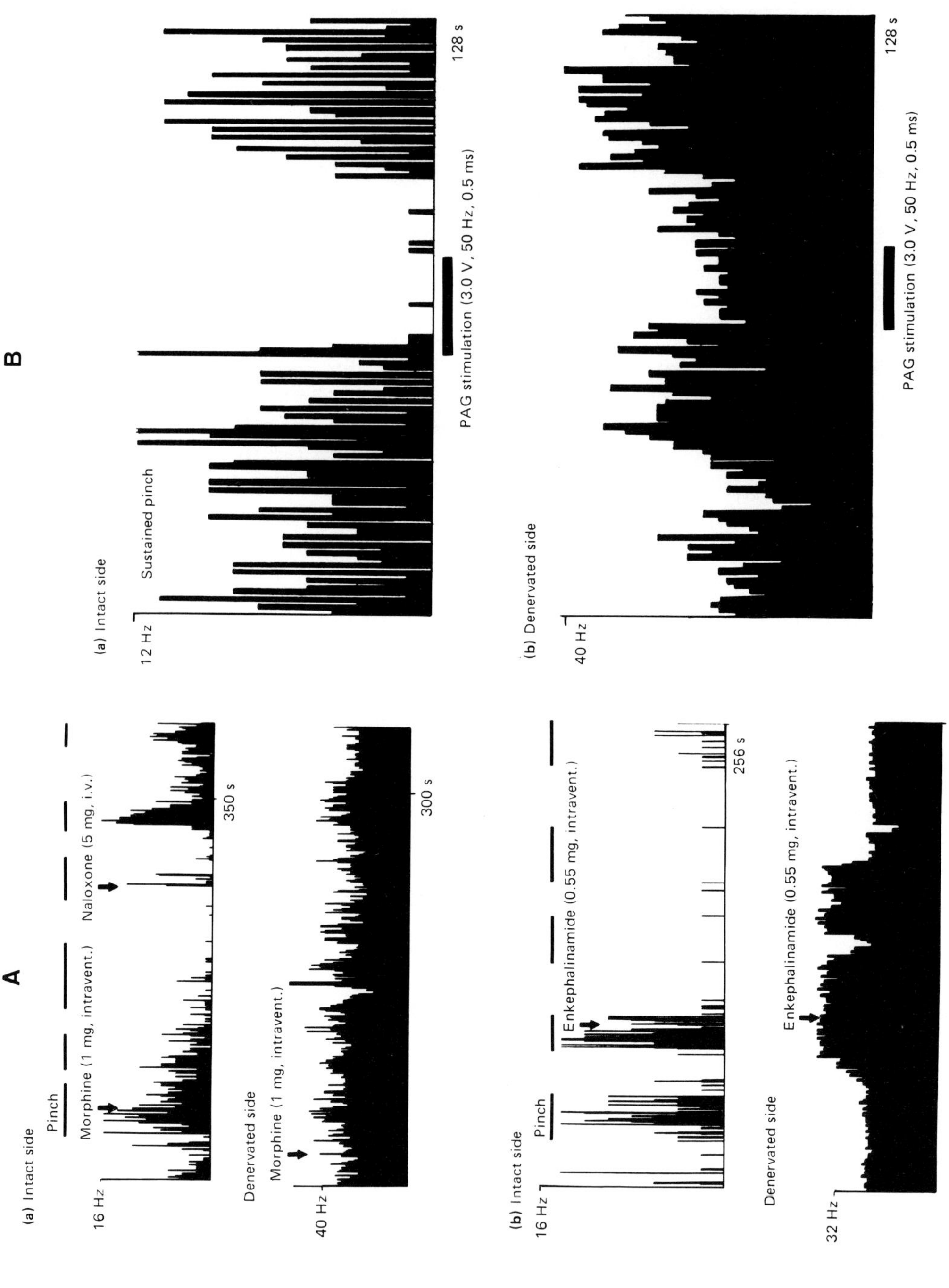
A
(a) Intact side
Pinch
Morphine (1 mg, intravent.)
Naloxone (5 mg, i.v.)
16 Hz
350 s
Denervated side
Morphine (1 mg, intravent.)
40 Hz
300 s
(b) Intact side
Pinch
Enkephalinamide (0.55 mg, intravent.)
16 Hz
256 s
Denervated side
Enkephalinamide (0.55 mg, intravent.)
32 Hz
256 s
B
(a) Intact side
Sustained pinch
12 Hz
128 s
PAG stimulation (3.0 V, 50 Hz, 0.5 ms)
(b) Denervated side
40 Hz
128 s
PAG stimulation (3.0 V, 50 Hz, 0.5 ms)

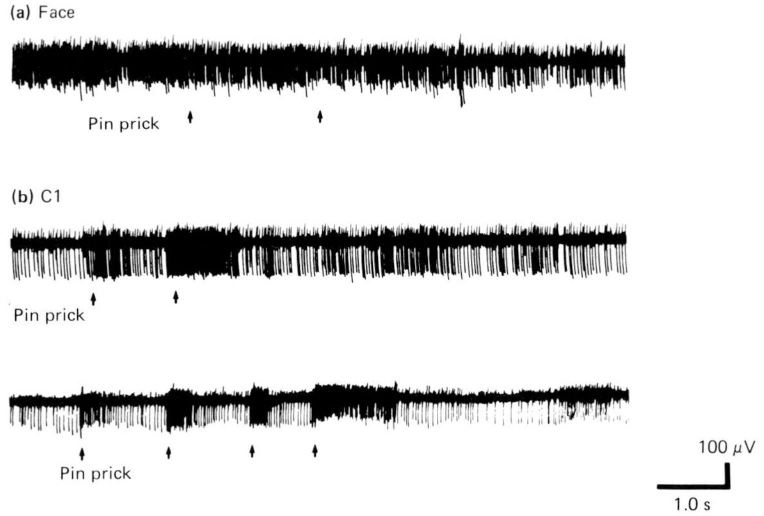

Fig. 5. A hyperactive neuron which responded to pain stimuli on the uppermost cervical skin (b), but not to stimuli on the face (a) on the 16th day after denervation.

as well (fig. 4). These spontaneous hyperactive neurons were distributed from the marginal zone (1st layer) or substantia gelatinosa (2nd layer) of STNcd superficially to the depth of the dorsal reticular subnucleus; however, they were predominant in the superficial layers (1st and 2nd layers) of the STNcd. Two of the hyperactive neurons of the denervated side showed more intensive firing responsive to the pain stimuli of the skin of the upper cervical region but not to the stimulation on the face (fig. 5).

Neuronal firing in the STNcd of the intact (right) side responsive to the facial pain stimulation was remarkably inhibited or abolished by the intraventricular administration of morphine or enkephalinamide

---

Fig. 4. Spike frequency/s histograms of the neuronal firings in the STNcds of the intact and denervated sides. **A** The facilitation of the firing responsive to painful stimuli in the intact STNcd was remarkably inhibited or abolished after intraventricular morphine (a) or enkephalinamide (b) injection, the inhibition being reversed by intravenous naloxone. The hyperactivity in the denervated STNcd was not influenced by either of the drugs. **B** The same kind of discrepancy in the effect of the PAG stimulation was seen between the neurons of the intact (a) and denervated (b) STNcds.

and also by the PAG stimulation. This inhibition was reversed by intravenous naloxone injection. On the contrary, continuous and spontaneous firing of the hyperactive neurons in the denervated STNcd were inhibited neither by intraventricular administration of these drugs nor by PAG stimulation (fig. 4A, B).

Discussion

The STNcd is usually divided into three layers; marginal zone (I), substantia gelatinosa (II) and magnocellular layer (III) [3, 4, 9]. Pain-perceptive WDRN and NSN are believed to be located in the I and II layers, and III is the zone where the touch sensation-perceptive LTMRN is mainly distributed. In the present study there were many WDRNs not only in these three layers of STNcd but also in the more ventrally located reticular subnuclei. *Yokota* [9] described the same finding that there are many pain-perceptive neurons, most being WDRNs, in the dorsal and ventral reticular subnuclei. According to these findings, he insisted these reticular subnuclei should be included into the STNcd.

Anderson et al. [1] described the deafferentation hyperactivity of the neurons in the STNcd after denervation of the peripheral trigeminal nerve. Spontaneous and continuous firings with high amplitude after ganglionectomy of the neurons observed in the present study is considered to be the same phenomenon as *Anderson's* description. The spinal trigeminal tract was ascertained to be degenerated in this study, which seemed to mean that the afferent input from peripheral to STNcd was abolished. Neurons with denervation hyperactivity were distributed in STNcd including the dorsal reticular subnucleus; however, they were predominantly located in the superficial layers of STNcd (I or II layers). This might have occurred as neurons in the superficial layers receive the afferent input more directly than deeper neurons. It seems to be interesting that the hyperactivity became more intensive in response to stimulation of upper cervical skin in 2 of the neurons. This is probably because STNcd is continuous with the dorsal horn of the upper cervical spinal cord.

The cats showed abnormal behavior after the ganglionectomy. The definitive explanation for this abnormal behavior is impossible, but it might be a result of an abnormal feeling on the face similar to anesthesia dolorosa. It is well known that trigeminal rhizotomy for pain relief in patients with trigeminal neuralgia not infrequently causes facial anesthesia dolorosa after rhizotomy [5, 7]. In the present study, the facilitation of a well-established peripheral or excess pain-inhibiting system by the administration of morphine or enkephalinamide and by PAG stimulation, did not suppress the deafferentation hyperactivity. In contrast, inhibition or abolition of pain-responsive neuronal firing of the intact STNcd was clearly demonstrated. These results are compatible with the clinical experience that facilitation of the opioid-mediated pain-inhibiting system is effective in relieving pain in patients with peripheral or excess pain, but not in patients with deafferentation pain. Therefore, the deafferentation hyperactivity produced in this experiment in the STNcd of the denervated side may have a close physiological relationship to the deafferentation pain of clinical patients.

References

1 Anderson, L.S.; Black, R.G.; Abraham, J.; Ward, A.A., Jr.: Neuronal hyperactivity in experimental trigeminal deafferentation. J. Neurosurg. *35:* 444–452 (1971).

2 Berman, A.L.: The brain stem of the cat, a cytoarchitectonic atlas with stereotaxic coordinates (University of Wisconsin Press, Madison 1968).

3 Carpenter, M.B.: Cytoarchitectual lamination in human neuroanatomy, pp. 222–229 (Williams & Wilkins, Baltimore 1977).

4 Carpenter, M.B.: The trigeminal nerve; in Neuroanatomy, pp. 352–362 (Williams & Wilkins, Baltimore 1977).

5 Hosobuchi, Y.; Adams, J.E.; Rutkin, B.: Chronic thalamic stimulation for the control of facial anesthesia dolorosa. Archs Neurol. *29:* 158–161 (1973).

6 Jasper, H.H.; Ajmone-Marsan, C.: A stereotaxic atlas of the diencephalon of the cat (National Research Council of Canada, 1961).

7 Peet, M.M.; Schneider, R.C.: Trigeminal neuralgia: a review of six-hundred and eighty-nine cases with follow-up study on sixty-five percent of the group. J. Neurosurg. *9:* 367–377 (1952).

8 Snider, R.S.; Niemer, W.T.: A stereotaxic atlas of the cat brain (University of Chicago Press, Chicago 1961).

9 Yokota, T.: Nociceptive neurons in the dorsal horn of the spinal cord and in the spinal tract nucleus of the trigeminal nerve. Adv. neurol. Sci. *26:* 843–856 (1982).

Shimpei Namba, MD, Department of Neurological Surgery, Okayama University Medical School, 2-5-1 Shikata-cho, Okayama City, 700 (Japan)

Proc. 9th Meeting World Soc. Stereotactic and Functional
Neurosurgery, Toronto 1985
Appl. Neurophysiol. *48:* 212–215 (1985)

Enhancement of Memory with Human Ventrolateral Thalamic Stimulation: Effect Evident on a Dichotic Listening Task

George A. Ojemann

University of Washington, Department of Neurological Surgery, RI-20,
Seattle, Wash., USA

Key Words. Thalamus · Memory · Stimulation · Dichotic listening · Stereotactic surgery · Thalamotomy

Abstract. Previous experience with left ventrolateral thalamic (VL) stimulation during visually presented language and verbal memory tasks has shown that stimulation at the time information enters memory increases the accuracy of subsequent recall. The present study investigated the effects of VL stimulation on an auditory dichotic listening task. A similar effect was identified with significantly more words presented during left VL stimulation subsequently correctly reported, compared to words presented in the absence of stimulation, or with right VL stimulation. No significant effects on the ratios of correct responses from opposite ears were observed.

Introduction

Identification of aphasia (usually transient) and verbal memory deficits (more often persisting) after left thalamotomy for dyskinesias provided some of the early evidence of a role for lateral thalamus in language and memory [2]. The nature of this role has been further defined in investigations of the effects of electrical stimulation of lateral thalamus on measures of language and memory. Language and memory share a common mechanism in left lateral thalamus, the 'specific alerting response' [1, 4, 5]. A diminished response in an individual patient is associated with an increased probability of both language and memory deficits after a VL lesion [1, 6]. A similar mechanism but specific to visuospatial material has been evoked from right VL [3].

A feature of the specific alerting response evoked from left VL is that stimulation at the time information enters memory increases the accuracy of later recall of that information [1, 4, 5]. Although this effect has been identified even when retrieval from memory occurred a week later [1], the effect has been investigated only for visually presented verbal information. The present study was directed at identifying such an effect in an auditory language task.

Methods

The task was a dichotic listening test consisting of 10 sets of 4 pairs of simultaneously presented words differing by only one speech sound. Word pairs were presented from a prerecorded audio tape at 0.5 s intervals, with an 8 s response period after each set. One word of each pair was heard by the right ear, the other by the left. After each set subjects reported all the words they heard. Upon completion of the 10 sets, the earphones were reversed (so words that were presented to the right ear are now presented to the left) and the test repeated. The test is scored as the number of reported correct words presented to the right or left ear. Subjects were adult patients undergoing left (9 cases) or right (5 cases) stereotactic VL thalamotomies for dyskinesias, who had not had previous thalamotomies, and who produced at least 20 correct responses on the dichotic test. Three patients had Parkinson's disease, 6 multiple sclerosis with intention tremor, 2 dystonia, and 1 each mild choreoathetosis, familial intention tremor and posttraumatic intention tremor. All subjects showed right ear dominance on those sets presented in the absence of stimulation (mean ratio of correct words presented to right/left ears for left thalamotomy cases 7.54, for right 7.53). Since ear dominance is thought to indicate language dominance, all cases are likely to be left dominant for language even though 1 case was left handed. During the thalamotomy, following insertion of a 1×3 mm electrode into the VL nucleus, the patient engaged in the dichotic task. Monopolar electrical stimulation through the thalamic electrode occurred during the presentation of a preselected half of the sets, using 2 s trains of 60 Hz, 2 ms total duration biphasic pulses from a constant current stimulator at a current level just below the threshold for reported sensation, a mean of 5.9 mA for left thalamotomies and 4.2 for right, between peaks of the biphasic pulses (the difference in current levels during right or left thalamotomy is not statistically significant). No stimulation occurred during the response period after each set. Statistical analysis used the Mann-Whitney U test and Wilcoxon matched-pairs signed ranks test [7].

Results

The total number of correct words reported for sets presented during left VL stimulation was significantly greater than for sets presented without stimulation (mean number with stimulation 19, without 16, with 6 cases having more correct words with stimulation, 2 less and 1 the same, $p < 0.05$). On the other hand, right VL stimulation decreased the total number of correct responses (mean with stimulation 16, without 19, 1 case more with stimulation, 4 less) but this effect is not statistically significant, although the difference between left and right thalamic stimulation is at a $p < 0.025$. There was no significant effect of stimulation of either thalamus on right/left ear ratio (left stimulation: 4 increased this ratio, 5 decreased it; right: 1 increased, 4 decreased). There was a suggestion that contralateral ear responses were more likely to be reported for sets with stimulation than for sets without (left thalamic stimulation increased the number of contralateral responses in 6 cases, decreased it in 3, while right thalamic stimulation increased it in 4 and decreased it in 1, an effect that is not quite statistically significant).

Discussion

The presence of the 'specific alerting response' effect of left VL stimulation on this dichotic auditory task would appear as an increased probability of correct responses for sets presented with stimulation. This was observed. As with visually presented verbal tasks, there was significant lateralization of this effect to left thalamus; right VL stimulation had no effect on this auditory verbal task. Thus the lateralized 'specific alerting response' effect of VL stimulation can be generalized to both visually and auditorily presented verbal processes. The lack of significant change in ear ratios also indicates that the major effect is most likely a general one for verbal processes, rather than specific to the auditory system.

Acknowledgements

Dr. *Catherine Mateer* assisted in initiating this study, Dr. *Doreen Kimura* supplied the dichotic tape, Dr. *Itzhak Fried* tested some of the patients. Supported by NIH Grants NS 17111, NS 21724 and NS 20482. Procedures for obtaining informed consent from the patients in this study conformed to the currently applicable US Public Health Service guidelines, and were reviewed annually by the University of Washington Institutional Review Board.

References

1 Ojemann, G.: Language and the thalamus: object naming and recall during and after thalamic stimulation. Brain Language *2:* 101–120 (1975).
2 Ojemann, G.: Subcortical language mechanisms. Stud. Neurolinguist. *1:* 103–138 (1976).
3 Ojemann, G.: Altering memory with human ventrolateral thalamic stimulation; in Ballantine, Myerson, Modern concepts in psychiatric surgery, pp. 103–109 (Elsevier, Amsterdam 1979).
4 Ojemann, G.: Brain organization for language from the perspective of electrical stimulation mapping. Behav. Brain Sci. *6:* 189–230 (1983).
5 Ojemann, G.; Blick, K.; Ward, A.A., Jr.: Improvement and disturbance of short-term verbal memory during human ventrolateral thalamic stimulation. Brain *94:* 225–240 (1971).
6 Ojemann, G.; Hoyenga, K.; Ward, A.A., Jr.: Prediction of short-term verbal memory disturbance after ventrolateral thalamotomy. J. Neurosurg. *35:* 203–210 (1971).
7 Siegel, S.: Nonparametric statistics for the behavioral sciences (McGraw-Hill, New York 1956).

George A. Ojemann, MD, Department of Neurological Surgery, RI-20,
University of Washington, Seattle, WA 98195 (USA)

Proc. 9th Meeting World Soc. Stereotactic and Functional
Neurosurgery, Toronto 1985
Appl. Neurophysiol. *48:* 216–221 (1985)

Stimulation of the Basal Nucleus of Meynert in Senile Dementia of Alzheimer's Type

A Preliminary Report

I.M. Turnbull[a], *P.L. McGeer*[b], *L. Beattie*[c], *D. Calne*[c], *B. Pate*[d]

[a] Division of Neurosurgery, [b] Kinsmen Laboratory of Neurological Research, [c] Department of Medicine, [d] Department of Pharmaceutical Sciences, University of British Columbia, Vancouver, Canada

Key Words. Alzheimer's disease · Brain stimulation · Basal nucleus of Meynert · Stereotactic surgery

Abstract. The basal nuclei of Meynert are the principal sources of cholinerigic innervation of the cerebral cortex. It has been hypothesized that the depressed cortical glucose metabolic activity in senile dementia of Alzheimer's type (SDAT) may result primarily from diminished activity and loss of these cells. The present study was designed to test the hypothesis that electrical stimulation of the basal nuclei would bring about clinical improvement and increase cortical glucose metabolic activity in SDAT. An electrode was implanted in September 1984 into the left basal nucleus of a 74-year-old man with SDAT. Repetitive cycles of stimulation for 9 months since have had no definite effect clinically but a follow-up positron emission tomography scan shows that cortical glucose metabolic activity was preserved in the ipsilateral temporal and parietal lobes while it declined elsewhere in the cortex.

Introduction

The basal nucleus of Meynert contains large cholinergic cells that innervate the cerebral cortex but not the hippocampus [1, 3, 4, 7, 8]. Loss [1, 7, 8] or atrophy [9] of these large cells is a conspicuous feature of senile dementia of the Alzheimer's type (SDAT). Another feature which may be linked to this loss is decreased cerebral glucose metabolism as revealed by positron emission tomography (PET) scanning using the glucose analog 2-^{18}fluorodeoxyglucose (FDG) [2, 7]. The present study was undertaken to evaluate the possibility that electrical

The basal nucleus lies under the globus pallidus, lateral to the hypothalamus and optic tract and medial to the posterior limb of the anterior commissure. Part of it lies dorsal to the anterior perforated substance [3, 4, 7, 8, 10]. It is about 2 mm thick and has medial-lateral and anterior-posterior (A–P) diameters of roughly 10 mm. For electrode implantation, a lateral approach would require traversing the Sylvian fissure. An approach from above would expose the electrode to only the 2 mm thickness of the nucleus. The approach chosen was selected to pass through the nucleus in its A–P diameter while minimizing the risk of contacting either the penetrating arteries in the subarachnoid space or the optic tract.

A cadaver operation under ventriculographic control using the Todd-Wells stereotactic device was performed on a recently deceased elderly person whose brain was moderately atrophic. A needle was directed through the frontal pole to a target 8 mm behind the anterior commissure, 11 mm lateral to midline and 5 mm below the intercommissural line. Target localization was confirmed histologically after India ink was injected. The trajectory passed through the white matter and the nucleus accumbens. Air introduced into the ventricles and subarachnoid space accumulated under the frontal lobe making it clear that an operative approach would have to be sufficiently superior to allow penetration of the frontal pole rather than the orbital surface. By using the Brown-Robert-Wells (BRW) apparatus, we could operate without introducing air and could visualize the brain-subarachnoid space interface thereby defining the Z-axis.

Case Report

A 74-year-old had a 4-year history of progressive loss of recent memory. At times he would become confused and unable to recognize family members. He lived at home with his wife who, with the help of community services, kept him busy with recreations such as bowling and bingo. On examination, he was unable to recall anything after being briefly distracted, even an event like a key being hidden under a piece of paper. He made some mistakes naming objects, but his ability to do mental arithmetic was preserved. When he saw his image recorded at a previous session on a television monitor, he remarked, 'that man looks like my dad'.

He was evaluated with psychological tests and a CT scan, a MRI scan and a PET scan with FDG [6]. The first two showed moderate cortical atrophy, and the latter a widespread diminished utilization of glucose in the cerebral cortex consistent with a mild to moderate case of SDAT. A detailed consent form for the experimental surgical treat-

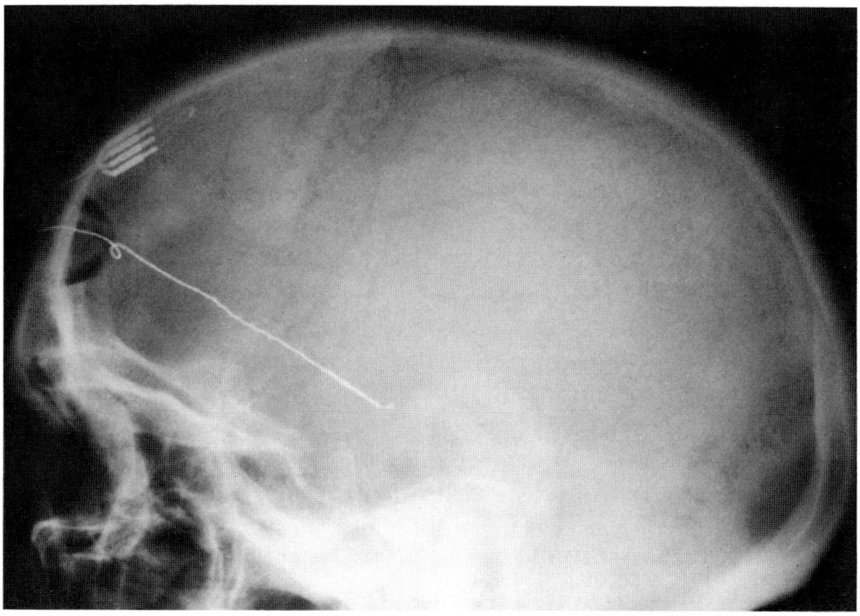

Fig. 1. Electrode implanted in basal nucleus of Meynert.

widespread diminished utilization of glucose in the cerebral cortex consistent with a mild to moderate case of SDAT. A detailed consent form for the experimental surgical treatment was signed by his wife after much discussion with the patient and their two sons [5]. Using the BRW apparatus, we implanted a flexible electrode (Medtronic) in September 1984, by way of a small frontal craniotomy placed above and lateral to the frontal sinus. A biopsy was taken which revealed numerous senile plaques, some neurofibrillary tangles and amyloid in the walls of small cerebral arteries indicating the diagnoses of SDAT and congophilic angiopathy.

A planned trial of percutaneous stimulation and recording from the basal nucleus could not be undertaken as the electrode extension was broken off where it emerged from the scalp when the patient removed his head dressing the day after implantation. A CT scan done on the second postoperative day revealed the electrode's tip to be within a millimeter of its intended position, 8 mm behind AC, 11 mm lateral to midline and within 2 mm of the base of the brain (fig. 1). The stimulation system was internalized with an ITREL (Medtronic) programmable pulse generator which was activated 2 days later under EEG control. No behavioral effects were noted when the system was activated and pulse intensity and rate were gradually increased. EEG spectral analysis techniques identified the pulse arriving in the brain. A lateral radiograph of the skull taken at this time revealed that the electrode had been retracted when the system was internalized, so that we had in fact been stimulating the nucleus accumbens. The electrode was replaced

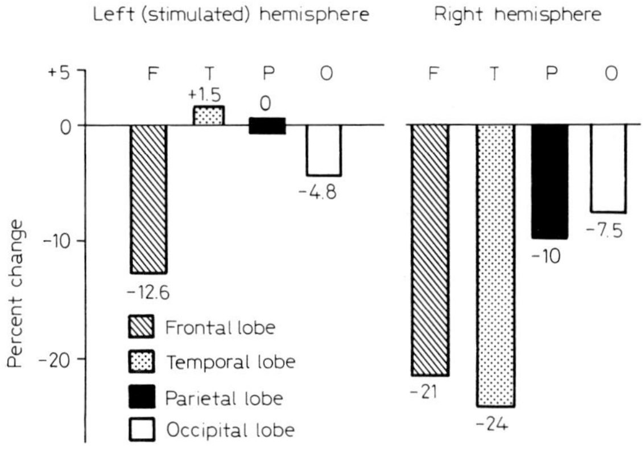

Fig. 2. Percent change from scan 1 to scan 2 in local glucose metabolic rate in various cortical areas of a person with Alzheimer's disease who had a stimulating electrode implanted in the left medial basal forebrain between scan 1 and scan 2.

once again using the BRW system for localization. It was reactivated a second time under EEG control and the parameters of stimulation have been changed from time to time over the ensuing 8 months.

The stimulation is bipolar over a distance of 3 mm judged to be in the center of the nucleus. We are currently stimulating at 3 V, 50 Hz with a pulse width of 210 ms. The cycle is on for 15 s and then off for 12 min day and night.

We have not been able to identify any response to stimulation clinically, even when the amplitude and frequency have been temporarily increased to high levels. He remains at home and there has been a little intellectual deterioration.

An initial PET scan was done in May 1984 followed by a repeat PET scan in November 1984, shortly after stimulation had commenced. A comparison of the two scans showed that glucose utilization in the contralateral frontal, temporal and parietal lobes had diminished 21, 24 and 10% respectively between the first and second scans. However, glucose utilization in the ipsilateral frontal lobe had diminished only 12%, in the parietal lobe was unchanged, and in the temporal lobe activity had increased by 1.5%. For the right occipital lobe it has declined by 7.5% and 4.1% in the left (fig. 2).

Discussion

While no conclusion regarding therapeutic value can be drawn from this single case, we have demonstrated that the basal nucleus of Meynert can be approached, entered and stimulated by an electrode over a prolonged period of time to the levels described without causing epilepsy or any other untoward reaction. Our inadvertant stimulation of the nucleus accumbens would suggest that the same applies to that area, at least in the short term.

No improvement in memory or cognition was noted. However, if the FDG results provide any indication, such a result would not be expected. It may be that the stimulation only served to arrest deterioration in cortical glucose metabolism in the left temporal and parietal areas, and to a partial extent in the left frontal area. Due to the placement of the electrode, no effect on the left hippocampal area could be expected, even though this area might have the greatest influence on short-term memory. The resolution of the PET apparatus is such that reliable data on areas as small as the hippocampus are hard to obtain and so objective data on glucose metabolic rate are not available for that area.

SDAT is a progressive disease. There is a relationship between the severity of symptoms and the reduction of glucose metabolic rate in the cortex. The case being studied showed typical deterioration except in the areas being stimulated, but not in clinical symptoms. It may be, therefore, that in this case some slowing down of clinical deterioration was achieved. Since the procedure was without adverse effect, further clinical studies would appear to be warranted.

Acknowledgements

The authors wish to thank the UBC TRIUMF PET team for carrying out the PET scans as well as the Mr. & Mrs. P.A. Woodward's Foundation and the B.C. Medical Services Foundation for financial support.

References

1 Davies, P.; Maloney, A.J.F.: Selective loss of central cholinergic neurons in Alzheimer's disease. Lancet *ii:* 1403 (1976).

2 Foster, N.L.; Chase, T.N.; Fedio, P., et al.: Alzheimer's disease: focal cortical changes shown by positron emission tomography. Neurology *33:* 961–965 (1984).

3 Johnston, M.V.; McKinney, M.; Coyle, J.T.: Evidence for cholinergic projection to neocortex from neurons in basal forebrain. Proc. natn. Acad. Sci. USA *76:* 5392–5396 (1979).

4 Kimura, H.; McGeer, P.L.; Peng, J.H.; McGeer, E.G.: The central cholinergic system studied by choline acetyltransferase immunohistochemistry in the cat. J. comp. Neurol. *200:* 151–201 (1981).
5 Kolata, G.: Alzheimer's research poses dilemma. Science *215:* 47–48 (1981).
6 Martin, W.R.W.; Beckman, J.H.; Calne, D.B., et al.: Cerebral glucose metabolism in Parkinson's disease. Can. J. neurol. Sci. *11:* 169–173 (1984).
7 McGeer, P.L.; McGeer, E.G.; Suzuki, J.; Dolman, C.E.; Nagai, T.: Aging, Alzheimer's disease, and the cholinergic system of the basal forebrain. Neurology, Cleveland *34:* 741–745 (1984).
8 Nagai, T.; McGeer, P.L.; Peng, J.H.; McGeer, E.G.; Dolman, C.E.: Choline acetyltransferase immunohistochemistry in brains of Alzheimer's disease patients and controls. Neurosci. Lett. *36:* 195–199 (1983).
9 Pearson, R.C.A.; Sofroniew, M.V.; Cuello, A.C., et al.: Persistence of cholinergic neurons in the basal nucleus in a brain with senile dementia of the Alzheimer's type demonstrated by immunohistochemical staining of choline acetyltransferase. Brain Res. *265:* 375–379 (1983).
10 Van Buren, J.M.; Borke, R.C.: Variations and connections of the human thalamus. 2. Variations of the human diencephalon (Springer, New York 1972).

Ian M. Turnbull, MD, 700 West 10th Avenue, C Floor/Room 305,
Vancouver, BC V5Z 4E5 (Canada)

Proc. 9th Meeting World Soc. Stereotactic and Functional
Neurosurgery, Toronto 1985
Appl. Neurophysiol. *48:* 222–225 (1985)

The Spread of Somatosensory-Evoked Potentials Within the Nervous System

A. Sólyom, S. Tóth, I. Holczinger, J. Vajda, Z. Tóth, R. Kálmánchey

National Institute of Neurosurgery, Budapest, Hungary

Key Words. Somatosensory-evoked potentials · Sensory-motor cortex · Subcortical structure · Chronic deep electrodes

Abstract. Four thalamic and cortical recordings were carried out in 5 patients. The thalamic-evoked potentials were typical and revealed a triphasic complex, but their latencies showed a relatively high standard deviation. They could be divided into two groups according to their latencies, both of which had low SD. These data suggested that there could be two types of latency of thalamic SEP, because the 4 patients' body sizes were very similar. More detailed surface, cortical and depth recordings are needed to resolve these questions.

The sources of human short latency SEP components remain somewhat uncertain despite many previous studies using various electrode montages and locations. Very few direct recordings have been carried out from the human cortex and subcortical structures on patients with chronic deep electrodes. Direct recordings from the thalamus [1–3, 5–8] and the cortex [2, 4] have been discussed but failed to provide definite results and conclusions.

Methods and Materials

A pair of cup stimulating electrodes were attached over the contralateral median nerve just proximal to the wrist with the cathode about 2 cm proximal to the anode. The stimuli were 0.2 ms rectangular pulses and were adjusted to produce a small twitch of the thumb. Input from the recording electrodes was led to a Medicor 440 differential amplifier and the output was summated by Myoproc V.3 averager. An analysis time of 30 or

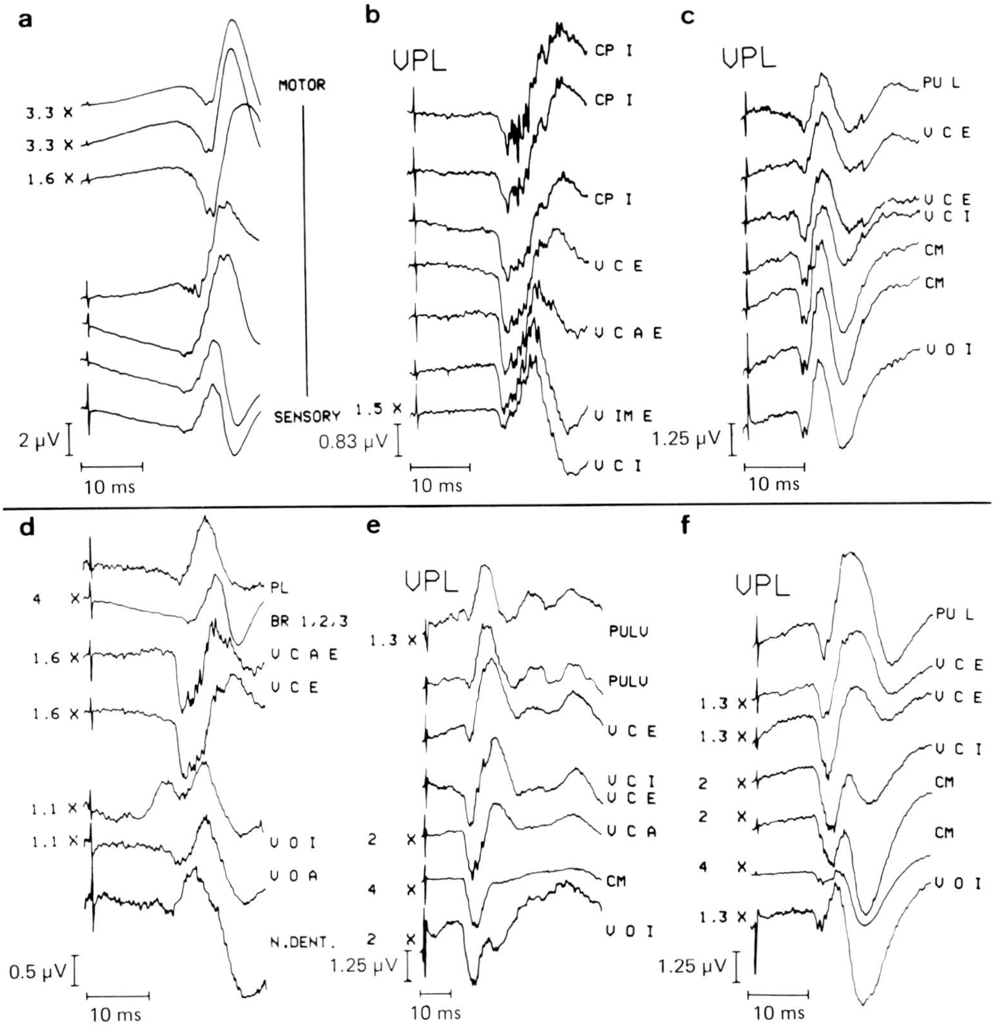

Fig. 1. a Distribution of somatosensory-evoked potentials from electrodes placed immediately in the subcortical white matter. **b, c, e, f** Activity in the primary receiving nucleus of thalamus (VPL) at about the same time (at their negativity) that the peak of widespread negativity was seen on the scalp or preceding it by 1–3 ms. The initial large first positivity was coincident with the scalp P 15 in 3 patients. The N wave showed a slight polarity inversion in 3 cases **(b, e, f)**. The negative potential might have been due to depolarization of VPL neurons by the lemniscal volley. **c** The short latency P1/N1/P2 complex suggested a synchronized afferent volley, as would be expected from the lemniscal system **(f)**. **d** Depth recorded somatosensory-evoked potentials from different sites of the nervous system on the same patient.

60 ms was used with all patients at 1 ms delay. The horizontal resolution was 20 or 40 ms. Negativity showed an upward deflection. The technique of insertion of depth electrodes was published in detail elsewhere [9, 10]. Routinely, 1,024 responses were averaged at a stimulus rate of 3-5 sec using 10 Hz low and 10 kHz high filters.

SEPs were recorded in 4 patients with parkinsonism and in 1 patient with depression. Both monopolar (common reference Fz) and bipolar montages were carried out, and each active point of the electrodes was recorded.

Results and Conclusions

Characteristic and relatively consistent wave forms were present in the thalamic ventrobasal complex (fig. 1). In all cases VPL showed a triphasic complex, a positivity peaking at 13.8 ± 3.21 ms, larger negativity at 18.28 ± 3.97 ms and a positivity at 23.8 ± 5.7 ms. If the 4 patients were divided into two groups the following latencies could be found. In the first group: P1 14 ± 0.74 ms, N1 22.11 ± 1.09 ms, and P2 29.4 ± 2.0 ms. In the other one: P1 11.25 ± 1.25, N1 14.45 ± 1.05 ms and P2 18.37 ± 0.7 ms. Only in 1 patient was a monophasic positive wave of short latency in CM (fig. 1e). No polarity reversal of the first positivity was observed in the present recordings within the VPL. The initial positive wave was followed by a slower negative potential in the thalamus and 3 of them showed phase reversal (fig. 1b, e, f). These data were similar to other authors' results but there are some controversial points [1-3, 5-8]. We conclude that the thalamic first positive deflection must have been of medial lemniscal origin and the first negative wave was attributable to synaptic potentials of thalamic relay neurons [7]. The thalamic and lemniscal activity could generate more complex potential forms and the monophasic wave needed a special electrode location ('killed end' recording).

In our cortical recordings, so-called white matter electrodes, the most common response consisted of a small positive deflection and a major negative potential (P 19.54 ± 1.26 ms, N 24.97 ± 1.49 ms). The rise phase of the initial deflection could show one or more identations giving a 'polyspike' appearance in all cases (fig. 1a). Only 1 patient of 4 showed polarity reversal across the central fissure. The latter finding might have been due to technical circumstances because the points of reference were the coronal suture and the external auditory meatus in the case of cortical electrode, so the cortical electrode might have crossed the central sulcus, causing this phenomenon.

No polarity reversal was observed in the recordings of the authors [2, 4]. Peak major N had its highest amplitude under the precentral gyrus in 3 cases and only 1 patient showed higher amplitude under the postcentral gyrus. We could see definitely in 1 patient (fig. 1a) that there are differences in form of the SEPs in the precentral and postcentral strips of human cortex.

References

1 Allison, T.; Hume, A.L.: A comparative analysis of short-latency somatosensory evoked potentials in man, monkey cat and rat. Expl Neurol. *72:* 592–611 (1981).
2 Celesia, G.G.: Somatosensory evoked potentials recorded directly from human thalamus and Sm I cortical area. Archs Neurol. *36:* 399–405 (1979).
3 Fukushima, T.; Mayanagi, Y.; Bouchard, G.: Thalamic evoked potentials to somatosensory stimulation in man. Electroenceph. clin. Neurophyisol. *40:* 481–490 (1976).
4 Kelly, D.L.; Goldring, S.; O'Leary, J.L.: Averaged evoked somatosensory responses from exposed cortex of man. Archs Neurol. *13:* 1–9 (1965).
5 Larson, S.J.; Sances, A. Jr.: Averaged evoked potentials in stereotaxic surgery. J. Neurosurg. *28:* 227–232 (1968).
6 Strassburg, H.M.; Thoden, U.; Mundinger, F.: Mesencephalic chronic electrodes in pain patients. An electrophysiological study. Appl. Neurophyisol. *42:* 284–293 (1979).
7 Suzuki, I.; Mayanagi, Y.: Intracranial recording of short latency somatosensory evoked potentials in man: identification of origin of each component. Electroenceph. Clin. Neurophysiol. *59:* 286–296 (1984).
8 Thoden, U.; Doerr, M.; Dieckman, G.; Krainick, J.U.: Medial thalamic permanent electrodes for pain control in man: an electrophysiological and clinical study. Electroenceph. clin. Neurophysiol. *47:* 582–591 (1979).
9 Tóth, S.; Vajda, J.: Multitarget technique in Parkinson surgery. Appl. Neurophysiol. *43:* 109–113 (1980).
10 Tóth, S.; Vajda, J.; Zaránd, P.; Sólyom, A.: Recent developments of neurobiology in Hungary, vol. VIII, pp. 73–91 (Akademia, Budapest 1979).

A. Solyom, MD, National Institute of Neurology, Amerikai u. 57,
Budapest XIV (Hungary)

Proc. 9th Meeting World Soc. Stereotactic and Functional Neurosurgery, Toronto 1985
Appl. Neurophysiol. *48:* 226–233 (1985)

An Animal Model for Neuron-Specific Spinal Cord Lesions by the Microinjection of N-Methylaspartate, Kainic Acid, and Quisqualic Acid

Madhavan Pisharodi, Haring J.W. Nauta

Division of Neurosurgery, University of Texas Medical Branch, Galveston, Tex., USA

Key Words. Lesioning methods · Neuron-specific lesions · Dorsal root entry zone lesions

Abstract. It has been shown that N-methylaspartate (NMA), kainic acid (KA), and quisqualic acid (QA) can produce preferential neuronal damage in various parts of the striatum, hippocampus, and thalamus with relative sparing of axons in transit. Thus far, the evidence that axons in transit escape destruction has been based largely on histological observations. To test the functional integrity of axons in passage, we made unilateral lesions with these agents in the cervical spinal cord of rats and compared the subsequent functional deficits with those seen after spinal cord hemisections.

Observations were made in 14 rats. In each case, a laminectomy at the C6-C7 level was performed under general anesthesia. Animals receiving microinjections of KA, QA, or NMA showed motor and sensory deficits only in the ipsilateral forepaw and remained able to use the hindpaws normally. By contrast, animals undergoing spinal cord hemisection developed obvious motor deficits in the ipsilateral hindpaw in addition to the deficits in the forepaw. Histological observations of the spinal cords confirmed an extensive gray matter destruction with relative preservation of the long tracts in animals injected with KA, QA, and NMA. In addition, it was noted that spinal cord neurons appear relatively less sensitive to KA and more sensitive to QA than neurons in the thalamus, striatum, or hippocampus. The possible application of these findings for the production of dorsal root entry zone lesions will be discussed.

Introduction

The production of location-specific lesions remains useful in the treatment of some types of functional disorders including chronic pain, movement disorders, seizure disorders, and spasticity. Methods now commonly used to produce lesions include electrolytic current, radiofrequency heat, and the laser. These methods can produce lesions

Table I. Neurotoxins capable of producing selective or preferential neuronal destruction

Transmitter cell-type specific lesions
a) 1-Methyl-4-phenyl-1,2,5,6-tetrahydropyrine (MPTP) – dopamine neurons [2,8]
b) 6-OH-dopamine – dopamine neurons (+ some damage to norepinephrine and serotonin neurons) [7]
c) 5,7-Dihydroxytryptamine – serotonin neurons [1]
d) Capsaicin – substance P neurons (?) [5,12]
e) Aziridium ion of ethyl choline – cholinergic neurons [10]

Receptor-specific lesions

Related to glutamate and/or aspartate receptors on cell bodies and dendrites [9,11,15,16]

a) Kainic acid
b) N-methylaspartate
c) Quisqualic acid
d) L-2-amino-4-phosphobutyric acid
e) Ibotenic acid

Terminal locus-specific lesions
By 'suicide retrograde axonal transport' of toxin back to cell body

a) Ricine lectin [17]
b) Doxorubicin [6]

which are well localized and predictable in both size and shape. However, they all share the disadvantage that *all* structures at the lesion site are affected, including neurons, axons in passage through the lesion area, and sometimes blood vessels passing through the lesion area. Such concomitant damage may produce unwanted deficits which might ultimately be avoided if more selective lesioning methods could be developed. Chemical agents hold promise for this purpose but, in contrast to the popularity of the radiofrequency, electrolytic, and laser lesioning methods, past experience with chemical methods has not been good. The injection of milliliter quantities of weak chemical toxins such as alcohol is known to produce lesions of unpredictable size, shape, and severity, and for these reasons have been largely abandoned. Recently, however, a number of potent neurotoxins have been discovered which work by very specific mechanisms and are capable of highly selective focal destructions (see references in table I). The production of more selective lesions by such new toxins offers at least potential advantages over presently popular methods, and should be evaluated for possible use in functional neurosurgery. Good localization can be obtained because these toxins are effective even when injected in nanoliter volumes. This represents over a thousandfold decrease in the injected volume required to produce lesions when compared to such weak, nonspecific toxins as alcohol. Table I shows a partial list of these newer, specific toxins and their selective lesioning characteristics.

The present experiments were undertaken to evaluate the lesioning capabilities of one family of neurotoxins thought to act by an interaction with excitatory amino acid transmitter receptors related to glutamate and/or aspartate receptors [9]. Since most neuronal cell bodies carry such receptors while axons in passage and blood vessels do not, these toxins are capable of producing neuron-specific, axon-sparing lesions [4, 11, 15, 16]. We evaluated their lesioning characteristics in the spinal cord with a specific interest in their potential application to the production of dorsal root entry zone (DREZ) lesions.

Methods

In each of 14 Sprague-Dawley rats, a laminectomy was performed at the C6 and C7 levels under pentobarbital anesthesia. In 12 of the rats, a unilateral microinjection was then made into the underlying cervical spinal cord. In each case, between 200 and 400 nl of toxin-bearing solution was slowly injected over a period of 30 min. The toxin was either 2.5 or 5% N-methylaspartate (NMA) (4 rats); 200 nm of quisqualic acid (QA) (4 rats); or 2 nm of kainic acid (KA) (4 rats). An additional 2 rats underwent unilateral spinal cord hemisection at the C6, C7 level. Following a survival period of 2 weeks, each animal was tested for neurologic deficits in the upper and lower extremities and then deeply reanesthetized with pentobarbital and perfused transcardially with 10% phosphate-buffered formalin. The entire brain and spinal cord was then removed and fixed for a period of 1 week in 10% formalin. The tissue was then transferred to 30% sucrose w/v in 10% formalin for another week. In each case, the brain and spinal cord was embedded in albumin and serially sectioned at 30 μm on a freezing microtome. A series of every twelfth section was then mounted on chrome alum-coated slides and stained with cresyl violet. An adjacent, every twelfth section series was then stained by the method of *Fink and Heimer* [3] for histological evaluation of axonal degeneration.

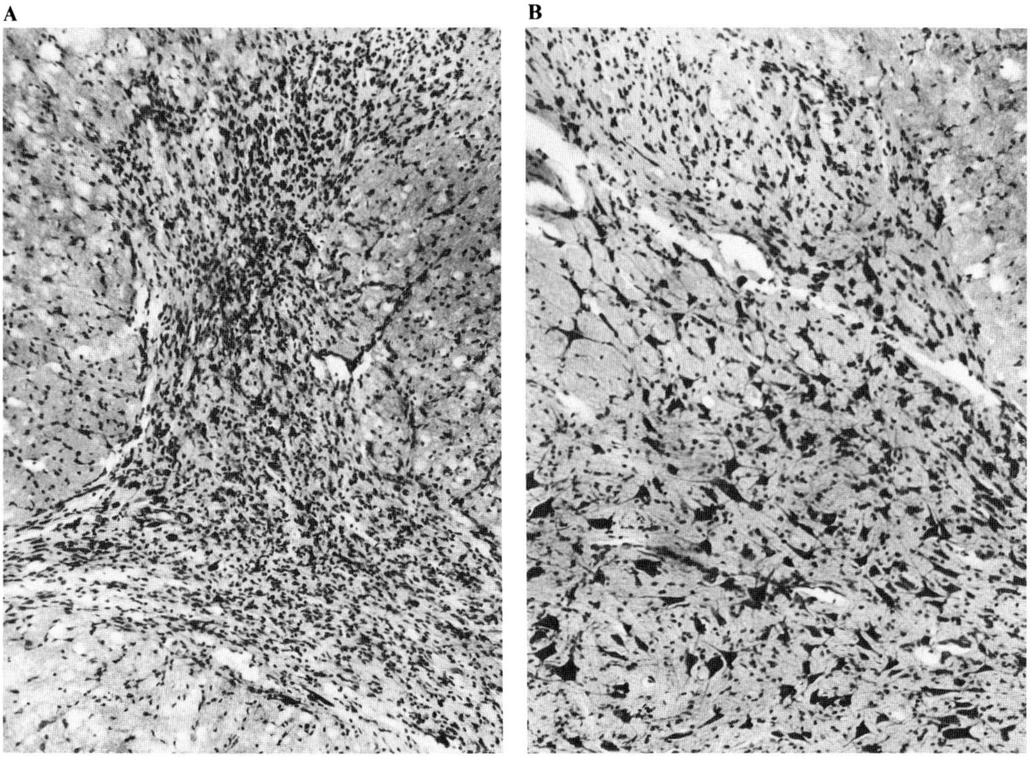

Fig. 1. This photomicrograph shows a typical gray matter lesion produced by QA. **A** It can be seen that there are no neurons in the gray matter and that there is extensive gliosis and neuronophagia. **B** The contralateral uninjected side shows normal numbers of neurons with preserved architecture of the dorsal and ventral horns. Cresyl violet. 30 μm section thickness. 59 × original magnification. Note that the fiber architecture of the dorsal and lateral funiculi remains intact even on the lesion side.

Results

All toxin-injected animals showed ipsilateral forepaw deficits but no detectable lower extremity deficits. The forepaw was typically held stiffly with the digits in flexion. Ulcerations on the skin over the digits were common although the animals appeared to use the extremity painlessly. In contrast, the lower extremity appeared normal: the digits were held normally and the extremity could be used normally in walking and in ladder climbing. The 2 rats that underwent spinal cord hemi-

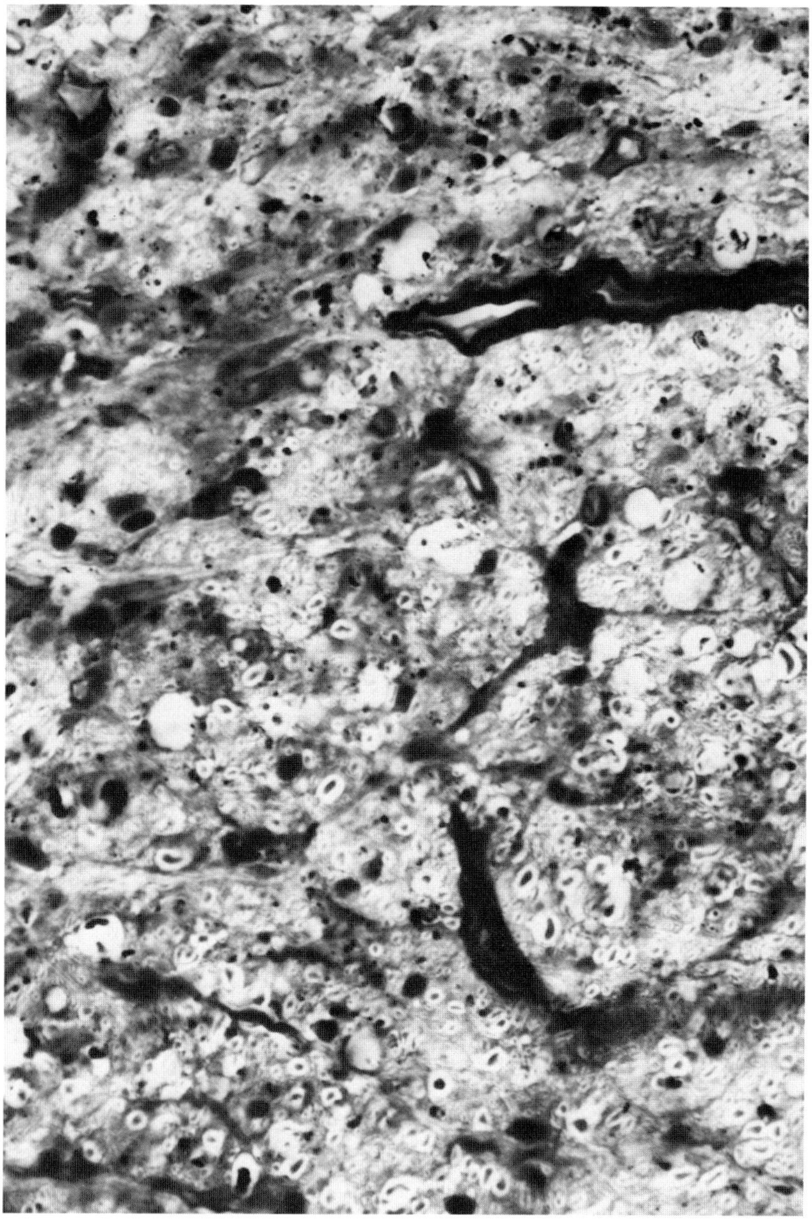

Fig. 2. This high power photomicrograph of a Fink-Heimer silver stained section through the lesion site shows preservation of axons even in the lesioned dorsal horn. 275 × original magnification.

section at the C6-C7 level showed both upper extremity and lower extremity deficits. The upper extremity deficits were similar to those described for the toxin-injected animals. However, the ipsilateral lower extremity typically was used clumsily in walking and, when ladder-climbing, the animal showed difficulty in finding the next rung with the affected limb.

Histological examination of the lesion site in the toxin-injected animals showed extensive gray matter damage with relative preservation of the adjacent axon bundles in the dorsal and lateral funiculus. When the lesion size for each agent was compared to that seen in the thalamus, striatum, or hippocampus following similar administrations [*Pisharodi and Nauta,* in preparation], QA seemed to show more activity in the spinal cord, while NMA and KA showed comparatively less activity. With each agent, all neurons appeared to undergo degeneration with neuronophagia, and no cell-type specificity was observed. Figure 1 shows an example of a neuron-specific, axon-sparing lesion in the spinal cord made with QU. The entire gray matter on the injected side is replaced by gliosis and no intact neurons were observed in the injection locus. The contralateral gray matter, however, appeared normal. The sections stained by the Fink and Heimer method for degenerating axons showed the expected degeneration of the propriospinal, spinoreticular, and spinothalamic tracts attributable to destruction of dorsal horn neurons, but showed only scant degenerating fibers in the dorsal columns rostral to the lesion and in the lateral funiculus caudal to the lesion. Intact axons were seen even within the lesioned dorsal horn itself (fig. 2).

Discussion

While it remains unproven whether the beneficial effects result from damage to the tract of Lissauer or to the neurons in the dorsal horn, DREZ lesions have been reported to relieve the phantom limb pain which often follows brachial plexus avulsion [14]. Several clinical series of patients treated with unilateral cervical DREZ lesions [13, 14] have reported deficits in the ipsilateral lower extremity that could be best explained by inadvertent damage to the lateral funiculus. If the beneficial effect of the DREZ lesion results from damage to the neurons of the dorsal horn, then the neuron-specific, axon-sparing lesioning properties of the substances evaluated here might offer an advantage over radiofrequency, electrolytic, or laser lesioning methods now in use. The principal advantage is that the toxins NMA, QA, and KA are all capable of producing localized neuronal damage while sparing blood vessels, axons in passage, and axons in contiguous fiber bundles.

Conclusions

It is possible to make highly localized, neuron-specific, axon-sparing lesions in the spinal cord by the injection of NMA, KA, or QA. Spinal cord neurons appear less sensitive to KA and NMA and more sensitive to QA than neurons in the thalamus, striatum, or hippocampus. There was no obvious neuronal subtype specificity observed in these lesions. Finally, lesioning by the toxins NMA, QA, and KA may eventually prove advantageous over lesioning methods of the dorsal horn by radiofrequency heat, electrolytic current, or laser because these toxins are capable of minimizing damage to blood vessels and adjacent fiber bundles in the dorsal columns and lateral funiculus.

Acknowledgements

This research was supported by Intramural and Departmental grants awarded to *Haring J.W. Nauta.* It is a pleasure to acknowledge the excellent technical assistance of Ms. *Marylee Terrell.* We thank Ms. *Beverly White* for her help in the manuscript preparation.

References

1 Baumgarten, H.G.; Bjorklund, A.; Lachemayer, L.; Nobin, A.: Evaluation of the effects of 5,7-dihydroxytryptamine on serotonin and catecholamine neurons in the rat CNS. Acta physiol. scand. *391:* 1–19 (1973).

2 Burns, R.S.; Chiueh, C.C.; Markey, S.; Ebert, M.H.; Jacobowitz, D.; Kopin, I.J.: A primate model of Parkinson's disease: selective destruction of substantia nigra, pars compacta neurons by N-methyl-4-phenyl-1,2,3,6-tetrahydropyrine. Proc. natn. Acad. Sci. USA *80:* 4546–4550 (1983).

3 Fink, R.P.; Heimer, L.: Two methods for selective silver impregnation of degenerating axons and their synaptic endings in the CNS. Brain Res. *4:* 369–374 (1967).

4 Hattori, T.; McGeer, E.G.: Fine structure changes in the rat striatum after local injections of kainic acid. Brain Res. *129:* 174–180 (1977).

5 Jancso, G.; Kiraly, E.; Jancso-Gabor, A.: Pharmacologically induced selective degeneration of chemosensitive primary sensory neurons. Nature, Lond. *270:* 741 (1977).

6 Koda, L.Y.; Kooy, D. van der: Doxorubicin: a fluorescent neurotoxin retrogradely transported in the central nervous system. Neurosci. Lett.: 1-8 (1983).

7 Kostrezewa, R.M.; Jacobowitz, D.M.: Pharmacologic actions of 6-hydroxydopamine. Pharmac. Rev. *26:* 199-288 (1974).

8 Langston, J.W.; Ballard, P.; Tetrud, J.W.; Irwin, I.: Chronic parkinsonism in humans due to a product of meperidine-analog synthesis. Science *219:* 979-980 (1983).

9 London, E.D.; Coyle, J.T.: Cooperative interactions at ^{3}H-kainic acid binding sites in rat and human cerebellum. Eur. J. Pharmacol. *56:* 287-290 (1979).

10 Mantione, C.R.; Fisher, A.; Hanin, I.: The AF 64A-treated mouse: possible model for central cholinergic hypofunction. Science *213:* 579-580 (1981).

11 Nadler, J.V.; Evenson, D.A.; Cuthbertson, G.J.: Comparative toxicity of kainic acid and other acidic amino acids toward rat hippocampal neurons. Neuroscience *6:* 2505-2517 (1981).

12 Nagy, J.I.; Vincent, S.R.; Staines, W.A.; Fibiger, H.C.; Reisine, T.D.; Yamamura, H.I.: Neurotoxic action of capsaicin on spinal substance P neurons. Brain Res. *186:* 435 (1980).

13 Nashold, B.S.; Bullitt, E.: Dorsal root entry zone lesions to control central pain in paraplegics. J. Neurosurg. *55:* 414-419 (1981).

14 Nashold, B.S.; Ostdahl, R.H.: Dorsal root entry zone lesions for pain relief. J. Neurosurg. *51:* 59-69 (1979).

15 Olney, J.W.: Neurotoxicity of excitatory amino acids; in McGeer, Olney, McGeer, Kainic acid as a tool in neurobiology, pp. 95-121 (Raven Press, New York 1978).

16 Schwarcz, R.; Hokfelt, T.; Fuxe, K.; Jonsson, G.; Goldstein, M.; Terenius, L.: Ibotenic acid-induced neuronal degeneration: a morphological and neurochemical study. Exp. Brain Res. *37:* 199-216 (1979).

17 Wiley, R.G.; Blessing, W.W.; Reis, D.J.: Suicide transport: destruction of neurons by retrograde transport of Ricine, ABRIN and modeccin. Science *216:* 889-890 (1982).

Madhavan Pisharodi, MD, Division of Neurosurgery, The University of Texas Medical Branch, Galveston, TX 77550 (USA)

Proc. 9th Meeting World Soc. Stereotactic and Functional Neurosurgery, Toronto 1985
Appl. Neurophysiol. *48:* 234–241 (1985)

Spinal versus Intraventricular Chronic Opiate Administration with Implantable Drug Delivery Devices for Cancer Pain

Y. Lazorthes, J.C. Verdie, R. Bastide, A. Lavados, D. Descouens

Neurosurgical University Clinic, CHU Rangueil, Toulouse, France

Key Words. Cancer pain · Opiate · Drug delivery systems · Intrathecal morphine

Abstract. Early publications have separately reported the efficacy, specificity and conservative character of direct spinal and intraventricular morphine analgesia in the treatment of intractable cancer pain. The objectives of this study are to compare efficacy and safety of these sites of local administration in order to determine the indication for each, the clinical effects of different opiates and the choice of various drug administration devices.

Material and Methods

Selection of patients was based upon strict clinical criteria: (1) chronic pain secondary to inoperable malignant tumors; (2) pain not relieved by medical treatment and in particular by the use of oral morphine; (3) bilateral midline or diffuse pain beyond the possibilities of percutaneous or open surgical interruption of nociceptive pathways; (4) absence of general risks of complications such as raised intracranial pressure, coagulation disturbances, cutaneous infection, septicemia; (5) consent from the patient and his family; (6) presence of favorable environment for ambulatory surveillance.

When the topography of pain was thoracic or subdiaphragmatic the clinical selection was confirmed by a trial involving a lumbar intrathecal injection of a small dose of morphine (1–3 mg). The percutaneous catheter was tunnelled if repeated injections of morphine or different opioids was intended. On the other hand, for pain of cephalic or diffuse topography, we began directly with intraventricular administration.

Thus, between September 1978 and April 1985, only 70 patients, i.e., approximately 1 in 3, were selected for chronic administration with an implanted device. We selected 52 patients for spinal administration (table I). The distribution of advanced cancers was as follows: pelvic 34, abdominal 13, cervicothoracic 5, (larynx 1, breast 2, lung 1, Kahler's disease 1). The topography of the pain was not always the same as that of the cancer. In summary, the 52 cases were suffering from subdiaphragmatic pain, usually in pelvis and legs, 5, cervicothoracic cancers were complicated by bone metastasis in the lower part of the body.

Table I. Clinical characteristics of the patients

Site	n	Sex m/f	Age		Topography of cancer					Topography of pain		
			range	mean	pelv.	abd.	thor.	cerv.	dif.	sub.	supra.	dif.
Spinal	52	30/22	34-82	60	34	13	4	1	–	52	–	–
Ventricular	18	12/6	43-80	64	–	2	8	5	3	2	14	2

pelv. = pelvic; abd. = abdominal; thor. = thoracic; cerv. = cervicocephalic; sub. = subdiaphragmatic; supra. = supradiaphragmatic; dif. = diffuse.

On the other hand, we have implanted 18 patients for intraventricular morphine administration (table I). The distribution of the primary malignant tumor was: abdominal 2 (stomach 1, pancreas 1), thoracic 8 (lung 7, esophagus 1), cervicocephalic 5 (tongue 2, maxillary 1, ear 1, larynx 1) and diffused bone metastasis 3 (breast 1, Kahler's disease 2). In all these patients, the topography of pain was supra diaphragmatic or diffuse, except in the 2 abdominal cancers, where the pain was epigastric.

The details concerning chronic administration, i.e., description of the drug administration devices and technique of implantation under local or neuroleptanalgesia, were reported in previous publications [2, 4, 5]. For spinal administration, we have implanted 43 'Unidose' reservoirs (Cordis) connected in 40 cases to an intrathecal lumbar catheter and in 3 cases to an epidural thoracic catheter. In the other 9 cases, the morphine infusion was performed with a micropump: 6 multibolus 'Secor' devices (Cordis) and 3 programmable 'DAD' devices (Medtronic) connected to an intrathecal lumbar catheter. For ventricular administration in the 18 cases we used a reservoir connected to a catheter placed in the frontal horn of the lateral ventricle close to the foramen of Monro.

The morphine administrated was a hyperbaric solution (7% dextrose) at the concentration of 5 mg/ml for spinal administration, and a normobaric morphine without preservative (at the concentration of 10 mg/ml) for intraventricular administration.

Results

Clinical evaluation of analgesia is based upon a multifactorial approach using the estimation of three criteria related to pain: (1) pain relief graded using a subjective linear scale; (2) consequences concerning the patient's activity, and (3) consumption of analgesic drugs.

Table II. Follow-up and daily doses of morphine

Administration	n	follow-up, days		Daily doses, mg/24 h		
		range	mean	range	mean	dextrose
Spinal	52	30–420	125	1–10	2.5	7%
Intraventricular	16	12–230	66	0.12–2	0.66	-

Table III. Percentage of good and excellent results: pain relief, functional activity, drug intake and overall analgesia evaluation ratio of major side-effects and tolerance

Administration	n	Results, % of good and excellent				Complications			
		Pain relief	activity	drug	overall analgesia	side-effects		tolerance	
						n	%	n	%
Spinal	52	81	67	88	75	3	6	3	6
Intraventricular	18	89	56	94	83	2	11	0	0

Finally, the overall analgesia corresponds to a summary of these three factors. The correlation provides a comparative 'quantitative' evaluation in any given patient. Unexpected side effects due to direct and chronic administration of intrathecal morphine, such as central depression or tolerance, were monitored and noted as well as complications due to the implanted device. One of us *(A.L.)* had the responsibility of teaching the patient and the family members and keeping in contact with them and the general physician during ambulatory surveillance at home.

Chronic Spinal Administration.

Follow-up and doses of hyperbaric morphine are summarized in table II. All patients had 50% pain relief and 42 patients (81%) had from 50% to 100% analgesia (table III). The daily activity was significantly improved in 35 cases (67%). The consumption of analgesics was reduced and limited to nonopiate drugs in 46 cases (88%). Overall, there were 39 cases with good to excellent results (75%) with a mean follow-up of 4 months.

We have observed 3 cases of central depression with drowsiness, myosis and respiratory disturbances. The first 2 occurred during the initial screening test: after an injection of 5 mg normobaric morphine in 1 case at the Th12 intrathecal space and in the other case at Th6 epidural space. These two spontaneously reversible complications required neither intubation nor injection of naloxone. The third complication occurred progressively in an ambulatory patient implanted with a pump programmed with a continuous flow of 3.1 mg/day. The somnolence and respiratory depression were immediately reversed by naloxone. The patient was secondarily reprogrammed to a bolus delay prescription of 2.5 mg/day without further incident.

A tolerance phenomenon developed in 8 cases, and was significant in 3 patients. However, it was not necessary in any patient to increase doses by more than 4 times the initial therapeutic doses.

In 2 patients, local infections occurred and it was necessary to remove the implant. In another case with purulent meningitis, recovery occurred spontaneously after intrathecal injection of antibiotics via the implanted reservoir.

Chronic Intraventricular Administration.

Follow-up and doses of normobaric morphine used are summarized in table II. 16 patients (89%) had 75% or more pain relief. Functional activity was improved in 10 patients (56%). Drug intake was reduced in 17 patients (94%). Overall there were 15 cases of good to excellent results (83%) with a mean follow-up of more than 2 months.

Until now we have not observed any significant tolerance phenomenon except in 2 cases where we have had to moderately increase the doses from 0.5 to 2 mg/day. On the other hand, there were 2 major side effects. In the first case, after administration of 1 mg, the patient developed visual hallucinations and behavior disorders. The second, after 1.5 mg morphine, developed drowsiness, myosis and respiratory depression. These two central complications were immediately reversed by systemic naloxone administration with small effect on analgesia. In this series of 18 patients, we have observed only one complication due to local infection of the implant.

Discussion

For the two sites of local administration of very small doses of morphine, the analgesia was immediate (latency of the onset from 5 to 10 min), selective, intense or complete and of long duration irrespective of the location of pain. However, for single doses of morphine, the analgesic effects are more prolonged after intraventricular (1–8 days) than after intrathecal spinal administration (1–3 days). In the same way, after repetitive injections, the mean daily doses are smaller for intraventricular (0.66 mg) than for spinal delivery (2.5 mg), but mean follow-up is two times lower, and the series are not comparable (18 vs. 52 patients).

On the other hand, the topographic distribution of analgesia is different, metameric with a maximal caudal effect for spinal administration and diffuse for ventricular administration. In summary, the efficacy of the two sites is comparable, but the distribution of analgesia is more limited to the inferior half of the body after lumbar spinal delivery [3, 5, 6, 8–11, 13, 14].

Among the 52 patients treated with spinal morphine, only 5 cases (table I) have thoracic or cervical cancer, but the topography of the pain was always subdiaphragmatic because these 5 patients complained of painful lumbosacral and iliac bone metastasis. We must point out that 1 case (larynx cancer) presented also cervicothoracic bone metastasis, only partially improved after lumbar intrathecal morphine administration.

Paradoxically, the risks of central respiratory depression are relatively high after intraventricular administration of low doses of morphine [6, 7, 12, 14] and can be immediately reversed by naloxone. But all these patients have already received morphine systematically and as a result must have reduced sensitivity of opiate receptors [5, 6, 12]. Minor and transient side effects, like nausea, vomiting, skin reactions and itching, occurred with the same rate in both [6, 8]. Transient urinary retention is more specific for spinal administration [2, 6, 10], whereas reversion behavior disorders or dysphoria were significantly reported after intraventricular infusion [7, 14].

By contrast, development of tolerance is not a serious problem [2, 5–7, 9–11]. So, in practice for cancer pain of the lower part of the body (pelvis and lower limbs), we always start with a percutaneous intrathecal lumbar trial. During a few days, we try progressively a placebo (saline solution) and different doses between 1 and 5 mg of hyperbaric morphine (> 4,8). If we do not observe significant analgesia with the maximal dose, we do not select the patient for chronic spinal administration, but in some cases and particularly for upper abdominal cancer pain (2 cases in our series), we decided on chronic intraventricular administration.

Since the objective is to offer these patients the possibility of a secure and comfortable ambulatory treatment, the choice of the drug delivery device depends on different criteria and in particular on quality-safety-cost ratio [4]. For chronic cancer pain treatment, the administration 'on demand' by intermittent bolus appears to be more effective than continuous infusion. The implantable pumps with nonprogrammable continuous flow are not adapted to this type of treatment, because it is not possible to stop the infusion in an emergency without emptying the reservoir and not easy to modify the prescription without changing the concentration of the morphine solution. The programmable and implantable drug administration devices offer the possibility of accurate prescription, but are at the present time too expensive, especially for the limited life expectancy patients. The most usual solution is the implantation of a small silastic reservoir, allowing one predetermined dose administration and allowing repeated percutaneous bolus injection. The optimal alternative will be, in the future, the development of multidose reservoirs, mechanically operated 'on demand' by transcutaneous action. These devices will have a sufficient capacity to offer greater autonomy and a side-port access, allowing administration of different drugs or control of the catheter.

The future of this conservative and noninvasive method also depends on the use of new opioids activating different opiate receptors. We have tried in 12 cases during the percutaneous intrathecal spinal screening, administration of pentazocine (5 mg) and in 5 cases of 1,13- or 1,10-amine dynorphin (100–200 μg). Our preliminary results are not definitive, and morphine remains the most effective agent for local administration.

Conclusions

According to ethical and clinical criteria, we conclude that chronic intrathecal lumbar spinal administration of small doses of hyperbaric (dextrose 7%) morphine is indicated for intractable cancer pain limited to the lower part of the body. After failure of spinal analgesia or for cervicothoracic or diffuse cancer pain, chronic intraventricular administration must be chosen. In practice, these two sites of local opiate administration are complementary. The efficacy and safety of the results confirm the role of this conservative and noninvasive method in the ambulatory treatment of cancer pain.

References

1 Lazorthes, Y.; Gouardères, C.; Verdié, J.C.; Montsarrat, B.; Bastide, R.; Campan, L.; Cros, J.: Analgésie par injection intrathécale de morphine. Etudé pharmacocinétique et application aux douleurs irréductibles. Neurochirurgie *26A:* 159–164 (1980).

2 Lazorthes, Y.; Cros, J.; Verdié, J.C.; Lagarrigue, J.; Bastide, R.; Boetto, S.: Morphine intrarachidienne chronique dans le traitement des douleurs d'origine néoplasique. Méd. Hyg. *40:* 1983–1989 (1982).

3 Lazorthes, Y.; Siegfried, J.; Gouardères, C.; Bastide, R.; Cros, J.; Verdié, J.C.: Periventricular grey matter stimulation versus chronic intrathecal morphine in cancer pain; in Bonica, Advances in pain research and therapy, vol. 5, pp. 467–475 (Raven Press, New York 1983).

4 Lazorthes, Y.; Verdié, J.C.; Bastide, R.; Caute, B.; Clemente, G.: Les systèmes implantables pour administration épidurale et intrathécale d'opioïdes; in Besson, Lazorthes, Spinal opioids and the relief of pain: basic mechanisms and clinical applications (Inserm, Paris 1985).

5 Lazorthes, Y.; Bastide, R.; Verdié, J.C.; Clergue, M.L.; Lavados, A.; Caute, B.; Cros, J.: Chronic spinal administration of opiate: application in the treatment of intractable cancer pain; in Besson, Lazorthes, Spinal opioids and the relief of pain: basic mechanisms and clinical applications (Inserm, Paris 1985).

6 Leavens, M.E.; Hill, C.S.; Cech, D.A.; Weyland, J.B.; Weston, J.S.: Intrathecal and intraventricular morphine for pain in cancer patients: initial study. J. Neurosurg. *56:* 241–245 (1982).

7 Lobato, R.D.; Madrid, J.L.; Fatela, L.V.; Rivas, J.J.; Reig, E.; Lamas, E.: Intraventricular morphine for control of pain in terminal cancer patients. J. Neurosurg. *59:* 627–633 (1983).

8 Nurchi, G.: Use of intraventricular and intrathecal morphine in intractable pain associated with cancer. Neurosurgery *15:* 801–803 (1984).

9 Onofrio, B.M.; Yaksh, T.L.; Arnold, P.G.: Continuous low-dose intrathecal morphine administration in the treatment of chronic pain of malignant origin. Mayo Clin. Proc. *56:* 516–520 (1981).

10 Penn, R.D.; Paice, J.A.; Gottschalk, W.; Ivankovich, A.D.: Cancer pain relief using chronic morphine infusion: early experience with a programmable implanted drug pump. J. Neurosurg. *61:* 302–306 (1984).

11 Poletti, C.E.; Cohen, A.M.; Todd, D.P.: Cancer pain relieved by long-term epidural morphine with permanent indwelling systems for self-administration. Neurosurgery *55:* 581–584 (1981).

12 Roquefeuil, B.; Benezech, J.; Blanchet, P.; Batier, C.; Frèrebeau, P.; Gros, C.: Intraventricular administration of morphine in patients with neoplasic intractable pain. Surg. Neurol. *21:* 155–158 (1984).

13 Saunders, R.L.; Coombs, D.W.: Dartmouth-Hitchcock Medical Center experience with continuous intraspinal narcotic analgesia; in Schmidek, Sweet, Operative neurosurgical techniques, vol. 2, pp. 1211–1212 (Grune & Stratton, New York 1983).

14 Thiebaut, J.B.; Blond, S.; Farcot, J.M.; Thurel, C.; Matge, G.; Schach, G.; Meynadier, J.; Buchheit, F.: La morphine par voie intraventriculaire dans le traitement des douleurs néoplasiques. Méd. Hyg. *43:* 636–646 (1985).

15 Wang, J.K.: Intrathecal morphine for intractable pain secondary to cancer of pelvic organs. Pain *21:* 99–102 (1985).

Y. Lazorthes, MD, Neurosurgical University Clinic, CHU Rangueil,
Chemin du Vallon, F-31052 Toulouse (France)

Proc. 9th Meeting World Soc. Stereotactic and Functional
Neurosurgery, Toronto 1985
Appl. Neurophysiol. *48:* 242–246 (1985)

Further Experience in Stereotactic Pontine Tractotomy

Edward Hitchcock, M.C. Kim, M. Sotelo

Department of Neurosurgery, University of Birmingham, Midland Center for Neurosurgery, Smethwick, Warley, Birmingham, UK

Key Words. Pons · Stereotactic surgery · Pain · Tractotomy · Spinothalamic tractotomy

Abstract. The problem with percutaneous and even stereotactic cordotomy is the difficulty in obtaining sufficiently high analgesic levels without autonomic complications, although the problem seemed to apply to relatively few patients since percutaneous and stereotactic spinal procedures achieved sufficiently high analgesic levels to encompass most patients' pain. There is a group of patients, however, with high pain in the shoulder and neck where conventional percutaneous and stereotactic spinal procedure are dangerous. From the standpoint of achieving high levels of analgesia with a low incidence of dysaesthesia, pontomedullary lesions appear to have advantages.

Stereotactic pontine spinothalamic tractotomy was first performed in 1970 and 7 patients were reported in 1973 [2]. At that time it was advocated as a suitable procedure for selected patients where high analgesic levels were necessary and/or where the risk of severe autonomic complications was high. Six of the first 7 patients were in a terminal state due to malignant disease. Four had chest and arm and 2 pelvic and leg pain. Only 3 patients survived for more than 3 months and 1 had recurrent pain at 3 months. All patients achieved immediate and sustained relief although mostly succumbing within the first few weeks to their primary disease.

When the procedure was first introduced no stereotactic brain atlas was available and a simple brain stem coordinate atlas was produced from anatomical atlases and prepared specimens. This used a coordinate system based on the fourth ventricular floor and a line drawn at right angles to it directed to the fastigium (the fastigal line).

Subsequently these coordinates were used by *Afshar* et al. [1] in a stereotactic brain stem atlas which has been used and compared to the simpler brain stem coordinate atlas since 1978. Unfortunately the latter atlas has a 10 mm gap in the representation of the spinothalamic tract around the fastigial plane, which is unfortunate, as this particular level is clearly the most desirable because of the short distance between target and basic coordinate planes. The use of the fastigial line is open to some objection since the fastigium has probably greater variability than other angles and coordinates. Furthermore the fastigium is a complex ventricular shadow since it is a bilateral recess rather than the single recess so frequently represented. It serves, however, as a useful rostrocaudal marker. *Hitchcock* et al. [3] examined the relationships of the third and fourth ventricles and found that the angle between the AC/PC and the aqueductal line, the commissural angle [C], the aqueductal angle [Aq] between the aqueductal line [Aq L] and the fourth ventricular line and the ventricular angle between the AC/PC line and the fourth ventricular line were independent of the ventricular size. However, the fastigial angle [F] (between the AC/PC and the fastigium) and the floor angle [Fl] (between the AC/PC and the point on the floor of the fourth ventricle at right angles to the fastigium) depended on the height of the fastigium and ventricular size. Measurements of 83 ventriculograms nevertheless showed that the standard deviations for the two measurements were comparable to that of the other angles. Our floor angle of 71.6 is in good agreement with the 72° of *Spiegel and Wycis.*

Since 1978, 9 stereotactic pontine spinothalamic tractotomies have been performed in the Department of Neurosurgery, University of Birmingham. These were in patients with intractable severe upper body pain due to cancer. There were 4 men and 4 women aged 46, 47, 55, 61, 62, 69, 73 and 77 years. Three women had breast cancer, 1 had a chondrosarcoma of the shoulder, and the 4 men had lung cancer, 1 (CG) had chest pain form metastatic scrotal cancer. All (except for CG) had brachial plexus invasion with characteristic severe pain frequently with dysaesthetic phenomena. All were unrelieved by opiates or other strong analgesics without serious side effects of confusion or drowsiness. The average duration of preoperative pain was 19.3 months and at the time of referral most of these patients were in frail and debilitated states. Two patients with lung cancer were in terminal states and died from their primary disease, respectively 6 and 28 days later.

Table I

Results	Percutaneous high cervical cordotomy [*Ischia* et al., 1985]	Stereotactic pontine tractotomy [*Hitchcock* et al., 1973, 1985]
	metastatic lung cancer %	metastatic breast and lung cancer, %
Pain relief	44	100
Low analgesic level	9	0
Deaferentation pain	9	0
'Mirror' pain	51	0
Motor paralysis Transient	30	20
Permanent	4	0
Facial weakness	–	15
VIth nerve palsy	–	7

Method

The procedure has been refined since the first report [2] with modification of the stereotactic instrumentation and lately the use of CT coordinates; in other respects it remains unchanged. The stereotactic instrument is fixed to the skull and the patient placed in a comfortable sitting position with the instrument fixed to the operating table. Local anaesthesia is used throughout, sometimes supplemented with intravenous diazepam. Target coordinates are based on a pontine coordinate atlas and conventional anatomical transverse sections are referred to throughout the procedure. Targets are selected in reference to the fourth ventricular floor angle and fastigial angle. These planes are defined either from water-soluble contrast ventriculography via a frontal burr hole or from reconstructed CT scans using the SCID technique (stereotactic CT scan interface device). A posterior fossa burr hole is made and the Radionics (0.8 × 1 mm) electrode advanced to the target. The usual track is via cerebellum and inferior cerebellar peduncle, trigeminal nucleus and tract and facial nucleus. Commonly the cochlea and vestibular nuclei are traversed. Stimulation at these sites confirms correct electrode passage and if satisfactory responses are obtained at target a radiofrequency lesion is made whilst testing for depth and extent of analgesia with a pin. If no satisfactory responses are obtained, another trajectory is chosen 2 mm lateral or medial to the original target. The method is described in greater detail by *Hitchcock* et al. [4].

Results

Complete pain relief was obtained in all patients and a satisfactory extent of deep analgesia which enclosed the pain area (table I). The single post-operative death 6 days later occurred because of electrode insulation failure resulting in a large stem lesion. This patient had a serious preoperative dyspnoea due to pneumonectomy and advancing lung cancer.

Six patients achieved complete pain relief until death at periods of 1, 1, 3, 4, 6 and 10 months later. One patient (MR) developed pain recurrence 3 months postoperatively and the procedure was repeated. This resulted in complete pain relief for 6 months when she developed contralateral pain due to extension of the tumour into the cervical spine.

Discussion

The original criteria for patient selection were severe respiratory inadequacy, frailty and high cervicothoracic pain. The large majority of other patients are treated by other techniques including cordotomy. There is no evidence for regarding percutaneous cordotomy as inadequate in dealing with cervicothoracic pain and the criteria for selection for pontine tractotomy can now be widened. *Ischia* et al. [5] noted that after percutaneous cordotomy only 44% of patients with Pancoast tumour remained pain free until death and only 19% of patients surviving more than 3 months. In 9% the analgesic level was too low, 8% had deafferentiation pain and 53% had 'mirror' pain of sufficient severity to require analgesics. The incidence of 'mirror' pain was exceptionally high (72%) in patients with thoracic pain. None of the patients following pontine tractotomy either in the present series of patients or in those reported earlier have had 'mirror' pain postoperatively and in itself this favours consideration of pontine tractotomy rather than percutaneous cordotomy. Of the present series of 8 surviving patients, 6 achieved complete pain relief until death or last follow-up - the long period of more than 4 years. *Ischia* et al. [5] report transient paresis in 30%, and 4% patients had permanent ipsilateral paresis or paralysis. In the admittedly smaller series of pontine tractotomies of the 16 patients from both 1973 and the present series, 19% had transient paresis usually for only a few days and none had a permanent paresis or paralysis. The major complications of pontine tractotomy, admittedly transient, was facial weakness in 2 patients and sixth nerve weakness in 1 patient. Against these advantages must be set the limited availability of stereotactic experience and instrumentation for an exceptionally precise technique.

Acknowledgements

My thanks to *Veronica Turner* for typing the manuscript.

References

1 Afshar, F.; Watkins, E.S.; Yap, J.C.: Stereotactic atlas of the human brainstem and cerebellar nuclei, pp. 80–88 (Raven Press, New York (1978).
2 Hitchcock, E.R.: Stereotaxic pontine spinothalamic tractotomy. J. Neurosurg. *39:* 746–752
3 Hitchcock, E.R.; Oppitz, P.; Donaldson, A.A.: Relationships between portions of the third and fourth ventricles. An aid to stereotactic accuracy for posterior fossa stereotaxy. Neuroradiology *15:* 197–199 (1978).
4 Hitchcock, E.R.; Sotelo, M.G.; Kim, M.C.: Analgesic levels and technical method in stereotactic pontine spinothalamic tractotomy. Acta neurochir. (1985).
5 Ischia, S.; Ischia, A.; Luzzani, A.A.; Toscano, D.; Steel, A.: Results up to death in the treatment of persistent cervicothoracic. Pancoast and thoracic malignant pain by unilateral percutaneous cervical cardotomy. Pain *21:* 339–355 (1985).
6 Spiegel, E.A; Wycis, H.T.: Stereoencephalotomy (thalamotomy and related procedures). I. Methods and stereotaxic atlas of the human brain (Grune & Stratton, New York 1952.

E. Hitchcock, MD, Department of Neurosurgery, University of Birmingham, Midland Center for Neurosurgery, Holly Lane, Smethwick, Warley, Birmingham (UK)

Proc. 9th Meeting World Soc. Stereotactic and Functional
Neurosurgery, Toronto 1985
Appl. Neurophysiol. *48:* 247–251 (1985)

Woroschiloff's Locating Device for Interventions on the Spinal Cord and Its Influence on Spinal Stereotaxis

P. Nádvorník

Department of Neurosurgery, Comenius University, Bratislava, CSSR

Key Words. Spinal cord · Stereotactic surgery

Abstract. 111 years ago the first locating device for the spinal cord was constructed, which became the basis for the contemporary spinal cord stereotaxy. Woroschiloff invented this device to operate stereotactically in different spinal cord segments. Nowadays only the fixation of the spinal cord stereotactic device to the wound retractor has changed from his concept, and control of the surgical instrument has been improved in three perpendicular planes corresponding to the special stereotactic maps of the human spinal cord.

No significant inventions come into existence without precursors, even through original work and ideas may be forgotten by that time. It applies also in clinical stereotaxy, which *Spiegel and Wycis* [6] started and soon was extended further. They based their apparatus on the first brain stereotactic device which was constructed for experimental procedures by *Clarke and Horsley* [1]. It was originally used for the research of cerebellar activity, and the stereotaxy of other brain structures developed later.

From the historical point of view, however, aimed procedures on the deep structures of the central nervous system by means of a device, which anticipated the principles of stereotaxy, started in the spinal cord. *Dittmar* [2], an assistant in the Physiological Institute of Prof. Ludwig in Leipzig, who investigated the vasoconstrictor pathways in the spinal cord, was occupied with the idea of such an apparatus.

At that time, *Woroschiloff* [7] from the same institute constructed for this purpose a special fixation and locating device (fig. 1). A fixa-

a

b

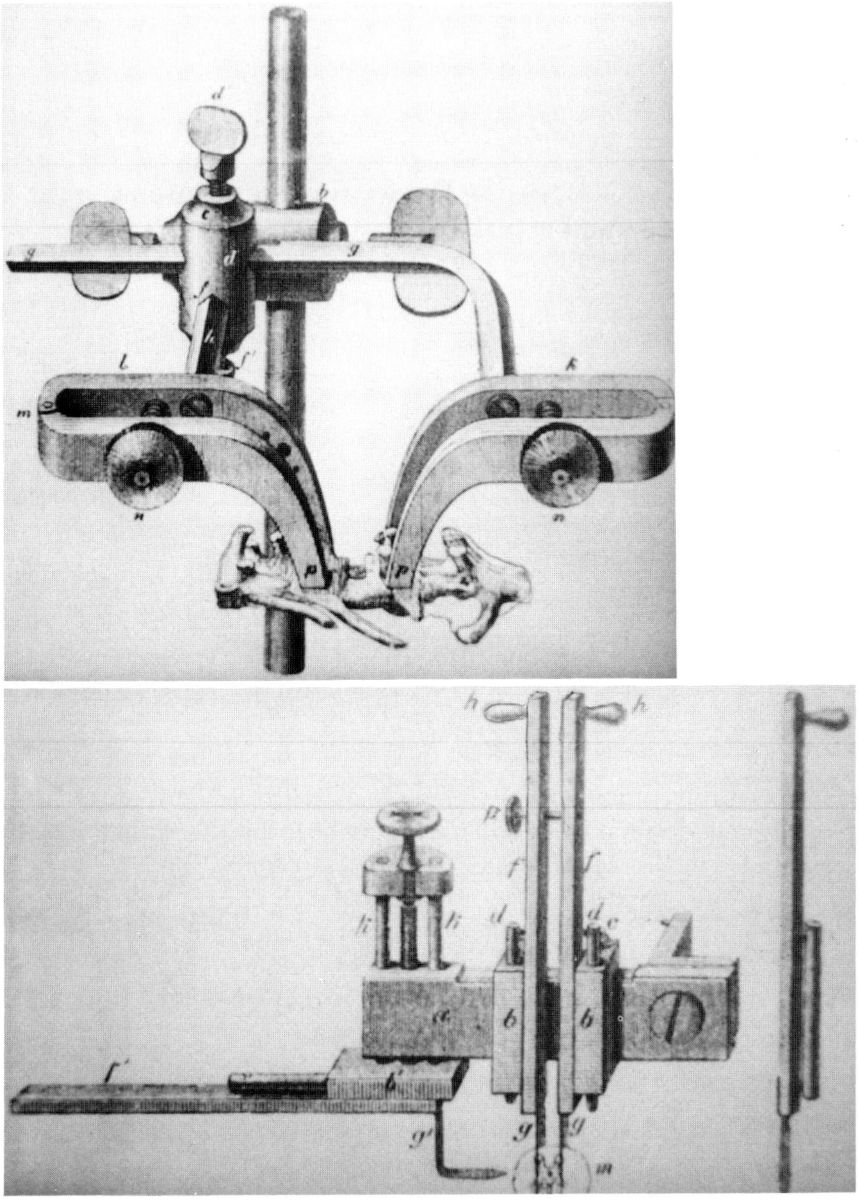

Fig. 1. Original Woroschiloff's device showing **(a)** fixator and **(b)** manipulator.

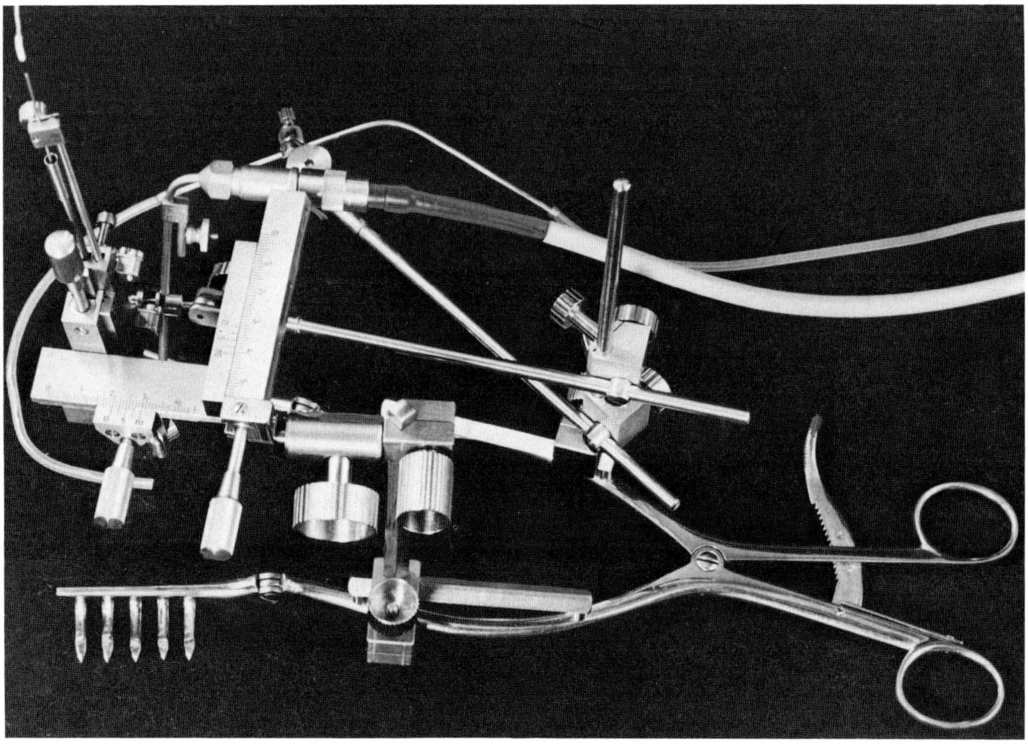

Fig. 2. New spinal cord stereotactic apparatus.

tion frame was connected with two clamps, which were firmly attached by screws to the spinous processes on both sides of the laminectomy. A block was fastened to the clamps in the longitudinal axis to control the motion of two fine knives in the vertical and horizontal directions. Thus, it was possible to perform precisely localized lesions separately in each half of the spinal cord.

Later the knives were replaced by electrodes, which enable the study of motor pathways and vegetative spinal cord centers by means of electrostimulation. The localization of the electrode and/or the extent of the lesion had to be controlled by section and histology.

Table I. Stereotactic procedures on the spinal cord, 1970–1984

Segment	Pain	Spasticity	Bladder
C_{1-2}	66		
Th_{5-8}		4	
L_{1-5}		15	
S_{2-3}			3

At that time, another device, fixed to the skull, was developed by anatomist *Zernov* [8] in Moskow for identification of the location of subcortical brain structures. He elaborated the first coordinated maps of the brain structures as a basis for topometric anatomy.

Woroschiloff's device was forgotten together with the stereotaxy of the spinal cord. Clinical spinal cord stereotaxy was introduced by *Hitchcock* [3] for surgery on the cervical spine, which was reached by a stereotactic apparatus attached to the head of the patient. Three years later the surgery was carried out also in the lumbar enlargement, or in the other segments of the spinal cord, by means of a special device which resembles Woroschiloff's system and relies on the model maps of the spinal cord [5, 9]. The original simple apparatus for experimental purposes [4] was improved by *Nádvorník* et al. [5].

The latest model of this device (fig. 2) is adjusted for precise interventions on the surgically exposed spinal cord. The stereotactic device is fixed to the wound retractor, and the functional electrode is attached to a system of mobile segments controlled in three perpendicular planes. The apparatus is completed by suction, cold light and magnifying glass.

88 procedures in various spinal cord segments have been performed in our own clinic, mostly for pain and spasticity (table I).

The basis of the spinal cord stereotaxy is the spinal cord stereotactic device whose principles were discovered 111 years ago.

References

1 Clarke, R.; Horsley, V.: On method of investigating the deep ganglia and tracts of the central nervous system (cerebellum). Br. med. J. *ii:* 1799–1800 (1906).

2 Dittmar, C.: Über die Lage des sogenannten Gefässcentrums in der medulla oblongata. Ber. sächs. Ges. Wissenschaften, Leipzig *25:* 449–469 (1873).

3 Hitchcock, E.: Stereotaxic spinal surgery. A preliminary report. J. Neurosurg. *31:* 386–392 (1969).

4 Nádvorník, P.: Pokusná stereotaktická studie míšního mikčního centra u králika. Čs. Fyziol. *9:* 567–568 (1960).

5 Nádvorník, P.; Fröhlich, J.; Ježek, V.; Šramka, M.: New apparatus for spinal cord stereotaxis and its use in the microsurgery of lumbar enlargement. Confinia. neurol. *34:* 311–314 (1972).

6 Spiegel, E.A.; Wycis, H.T.; Freed, H.: Thalamotomy. Neuropsych. aspects. N.Y. St. J. Med. *49:* 2273–2274 (1949).

7 Woroschiloff, C.: Der Verlauf der motorischen und sensililen Bahnen durch das Lendenmark des Kaninchens. Ber. sächs. Ges. Wissenschaften, Leipzig *26:* 248–304 (1874).

8 Zernov, D.V.: Encephalometer. Pribor dl'a opredelenija položenija častej mozga u živogo čeloveka. Trudy fizikomed. Obšč., Moskva *2:* 70–80 (1889).

9 Zlatoš, J.; Čierny, G.; Nádvorník, P.: A contribution to the topometry of the spinal cord. Confinia. neurol. *33:* 342–349 (1971).

P. Nádvorník, MD, Department of Neurosurgery, Limbova 5,
CSSR-83305 Bratislava (Czechoslovakia)

Proc. 9th Meeting World Soc. Stereotactic and Functional
Neurosurgery, Toronto 1985
Appl. Neurophysiol. *48:* 252–257 (1985)

Problems with Retrogasserian Glycerol in the Treatment of Trigeminal Neuralgia

William H. Sweet, Charles E. Poletti

Massachusetts General Hospital, Boston, Mass., USA

Key Words. Analgesia · Corneal sensation · Glycerol · Trigeminal neuralgia

Abstract. Following glycerol injections for trigeminal neuralgia. Håkanson, Lunsford, Apfelbaum, Beck and Lobosky and Dieckmann, among others, report that few patients have sensory loss and dysesthesia and a high percentage have sustained gratifying relief. Such was not our experience or that of Laitinen, Price, Siegfried, or Takusagawa, among others. Our own disappointing results re initial failures to achieve relief, significant sensory loss including corneal anesthesia and some dysesthesias in 77 patients are described.

A puzzling discrepancy distinguishes the reports on the results of using glycerol to treat trigeminal neuralgia. The originator of the method, *Håkanson* [6, 7] and his tutee, *Lunsford* [8, 9], have given us accounts of the largest series of respectively 100 and 112 patients. *Håkanson* [6] in his original article noted that the injection of up to 0.4 ml of glycerol 'does not produce any appreciable sensory deficit, so there is no need for repeated examination of the facial sensibility during the course of the procedure'. 'Following the injection, about 60% of previously untreated patients noted a slight numbness.' 'None of the patients complained of painful dysesthesias.' Similarly, *Lunsford and Bennett* [9] had only 2 patients develop a facial sensory loss greater than 50% as compared to the unaffected side. Both had 'reduced corneal sensation'. 'Eight percent developed minor dysesthesias.'

Results of Our Glycerol Injections

Objective Sensory Loss

Early in our experience [10] with the procedure it became apparent that we were producing substantial sensory losses and we began to check facial sensation after injection of each drop (0.05 ml). When analgesia was produced in the areas of the trigger zones or in the first trigeminal division or 0.4 ml had been introduced, we stopped. If first division analgesia occurred, the glycerol was poured back into the posterior fossa after 10 min. However, since in 1 patient so treated the corneal anesthesia has persisted we have been leaving the glycerol in the trigeminal cistern only 5 min. Of 77 patients, only 19 received the full 0.4 ml, indicating that the desired or a V_1 analgesic area had developed with less than 0.4 ml in about 58; 5 had the required analgesia after only 0.15 ml. The initial loss usually fades substantially. It was assessed in the 18 areas into which the trigeminal skin and mucosa have been divided, i.e., V_1-forehead, upper eyelid, bridge of nose; V_2-lower half of nose, lower eyelid, cheek, upper lip skin, nasal mucosa, upper lip mucosa, upper gum, hard palate; V_3-temple, front wall ear canal, lower lip skin, lower lip mucosa, lower gum, floor of mouth, tongue. Analgesia continued in at least 2 of these areas in 44 or 57% of the cases. In 5, a portion of the analgesic zones was also anesthetic to finger touch. In 11 more patients there were at least 2 hypalgesic areas graded by the patient at less than 5/10, and in 11 other patients there were such areas graded at 5–8/10. In only 11 patients were there no hypalgesic areas on the day after injection, but most of these had had some sensory loss right after the injection. The discrepancies in our findings and those in the *Håkanson* and *Lunsford* series may relate to more detailed examinations the day after injection.

Corneal Sensation

On the first day after injection, 21 (27%) of the 77 patients had significantly decreased corneal sensation. Of these, 14 patients had decreased corneal sensation 1–4/10; their injectates varied from 0.15 to 0.4 ml. The remaining 7 patients, with injectates from 0.2 to 0.3 ml, lost all corneal sensation. In 4 of these 7 patients there was some recovery of corneal sensation within 1–12 months (average 6 months); in 1 it remained 0 at 4½ months; in 2 we have no follow-up.

A delayed loss of corneal sensation occurred in 1 patient. On the

Table I. Results re original pain

	Patients n	Failure to secure relief 1st injection %	Recurrences requiring medication %	Recurrences requiring re-op or re-inj %	Follow-up
Håkanson, 1983 [7]	100	4	19	15	1–6 y avg. 2 y
Lunsford, 1985 [8]	62	26	19	28	3–18 m avg. 12 m
Sweet et al., 1985 [10]	77	13	5	12	1–67 m avg. 26 m

Perhaps our sensory losses will be followed by fewer recurrences.

first postinjection day this patient had 5/10 corneal sensation. *Fraioli* et al. [5] had had a similar patient who by 3 months postoperatively developed a complete trigeminal anesthesia including the cornea. In contrast, *Håkanson* [6, 7] and *Lunsford* [8, 9] have not noted any loss of corneal sensation in any of their patients.

Controllability of Lesion Site

The path taken by the glycerol once it leaves the needle tip and hence the exact lesion site cannot be predicted as with RF heating. It has proven especially difficult for us to make a third division lesion.

Dysesthesias

Thirty-seven percent (28/77) of our patients complained of dysesthesias following the glycerol rhizotomy. These were mild and tended to improve in 16 patients (21%), but were bad enough to require medication in 9 (12%) and were a major source of distress in 3 more. Thirty-three had had both an RF lesion and a glycerol injection for their pain. The RF lesion was done first in 27 and glycerol first in the remaining 6. Five preferred the new sensations (or lack of them) after the glycerol; 13 preferred those after the RF lesion; 8 never relieved of the original pain naturally preferred the RF lesion. Seven patients saw little difference between the 2 procedures. Of the patients who preferred the RF lesions, 5 had only 0.15–0.25 ml glycerol and 8 had 0.3–0.4 ml. Hence the use of minimal amounts of glycerol does not assure lesser dysesthesias.

Experiences of other neurosurgeons include 3 recent encouraging accounts [1, 3, 4]. *Dieckmann* et al. [4] have given the method a thorough trial in 164 patients with facial pain. Of 51 patients with trigeminal neuralgia followed 1–4 years, 78% were pain free and 14% had minor pain controlled if needed by medication. Forty percent of the patients had minor well-tolerated 'numbness' associated with mild hypesthesia or hypalgesia in some areas. Only 1 developed a lasting 'painful dysesthesia'. Likewise, of *Beck and Lobosky's* [3] 33 patients with trigeminal neuralgia, only 1 developed permanent anesthesia and analgesia with loss of corneal reflex and 75% were pain free followed up to 3 years. *Apfelbaum* [1] is so pleased with the results of his glycerol injections that he has essentially stopped making RF lesions for trigeminal neuralgia. Although he notes that sensory loss is usually 'minimal to moderate' he has had 1 patient with total anesthesia including the cornea.

Other capable neurosurgeons have been much less satisfied with their results. Thus, *Fraioli* et al. [5], *Laitinen* [pers. commun., 1985], *Price* [pers. commun., 1985] and *Siegfried* [pers. commun., 1985] each after 20–30 operations have given up this method because of some combination of too many initial failures, later recurrences, major sensory losses and/or dysesthesias.

Specifically, *Price* had, at 3 years, 8 failures out of 14 re pain relief. Corneal anesthesia in 1, dysesthesias in 3, and 2 severe sensory deficits in another group of 6 patients comprise his bases for discouragement. *Takusagawa* et al. [11] described 'hopeful results' in their abstract. However, the paper they gave at the International Congress, reporting 122 cases of 'tic pain', listed only 58% pain free at 1–3 years' follow-up, 30% with 'unpleasant dysesthesias', 2 patients with frank anesthesia dolorosa and 3 with keratitis. They were discontinuing the procedures.

Discussion

Lunsford [8] has suggested that the discrepancy in results is due to injections into the ganglion by those of us producing sustained sensory losses and dysesthesias. Our injections are usually behind the profile of the clivus as seen in the lateral view of the skull, are never carried out unless CSF drips from the needle just prior to placement of the syringe, and proceed only in the absence of significant resistance. We are inclined to suggest variations in the patients themselves as the explanation of some of the discrepant findings. Fearful that we might have some impurity in our 'pure' glycerol we have used supplies from 3 different sources without changing our results. Studies of *Baxter and Schacherl* [2] in 1962 and currently by *Vallat* [pers. commun., 1985] upon spinal intrathecal injections of glycerol into animals reveal severe destruction of rootlets.

In 1 of our patients at the end of 1 h of glycerol in the trigeminal cistern we extended her head, provoking within a few minutes a trochlear nerve palsy. We presume subdural flow of metrizamide along the clivus caused this sequel. The diplopia lasted about a year, which is we think clear-cut evidence of potential glycerol toxicity.

Conclusion

Pure glycerol is toxic to trigeminal nerve roots, at least in some patients. This toxicity can be controlled most safely by injection into the trigeminal cistern drop by drop with careful monitoring of sensation and elimination of the glycerol from the cistern when an appropriate level of sensory loss has been maintained for 5 min. We strongly urge all those doing the procedure to inform patients of the possibility of the sequelae several of us have described. Our experience here we feel does not currently justify using glycerol for trigeminal rhizotomies.

Acknowledgement

The authors wish to express their appreciation to the Neuro-Research Foundation for its support during the preparation of this manuscript.

References

1 Apfelbaum, R.I.: Discussion of Lunsford and Bennett. Neurosurgery *14:* 424–430 (1984).

2 Baxter, D.W.; Schacherl, V.: Experimental studies on the morphological changes produced by intrathecal phenol. Can. med. Ass. J. *86:* 1200–1205 (1962).

3 Beck, D.W.; Lobosky, J.M.: Treatment of trigeminal neuralgia and atypical facial pain by percutaneous injection of glycerol into the trigeminal cistern. Abstr. 8th Int. Congr. of Neurological Surgery, Toronto 1985, abstr. 230, pp. 143–144.

4 Dieckmann, G.; Veras, G.; Sogabe, K.: Retrogasserian glycerol injection or percutaneous stimulation in the treatment of typical and atypical trigeminal pain. Abstr. 8th Int. Congr. of Neurological Surgery, Toronto 1985, abstr. 227, p. 142.

5 Fraioli, B.; Ferrante, L.; Santoro, A.; Di Giugno, G.: Recent progress in the treatment of trigeminal neuralgia: glycerol into the trigeminal cistern and percutaneous Gasserian compression by means of Fogarty's catheter. Acta neurochir. *33:* suppl., pp. 507–510 (1984).

6 Håkanson, S.: Trigeminal neuralgia treated by the injection of glycerol into the trigeminal cistern. Neurosurgery *9:* 638–646 (1981).

7 Håkanson, S.: Retrogasserian glycerol injection as treatment of tic douloureux; in Bonica, Lindblom, Iggo, Advances in pain research and therapy, vol. 5, pp. 927–933 (Raven Press, New York 1983).

8 Lunsford, L.D.: Trigeminal neuralgia; in Wilkins, Rengachary, Neurosurgery, pp. 2351–2356 (McGraw-Hill, New York 1985).

9 Lunsford, L.D.; Bennett, M.H.: Percutaneous retrogasserian glycerol rhizotomy for tic douloureux. I. Technique and results in 112 patients. Neurosurgery *14:* 424–430 (1984).

10 Sweet, W.H.; Poletti, C.E.; Macon, J.B.: Treatment of trigeminal neuralgia and other facial pain by retrogasserian injection of glycerol. Neurosurgery *9:* 647–653 (1981).

11 Takusagawa, Y.; Wakiya, K.; Fukushima, T.: Treatment of trigeminal neuralgia by percutaneous Gasserian ganglion glycerol injection. Abstr. 8th Int. Congr. of Neurological Surgery, Toronto 1985, abstr. 229, p. 143.

W.H. Sweet, MD, Massachusetts General Hospital, ACC 312,
Boston, MA 02114 (USA)

Proc. 9th Meeting World Soc. Stereotactic and Functional Neurosurgery, Toronto 1985
Appl. Neurophysiol. *48:* 258–261 (1985)

Effectiveness of Radiofrequency Thermocoagulation in Recurrent Trigeminal Neuralgia after Previous Retrogasserian Rhizotomy

Y. Kanpolat, N. Avman, H.Z. Gökalp, E. Arasil, M. Selçuki, T. Mertol

University of Ankara Ibni Sina Medical Center, Department of Neurosurgery, Ankara, Turkey

Key Words. Retrogasserian rhizotomy · Radiofrequency thermocoagulation · Trigeminal neuralgia

Abstract. Between 1974 and 1984, 428 trigeminal neuralgia cases were treated by controlled radiofrequency thermocoagulation (RFTC). 29 had recurrent trigeminal neuralgia after intracranial surgery. 26 of the 29 patients were treated by retrogasserian rhizotomy and 3 by posterior fossa exploration. Among the 26 recurrent trigeminal neuralgia following retrogasserian rhizotomy, RFTC was effective in 23 cases (88.5%), and in 3 cases (11.5%) RFTC was effective for a short period. Repeated RFTC was unable to control the pain attacks which were later relieved by posterior fossa exploration and root section. Of the 3 recurrent trigeminal neuralgia following posterior fossa exploration, RFTC was effective in 2 cases (66.6%).

Introduction

The number of surgically treated recurrent trigeminal neuralgia (TN) patients in overall TN cases is considerably high. However, a successful technique has not yet been standardized in the treatment of the recurrent TN patients after previous intracranial surgery. In this paper, we shall give the results of controlled radiofrequency thermocoagulation (RFTC) application in 26 recurrent TN cases after retrogasserian rhizotomy (RGR) and on 3 current TN after posterior fossa exploration (PFE). Thus, we shall try to explain the role of RFTC in treating these patients.

Materials and Methods

Between 1974 and 1984, 428 TN cases were treated by the controlled RTFC method. 29 of these patients had either pain attacks or recurrent TN which had previously been treated by intracranial surgery. 26 of 29 cases had previously been treated by the middle fossa approach and RGR and 3 by PFE.

We shall first consider the 26 patients who previously had RGR and subsequently consider the remaining 3 cases. 17 cases of the first group were male and 9 were female, aged between 30 and 70 years (average 51). RGR was applied in this group – twice in 3 cases. In 21 of 26 patients, pain was relieved but later recurrent TN complaints were observed within the 3-month to 10-year period. RGR was effective in TN for an average of 40 months. In 5 patients however, RGR was ineffective.

All 26 cases were treated by RFTC described by *Sweet and Wepsic* [3]. A Radionics RF generator with cordotomy needle electrodes with a temperature-monitoring electrode system was used. In 26 cases, 34 procedures of electrode placement in the ganglion had been performed with success. In these procedures CSF was obtained in 19 patients. The required branches of the ganglion were reached in 25 patients, but efforts to reach the ophthalmic division in 1 patient were unsuccessful. In an exceptional case, the ophthalmic division of the ganglion was reached 10 mm above the clivus-petrosal apex junction.

Results

In the first application of RFTC, pain was relieved in all 26 cases. In 6 cases early recurrence of TN was observed. In 3, repeated RFTC failed to control the pain. These 3 patients were then treated by PFE and root section. It was observed that the trigeminal nerve was atrophic in all 3 cases. In 2, motor and sensory divisions were sectioned and in 1 the motor root was preserved. In 1 case repeated RFTC for early recurrence was effective for 4 years, and following the third repeated application no complaints have been observed. In the long-term follow-up of the 2 cases, pain attacks were controlled by minimal doses of carbamazepine and new applications were not required by the patients. In 3 cases late recurrence was observed within a 1- to 3-year period. The pain attacks were controlled by repeated RFTC.

Finally, during the 1- to 7-year follow-up of 26 cases, 21 were pain free (81%). In 2 cases RFTC was partially effective necessitating no new applications. Consequently, total effectiveness of RFTC in recurrent TN after RGR is found to be 88.5%, showing excellent results in 81%. At the end of 34 procedures carried out on 26 patients, only 2 showed decreased corneal reflexes and had temporary complications of trigeminal motor weakness. In the second group of 3 cases who had PFE, RFTC was carried out. During the 3- to 5-year follow-up, 2 cases were pain free, the success rate being 66.6%. The RFTC application as a last resort on a patient formerly treated with PFE and root section who had complaints of phantom pain was unsuccessful.

Discussion

The rate of recurrence of trigeminal pain in patients who had previous intracranial surgery was stated as 20% by *Latchaw* et al. [1], 13% by *Siegfried* [2] and 11% by *Tew* et al. [4]. Moreover, *Turner* [5] stated that RFTC was successful in recurrent TN patients who had had previous intracranial surgery. However, no discrimination has been made between the two groups of patients, that is, the ones with recurrent TN previously treated by intracranial surgery and the others who had not had any previous surgical treatment.

In our studies the success rate of RFTC in overall TN patients has been found to be 94%. Further studies between the two groups of patients mentioned above have shown that the rate of RFTC success is 88.5% in the former and 66.6% in the latter. Since the latter group comprised only 3 cases, we refrain from giving any definite result.

We would like to conclude that in the evaluation of our series, the application of RFTC in recurrent TN patients previously treated by intracranial procedures and specifically in patients with post-RGR history has proved to be successful. Moreover, the safety of RFTC as a great procedure in early or late recurrence convinces us of its superiority and preference over the other technics. On the other hand, in the case of recurrent TN, patients who had several peripheral and cranial surgeries and have still not been relieved of pain by repeated RFTC, we suggest the application of PFE and root section as a final step.

References

1 Latchaw, J.P.; Hardy, R.W.; Forsythe, S.B.; Cook, A.F.: Trigeminal neuralgia treated by radiofrequency coagulation. J. Neurosurg. *59:* 479–484 (1981).

2 Siegfried, J.: Percutaneous controlled thermocoagulation of gasserian ganglion in trigeminal neuralgia, experience with 1,000 cases; in Samii, Janetta, The cranial nerves, pp. 322–330 (Springer, Berlin 1981).

3 Sweet, H.; Wepsic, J.G.: Controlled thermocoagulation of trigeminal ganglion and rootlets for differential destruction of pain fibers. J. Neurosurg. *40:* 143-156 (1974).

4 Tew, J.M.; Tobler, W.G.; Loveren, H.V.: Percutaneous rhizotomy in the treatment of intractable facial pain (trigeminal, glossopharyngeal and vagal nerves); in Operative neurosurgical techniques, vol. 70, pp. 1038-1106 (Grune & Stratton, New York, 1982).

5 Turner, J.W.: The effectiveness of trigeminal thermocoagulation for recurrent paroxysmal trigeminal neuralgia after previous intracranial surgery. Acta neurochir. *30:* suppl., pp. 371-376 (1980).

Dr. Y. Kanpolat, University of Ankara Ibni Sina Medical Center, Department of Neurosurgery, Ankara (Turkey)

Proc. 9th Meeting World Soc. Stereotactic and Functional Neurosurgery, Toronto 1985
Appl. Neurophysiol. *48:* 262–266 (1985)

Therapeutic Approach to the Pancoast Pain Syndrome

S. Esposito, P. Bruni, A. Delitala, A. Canova, R. Hernandez, G.M. Callovini

Division of Neurosurgery, San Camillo Hospital, Rome, Italy

Key Words. Pain · Pancoast syndrome · Selective posterior radiculotomy · Morphine

Abstract. The incidence of the Pancoast syndrome ranges from 2 to 5% of patients with lung cancer. We treated 20 cases between 1979 and 1984 with 29 procedures including percutaneous cordotomy, selective posterior radiculotomy, decompressive laminectomy, central administration of opiates, and TENS. Selective posterior radiculotomy gave the best pain relief.

The Pancoast syndrome (PS) is an infrequent presentation for lung cancer [2]. We treated 20 cases between 1979 and 1984 referred from our main Department of Chest Diseases which admits almost 500 tumor patients per annum. The difficulty of relieving lung cancer pain is well known and discourages many neurosurgeons [1–12]. Reported therapeutic techniques include rhizotomy, open cordotomy, and alcohol or phenol blocks [5, 6]. Recently, selective posterior radiculotomy (SPR) has been introduced [15], and intrathecal and intraventricular administration of opiates have been advocated for pain relief [8–11]. Fifteen SPR procedures and 5 instances of central administration of opiates are included in our series.

Material and Methods

Our patients were all males with an average age of 59 years, previously treated with chemotherapy and radiotherapy but not surgery. 15 were in good physical condition with a life expectancy of over 6 months. 5 were ill with only a few months of expected life.

The patients were divided into two groups according to their pain symptoms. In the first group the pain was localized in the C8 to T2 distribution; in the second, pain extended up to the C4–C5 region. Clinical features and myelography suggested spinal cord involvement by cancer in 4 patients.

In Sindou's original report, ventrolateral section of the spinal cord rootlet is done with a minimal penetration (1–2 mm) into the region of Lissauer's tract. There is no risk of direct pyramidal tract damage but ischemic damage of the posterior horn is possible with consequent atonia of the upper limb. Consequently, we prefer to make the ventrolateral section not oblique. The analgesia is selective and the tactile, discriminative and proprioceptive sensations are preserved.

In patients with short survival, we used intrathecal administration of opiates (morphine and buprenorphine) [3, 8, 11]. A unidirectional low-pressure valve is placed between the reservoir and the lumbar or intraventricular catheters. Analgesia lasting from 24 to 52 h with variable morphine doses of 0.50–2 mg was obtained after 30–60 min. Pain was relieved by morphine in all cases [7].

Results

We have performed 29 therapeutic procedures in 20 patients as shown in table I. The 4 percutaneous cordotomies relieved pain for only 2–3 months. For this reason the SPR was performed extensively because of the wide distribution of pain. At 6 months' follow-up all but 1 patient in whom it was necessary to give morphine by intrathecal administration showed very good results.

The results after 6 months' follow-up can be considered satisfactory in those 7 patients who underwent SPR primarily. The persistence of a painful hypoesthesia in 2 patients necessitated the use of TENS. In 4 patients treated with SPR in combination with decompressive laminectomy, 3 obtained excellent results, while the other died of bronchopneumonia. In every case, decompressive laminectomy proved helpful in relieving spinal cord symptomatology and it allowed a pathological diagnosis. In 5 patients treated with intrathecal administration of morphine as a first procedure, 3 showed good results while the remaining 2 required the use of intraventricular administration of morphine with relief in 1 (table II).

Complications

Of the patients treated with percutaneous cordotomy, 1 suffered from homolateral hemiparesis and from ataxia of the upper limb, but deficits resolved after 3 weeks. All cases treated with SPR suffered for 2

Table I. Employed techniques in 20 cases of Pancoast syndrome

	First attempt	Second attempt	Third attempt
Percutaneous cordotomy	4	SPR (4)	Opiates (1)
SPR	7	TENS (2)	–
Decompressive laminectomy + SPR	4	–	–
Opiates	5 IT	2 IV	

Table II. Results after 6 months' follow-up

	Good	Fair	Poor
Percutaneous cordotomy	3[1]	–	1
SPR (first attempt)	5	2	–
SPR (second attempt)	3	1	–
Decompressive laminectomy + SPR	3	–	1[2]
Opiates IT	3	–	2
Opiates IV	1		1[2]

1 Only for 2–3 months.
2 Dead patients.

weeks from significant hypoesthesia and ataxia of the upper limb and the other affected roots. CSF leakage from the wound, successfully treated with continuous lumbar drainage, occurred in 3 patients. We had some difficulty with respiration in only 1 case, but it was controlled by naloxone. We used buprenorphine in 2 patients to reduce the respiratory risk. It is not possible to make a comparison of the two drugs because of the lack of data.

Discussion

Our choice of therapeutic approach was based on radicular pain topography, the patients' general status, extent tumors, and the number of roots involved. We preferred SPR when the patient's condition was good and the pain limited to a few roots. Percutaneous cordotomy was performed when the painful symptomatology was extensive. Though opinions vary, it is generally [1, 10, 14] agreed that a sufficiently high and stable analgesic level is difficult to obtain with cordotomy, in that such a high lesion is likely to produce a respiratory disturbance from reticulospinal involvement. For these reasons we used percutaneous cordotomy with extreme caution, making small radiofrequency lesions with 40 mA for 5 s on 2 or 3 occasions, but our results have been poor. In patients with a long life expectancy we preferred not to run the risk of respiratory complications, and instead of enlarging their cordotomy lesion, performed SPR as the second procedure. We have no experience with stereotactic mesencephalotomy, a very useful technique for cervicothoracobrachial pain syndrome in patients with respiratory risks. Although it can be performed bilaterally, postoperative complications such as anesthesia dolorosa occur.

References

1 Batzdorf, U.: Management of pain associated with Pancoast syndrome. Am. J. Surg. *15:* 638–646 (1979).
2 Berrino, S.: Epidemiology of Pancoast syndrome. Abstr. Sem. on Management of Superior Pulmonary Sulcus Syndrome (Pancoast Syndrome), Stresa 1981, pp. 14–15.
3 Esposito, S.; Canova, A.; Colangeli, M.: Posterior radiculotomies in the treatment of the lumbo-sacral pain syndrome. Acta neurochir. *53:* 132–133 (1980).
4 Frank, F.; Tognetti, F.; Gaist, G.; Frank, G.; Galassi, E.; Sturiale, C.: Stereotactic rostral mesencephalotomy in the treatment of malignant faciothoracobrachial pain. A survey of 14 treated patients. J. Neurosurg. *56:* 807–811 (1982).
5 Friedberg, S.R.: Neurosurgical treatment of pain caused by cancer. Med. Clins N. Am. *59:* 481–484 (1975).
6 Grant, F.C.; Wood, S.A.: Experiences with cordotomy. Clin. Neurosurg. *5:* 38–45 (1958).
7 Hosobuchi, Y.; Adams, J.I.; Linchitz, R.: Pain relief by electrical stimulation of the central grey matter in humans and its reversal by naloxone. Science *197:* 183–186 (1977).
8 Lazorthes, V.; Gouarderes, C.; Verdie, J.C.; Monsarrat, B.; Bastide, R.; Campan, L.; Alwan, A.; Cros, J.: Analgésie par injection intrathécale de morphine. Neurochirurgie *26:* 159–164 (1980).
9 Mazars, G.: La chirurgie de la doleur. Neurochirurgie *22:* suppl., p. 40 (1976).
10 Meglio, M.; Cioni, B.: The role of percutaneous cordotomy in the treatment of chronic cancer pain. Acta neurochir. *59:* 111–121 (1981).
11 Nurchi, G.: Use of intraventricular and intrathecal morphine in intractable pain associated with cancer. Neurosurgery *15:* 801–803 (1984).

12 Pagni, C.A.: Neurosurgical treatment. Status of the problem. Abst. Sem. on Management of Superior Pulmonary Sulcus Syndrome (Pancoast Syndrome), Stresa 1981, pp. 36-37.
13 Papo, I.: Spinal posterior rhizotomy in commissural myelotomy in the treatment of cancer pain. Advances in pain research and therapy, pp. 439-447 (Raven Press, New York 1979).
14 Rosomoff, H.L.: Percutaneous radiofrequency cervical corodotmy for intractable pain. Adv. Neurol. *4:* 683-693 (1974).
15 Sindou, M.; Goutelle, A.: Surgical posterior rhizotomies for treatment of pain; in Krayenbühl, Advances and technical standards in neurosurgery, pp. 147-185 (Springer, Wien 1983).
16 Tasker, R.: The merit of percutaneous cordotomy over the open operation; in Morley, Current controversies in neurosurgery, pp. 496-501 (1976).

S. Esposito, MD, Division of Neurosurgery, 'G. Lancisi' - San Camillo Hospital, I-00123 Rome (Italy)

Proc. 9th Meeting World Soc. Stereotactic and Functional
Neurosurgery, Toronto 1985
Appl. Neurophysiol. *48:* 267–270 (1985)

Cerebral-Evoked Responses Elicited by Direct Stimulation of the Lateral Spinothalamic Tract in the Human

T. Taira, K. Amano, H. Kawamura, T. Tanikawa, K. Kitamura

Department of Neurosurgery, Neurological Institute, Tokyo Women's Medical College, Tokyo, Japan

Key Words. Spinothalamic tract · Evoked potential · Noxious stimuli

Abstract. The authors recorded cerebral-evoked responses elicited by direct stimulation of the human lateral spinothalamic tract (LST) during percutaneous cordotomy to investigate central conduction of noxious stimuli. These responses consisted of four negative potentials, peak latency being 3.8 (N1), 8.4 (N2), 12.2 (N3) and 21.9 (N4) ms respectively. N1 showed wide distribution over the scalp and was considered to be of subcortical origin. N2–N4 were distributed in both the temporal and central area. The different distribution pattern of N2–N4 from conventional somatosensory-evoked potential suggested a different projection of LST from the medial lemniscus system.

Electrically stimulated signals in peripheral nerves are believed to be conducted mostly through the posterior column of spinal cord and medial lemniscus [3], while signals of noxious stimuli are found in the lateral spinothalamic tract. Little information concerned with the central conduction of noxious stimuli can be obtained from studies of conventional somatosensory-evoked potentials. The authors recorded cerebral-evoked responses elicited by direct stimulation of human LST during percutaneous cordotomy to investigate central conduction of noxious stimuli in humans.

Method and Materials

Evoked potentials were recorded in 12 patients aged 34–72 years (mean 52) who underwent percutaneous cordotomy for relief of cancer pain. Bilateral cordotomy was performed in 2 patients, and so 14 recordings were evaluated.

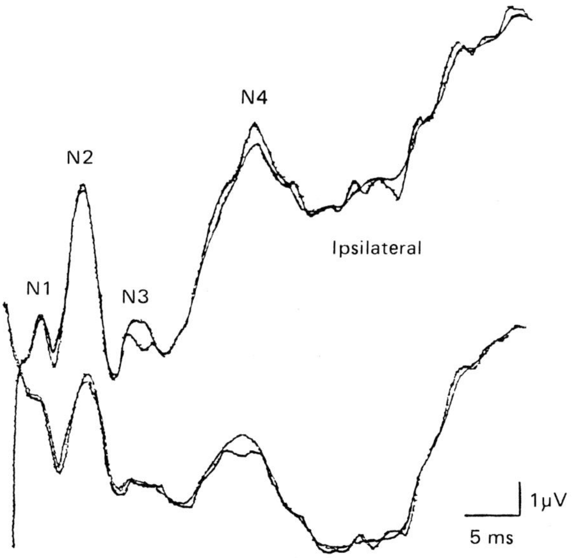

Fig. 1. Evoked potential elicited by direct stimulation of lateral spinothalamic tract in human. Four negative potentials are recorded within 50 ms.

A bipolar concentric electrode was introduced into the spinal cord at the C1-C2 level. Correct placement in the LST was confirmed with high frequency electrical stimulation (50 Hz, 1-2 V), which elicits painful sensation at the corresponding dermatome when the tip of the electrode is located in LST. Stimuli for the evoked potentials were delivered with a 0.5 ms square wave of 1-2 Hz. Stimulus intensity was 1-1.5 V. Recording electrodes were placed on the parietal scalp bilaterally, unless topographic distribution was studied. Reference and ground electrodes were placed on the forehead and earlobe respectively. Low and high cut filters were set at 10 and 500 Hz. One hundred responses within 50 ms were averaged.

Results

Four negative waves with peak latencies of 3.8, 8.4, 12.0 and 21.9 ms were recorded from the ipsilateral parietal electrode to the stimulation and named N1, N2, N3 and N4 respectively (fig. 1). N2 and N3 were sometimes recorded as one large negative deflection. N1 distributed widely over the scalp, while N2-N4 were prominent in the ipsilateral temporal and parietal area. N2 and N3 were sometimes recorded

Table I. Summary of peak latencies in each patient

Case	Patient	Disease	ipsilateral				contralateral				Stim. side
			N1	N2	N3	N4	N1	N2	N3	N4	
1	H.Y. 51 M	eso. ca.	3.8	9.0	13.0	21.0	3.9	9.5	13.3	21.0	Lt
2	K.S. 38 F	lung ca.	3.3	–	12.5	21.0	3.6	–	12.5	22.0	Rt
3	N.O. 34 M	rectum ca.	4.0	–	–	20.5	2.7	–	–	22.0	Rt
4	N.O. 34 M	rectum ca.	4.2	–	–	21.0	3.7	–	–	22.3	Lt
5	Y.K. 67 M	rectum ca.	4.0	–	11.0	20.5	3.4	–	10.6	–	Lt
6	Y.T. 56 M	hepatoma	4.0	8.4	12.2	24.1	–	8.5	12.8	24.0	Lt
7	H.I. 56 M	bladder ca.	–	–	12.5	20.2	–	9.0	12.7	19.1	Rt
8	S.K. 72 M	panc. ca.	3.6	–	13.0	–	–	–	–	–	Rt
9	S.N. 63 M	panc. ca.	3.6	–	11.5	24.0	3.5	9.5	–	27.6	Lt
10	K.S. 38 M	uter. ca.	3.0	–	10.7	23.5	5.5	–	10.0	–	Lt
11	T.S. 52 M	gastr. ca.	–	–	10.5	22.5	–	6.8	11.0	23.5	Rt
12	T.S. 59 M	pancr. ca.	3.0	8.0	–	18.5	3.0	8.0	–	20.5	Rt
13	H.K. 42 F	mam. ca.	4.0	–	14.0	22.0	4.0	6.8	14.0	22.0	Rt
14	H.K. 42 F	mam. ca.	5.5	8.0	–	25.0	5.0	8.5	–	24.5	Lt
		Average	3.83	8.35	12.0	21.9	3.83	8.33	12.1	22.6	
		SD	0.63	0.47	1.20	1.87	0.85	1.07	1.50	2.17	

on the contralateral side to the LST stimulation. N4 was constantly recorded bilaterally. A summary of peak latencies in each patient is shown in table I.

Discussion

Most studies concerned with human LST have been performed with anatomical methods [1]. Electrophysiological assessment of human LST was only documented by *Mayer* et al. [2].

The waveform of the LST stimulated evoked response was completely different from the conventional somatosensory-evoked potential elicited by median nerve stimulation. N1 had a short latency and distributed widely over the scalp, presumably representing a subcortical generator. The origin of N1 may be the brain stem or the thalamus. N2 and N3 were sometimes combined and recorded on the contralateral side. These may be cortical responses mediated via the brain stem reticular formation. N4 is usually recorded bilaterally. Mean peak latency of contralateral N4 was 0.7 ms longer than that of the ipsilateral response, but the difference is of no statistical significance. It is not obvious whether the contralateral N4 is mediated by brain stem or the corpus callosum.

References

1 Kuru, M.: Sensory paths in the spinal cord and brain stem of man (Kimura, Tokyo 1976).

2 Mayer, D.J.; Price, D.D.; Becker, D.P.: Neurophysiological characterization of anterolateral spinal cord neurons contributing to pain perception in man. Pain *1:* 51–58 (1975).

3 Nakanishi, T.; Shimada, Y.; Sakuta, M.; Toyokura, Y.: The initial positive component of the scalp-recorded somatosensory-evoked potential in normal subjects and in patients with neurological disorders. Electroenceph. clin. Neurophysiol. *45:* 26–34 (1978).

T. Taira, Department of Neurosurgery, Neurological Institute,
Tokyo Women's Medical College,
10 Kawada-cho, Shinjuku-ku, Tokyo 162 (Japan)

Proc. 9th Meeting World Soc. Stereotactic and Functional
Neurosurgery, Toronto 1985
Appl. Neurophysiol. *48:* 271–273 (1985)

Therapeutic Protocol in the Treatment of Trigeminal Neuralgia

S. Esposito, A. Delitala, P. Bruni, R. Hernandez, G.M. Callovini
Division of Neurosurgery, 'G. Lancisi' – S. Camillo Hospital, Rome, Italy

Key Words. Trigeminal neuralgia · Microcompression · Glycerol · Thermorhizotomy

Abstract. The ideal treatment of trigeminal neuralgia is still an open question. A recent large series reporting the results from the three available percutaneous techniques has been reviewed. Fifty consecutive cases, treated from January 1984 to January 1985, are reported. Microcompression was performed as the first approach in all cases. The other techniques were adopted only in case of failure of microcompression.

Many techniques for the treatment of essential trigeminal neuralgia have been proposed. At present, the safer and more used percutaneous operations are posterior selective thermorhizotomy [9], glycerol injection into the trigeminal cistern [4] and percutaneous microcompression of the Gasserian ganglion [7]. None of these techniques, including that of *Jannetta* [5], achieves a complete relief from neuralgia in all the cases without side effects.

Material and Methods

From January 1984 to January 1985, 50 patients with essential trigeminal neuralgia were admitted to our Division and selected for treatment with percutaneous microcompression of the Gasserian ganglion. Symptomatic and/or atypical neuralgias were excluded from the study. There were 31 female and 19 male patients; age distribution ranged from 48 to 82 years. In 35 cases only one branch was affected by neuralgia; 12 were complicated by a double branch distribution and in 3 patients a three branch neuralgia was present. All patients who had previously undergone surgical procedures were excluded. All patients had been treated with carbamazepine previously: 37 had a recurrence of pain due to tolerance to the drug, 13 were not able to endure pharmacological

Table I. Results after a mean follow-up of 6 months

<table>
<tr><th>Procedure</th><th>Cases
n</th><th>Pain-free
at 1st op.</th><th>Pain-free
at 2nd op.</th><th>Failure</th><th>Hypo-
esthesia</th><th>Painful
dys-
esthesia</th><th>Corneal
reflex im-
pairment</th></tr>
<tr><td></td><td></td><td>32</td><td>7</td><td></td><td></td><td></td><td></td></tr>
<tr><td>Micro-
compression</td><td>50</td><td colspan="2">78%</td><td>22%</td><td>49%</td><td>-</td><td>-</td></tr>
<tr><td>Glycerol</td><td>11</td><td colspan="2">77%</td><td>23%</td><td>39%</td><td>-</td><td>-</td></tr>
<tr><td>Thermo-
rhizotomy</td><td>3</td><td colspan="2">100%</td><td>-</td><td>66%</td><td>-</td><td>-</td></tr>
</table>

treatment due to side effects. Those patients who did not respond to the initial compression within a few days (18 cases) underwent a second compression; glycerol was injected as the third procedure if microcompression failed. Thermorhizotomy was performed only if the other two techniques failed.

Percutaneous microcompression was performed under neuroleptoanalgesia, with only a lateral radioscopic intermittent control, using a 14-gauge intravenous cannula as a guide to a No. 4 Fogarty catheter filled and inflated with 0.6 cm^3 water-soluble contrast media (Iopamiro 300); compression time was 5 min. The catheter and the teflon guide were drawn out together after the procedure. For the intracisternal glycerol injection procedure the technique described by *Hakanson* [4] was adopted. Patients who underwent thermorhizotomy were operated under light general intermittent anesthesia, with a continuous clinical monitoring of the corneal reflex [8]. The electrode tip was placed into the trigeminal posterior root (i.e. behind the root in the lateral view); radiofrequency was used to obtain a tip temperature of 60 °C for 55 s; if the sensibility testing was not satisfactory a second 65 s lesion was performed.

Results

Table I shows the results of the present study. All the cases were symptom-free at a mean follow-up of 6 months. Of the 50 patients treated with microcompression, 18 did not receive any relief from neuralgia within a few days and underwent a second compression, but only 7 obtained relief from neuralgia. Hypoesthesia was elicited in 24 cases. No complications, like painful dysesthesia or corneal reflex impairment, were obtained. Complete relief from neuralgia was obtained, with one or two compressions, in 39 cases. Glycerol injection was performed successfully in 8 of the remaining cases, while 3 cases underwent thermorhizotomy. In 1 case of microcompression a transient sixth nerve palsy was observed, but completely recovered after 1 month; in 1 case of glycerol injection a transient drowsiness, probably due to hyperosmolar diencephalic impairment, was observed.

References

1 Broggi, G.; Franzini, A.; Giorgi, C., et al.: Considerazioni sui risultati di 1,000 interventi consecutivi di termorizotomia trigeminale. Proc. 33rd Annual Meeting of the Italian Society of Neurosurgery, Ferrara 1984.

2 Fraioli, B.; Ferrante, L.; Santoro, A., et al.: Vantaggi e svantaggi della termocoagulazione, glicerolizzazione e compressione del ganglio di Gasser nel trattamento della nevralgia del trigemino. Proc. 33rd Annual Meeting of the Italian Society of Neurosurgery, Ferrara 1984.

3 Frank, F.; Sedan, R.; Cohadon, F., et al.: Le termocoagulazioni percutanee nel trattamento delle nevralgie trigeminali essenziali: rapporto sull'esperienza congiunta di Bologna, Marsiglia, Bordeaux in 965 pazienti trattati. Proc. 33rd Annual Meeting of the Italian Society of Neurosurgery, Ferrara 1984.

4 Hakanson, S.: Trigeminal neuralgia treated by the injection of glycerol into the trigeminal cistern. Neurosurgery *9:* 638–646 (1981).

5 Jannetta, P.J.: Microsurgical approach to the trigeminal nerve for tic douloureux. Prog. neurol. Surg. vol. 7, pp. 180–200 (Karger, Basel 1976).

6 Meglio, M.; Cioni, B.; D'Annunzio, V., et al.: Confronto dei risultati ottenuti nella terapia della nevralgia del trigemino con la microcompressione percutanea e con la termocoagulazione selettiva del ganglio di Gasser. Proc. 33rd Annual Meeting of the Italian Society of Neurosurgery, Ferrara 1984.

7 Mullan, S.; Lichtor, T.: Percutaneous microcompression of the trigeminal ganglion for trigeminal neuralgia. J. Neurosurg. *59:* 1007–1012 (1983).

8 Sindou, M.; Keravel, Y.: Termocoagulation percutanée du trijumeau dans le traitement de la nevralgie faciale essentielle. Resultats en fonction du siège de la thermolésion. Neurochirurgie *25:* 167–172 (1979).

9 Sweet, W.H.; Wepsic, J.G.: Controlled thermocoagulation of trigeminal ganglion and rootlets for differential destruction pain fibers. 1. Trigeminal neuralgia. J. Neurosurg. *39:* 143–156 (1974).

S. Esposito, MD, Division of Neurosurgery, 'G. Lancisi' - S. Camillo Hospital, I-00123 Rome (Italy)

Proc. 9th Meeting World Soc. Stereotactic and Functional
Neurosurgery, Toronto 1985
Appl. Neurophysiol. *48:* 274–276 (1985)

Stereotactic Mesencephalic Tractotomy in the Treatment of Pancoast Syndrome

F. Frank, C. Sturiale, G. Gaist, A.P. Fabrizi, R. Frank-Ricci

Division of Neurosurgery, Bellaria Hospital, Bologna, Italy

Key Words. Oculomotor palsy · Painful dysesthesias · Pancoast syndrome · Stereotactic mesencephalic tractotomy · Stereotactic surgery

Abstract. A series of 38 patients with Pancoast syndrome treated by means of stereotactic mesencephalic tractotomy (SMT) is presented. The immediate postoperative results were good in all patients with complete pain relief, and without any impairment of respiratory function (in contrast to percutaneous cervical cordotomy). After 1–7 months' follow-up the analgesic effect was unchanged in 33 (86.8%) out of 38 patients. Six patients (15.7%) showed recurrence of pain on the same side, while 4 patients (10.5%) presented contralateral pain. Immediate postoperative side effects of oculomotor palsy (18.4%) and dysesthesias (28%) remained unchanged at follow-up in 6 patients (16%). The intervention was well tolerated by all patients, and there was no mortality.

The authors have previously reported the success of stereotactic mesencephalic tractotomy (SMT) in the treatment of malignant cancer pain syndrome [2, 3]. *Mazers* et al. [4], *Nashold* [5], *Amano* et al. [1] and *Tasker* [7] have all repeatedly reported their experiences indicating the positive outcome of this surgical procedure. However, it is noteworthy to report the target discrepancies of these authors; therefore, it is difficult to compare their results. We have used the target suggested by *Mazars* et al. [4]. In this study we used SMT in the treatment of lung cancer-related pain syndromes (Pancoast syndrome).

Materials and Method

In the past 5 years, 38 patients were treated with SMT. In 4 cases, after 1 week the procedure was performed bilaterally. The immediate analgesic results were excellent in

Table I. Immediate side effects after SMT

Side effect	%	n
Oculomotor disturbances	18.4	7
Unpleasant dysesthesias	28.7	11

Table II. Clinical follow-up (1-7 months)

Side effect	%	n
Oculomotor disturbances	8	3
Anesthesia dolorosa	8	3
Pain recurrence	13.2	5

all the patients treated. Table I shows the immediate undesired side effects. 18.4% of the patients presented with Parinaud's syndrome and/or convergent strabismus, and 28% complained of unpleasant dysesthesias.

All the procedures were performed under local anesthesia, using the Riechert stereotactic frame (Fischer Inc., Freiburg i.Br., FRG) via a frontal approach.

Discussion

The authors consider SMT the treatment of choice in Pancoast syndrome. The alternative intervention, percutaneous cervical cordotomy according to *Rosomoff* et al. [6], carries a high risk of impaired respiratory function (Ondine syndrome and respiratory paralysis). In patients with compromised respiratory function, SMT is less hazardous, because the lesion is above the respiratory control centers in the brain stem.

The lesion site of SMT is, however, near the oculomotor centers, and the proprioceptive lemniscal pathways may be partially involved.

After 1-7 months' follow-up, gaze palsies were usually transient, with permanent damage in only 3 patients (8%). The dysesthesias are generally well tolerated by the patients, and only 3 patients (8%) complained of anesthesia dolorosa (table II). The analgesic results persisted in 86.8% of the cases treated.

Conclusions

The authors' experience shows that SMT is the procedure of choice in the treatment of Pancoast syndrome. The undesired side effects are usually transient; however, painful dysesthesias are worrisome because they are difficult to treat.

References

1 Amano, K.; Iseki, H.; Notani, M.: Rostral mesencephalic reticulotomy for pain relief. Report of 15 cases. Acta neurochir. *30:* suppl., pp. 391–393 (1980).
2 Frank, F.; Tognetti, F.; Gaist, G.; Frank, G.; Galassi, E.; Sturiale, C.: Stereotaxic rostral mesencephalotomy in treatment of malignant faciothoracobrachial pain syndromes. J. Neurosurg. *56:* 807–811 (1982).
3 Frank, F.; Frank, G.; Gaist, G.; Sturiale, C.; Fabrizi, A.: Rostral stereotactic mesencephalotomy in treatment of cancer pain: a survey of 40 treated patients. Acta neurochir. *33:* suppl., pp. 437–443 (1984).
4 Mazars, G.; Pansini, A.; Chiarelli, J.: Coagulation du faisceau spino-thalamique et du faisceau quinto-thalamique par stéréotaxie. Indications-résultats. Acta neurochir. *8:* 324–326 (1960).
5 Nashold, B.S., Jr.: Extensive cephalic and oral pain relieved by midbrain tractotomy. Confinia neurol. *34:* 382–388 (1972).
6 Rosomoff, H.L.; Krieger, A.J.; Kuperman, A.S.: Effects of percutaneous cervical cordotomy on pulmonary function. J. Neurosurg. *31:* 620–627 (1969).
7 Tasker, R.R.: Somatotopographic representation in the human thalamus, midbrain, and spinal cord; in Morley, Current controversies in neurosurgery, pp. 485–495, (Saunders, Philadelphia 1976).

F. Frank, MD, Division of Neurosurgery, Bellaria Hospital, via Altura 3,
I-40139 Bologna (Italy)

Proc. 9th Meeting World Soc. Stereotactic and Functional
Neurosurgery, Toronto 1985
Appl. Neurophysiol. *48:* 277–280 (1985)

A Method for Bulbospinal Trigeminal Nucleotomy in the Treatment of Facial Deafferentation Pain

Jose M. Siqueira

Hospital Felicio Rocho, Belo Horizonte, MG, Brazil

Key Words. Anesthesia dolorosa · Postherpetic pain · Subnucleus caudalis · Trigeminal nucleotomy

Abstract. Many types of facial pain are difficult to treat, such as postherpetic, post-traumatic, or pain following denervation procedures used in the treatment of trigeminal neuralgia (anesthesia dolorosa), all of which involve deafferentation of the spinal trigeminal nucleus.

A method for bulbospinal trigeminal nucleotomy in the treatment of facial deafferentation pain in 2 patients, 1 with severe facial pain following a complete traumatic lesion of the trigeminal nerve (anesthesia dolorosa) and other with postherpetic neuralgia, is described.

The patients were operated on under general anesthesia in the prone position. After a small posterior fossa craniectomy and C1-C2 laminectomy the dura was opened in the midline. Under the operating microscope the C2 posterior rootlets and the fourth ventricle were identified. In both patients the distance between the obex and the C2 posterior rootlets was 20 mm. A point 5 mm below and 6.5 mm lateral to the obex was delineated. This point was used as an upper limit when placing the radiofrequency lesions. An imaginary line was drawn between this point and the C2 posterior rootlets. This line corresponded to a region of the bulbospinal junction located lateral to the fasciculus cuneatus and posterior to the accessory nerve spinal rootlets. Using the

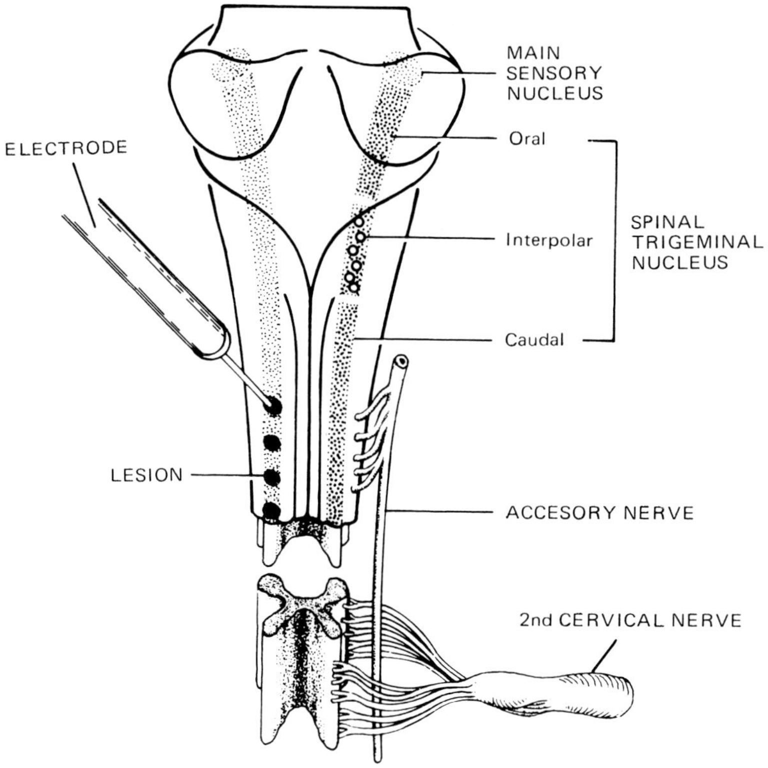

Fig. 1. Schematic representation of the surgical technique. See text for description.

same standard electrode as for percutaneous cordotomy, five radiofrequency lesions were made every 3 mm along this line at 30 mA and 30 s each [1–8].

A complete abolition of the pain was achieved in both patients. Until now, almost 1 year postoperatively, both patients are well and without pain.

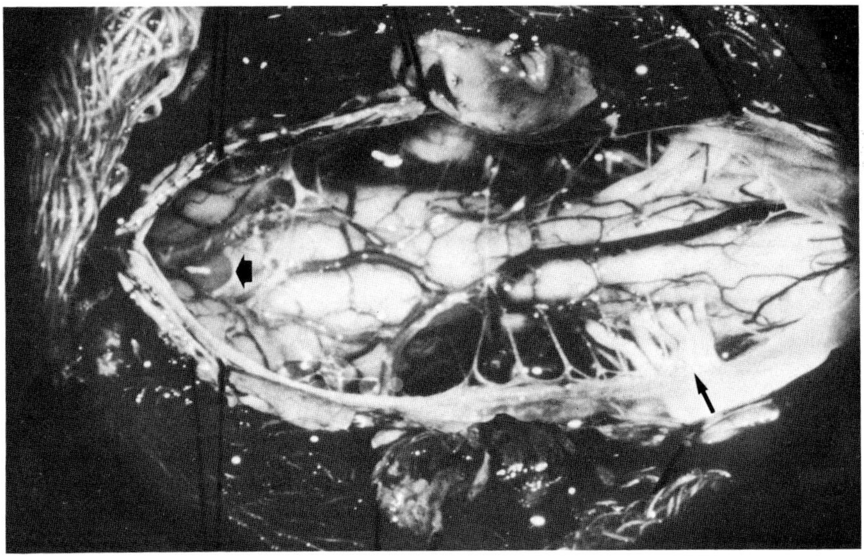

Fig. 2. Operative photograph showing the fourth ventricle and the second cervical posterior rootlets.

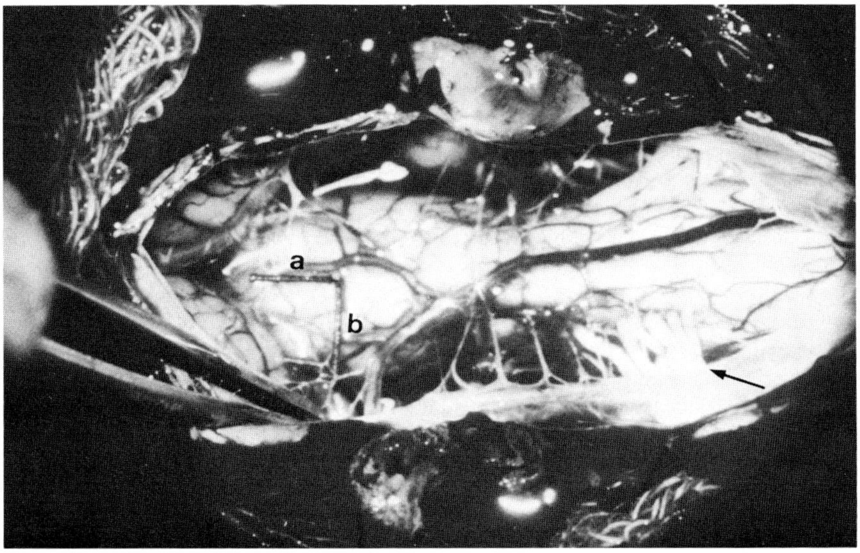

Fig. 3. Operative photograph showing a point 5 mm below (a) and 6.5 mm lateral (b) to the obex. The arrow points to the second cervical posterior rootlets.

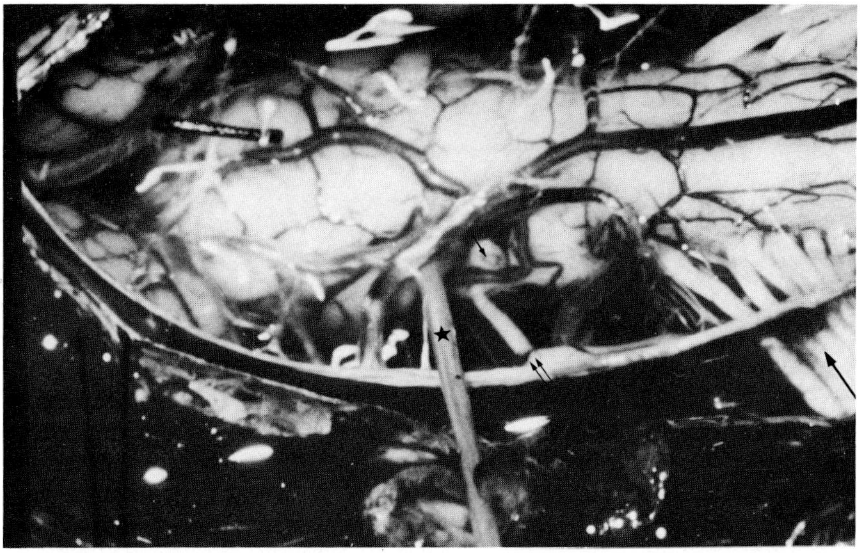

Fig. 4. The long arrow points to the second cervical posterior rootlets; the single small arrow points to a radiofrequency lesion. The two small arrows point to an accessory nerve spinal rootlet and the asterisk indicates the lesion electrode.

References

1 Anderson, L.S.; Black, R.G.; Abraham, J.; Ward, A.A., Jr.: Neuronal hyperactivity in experimental trigeminal deafferentation. J. Neurosurg. *35:* 444–452 (1971).

2 Brodal, A.: Neurological anatomy in relation to clinical medicine (Oxford University Press, New York 1981).

3 Friedman, A.H.; Nashold, B.S., Jr.; Ovelmen-Levitt, J.: Dorsal root entry zone lesions for the treatment of post-herpetic neuralgia. J. Neurosurg. *60:* 1258–1262 (1984).

4 Nashold, B.S., Jr.; Ostdahl, R.M.: Dorsal root entry zone lesions for pain relief. J. Neurosurg. *51:* 59–69 (1979).

5 Nashold, B.S., Jr.; Bullitt, E.: Dorsal root entry zone lesions to control central pain in paraplegics. J. Neurosurg. *55:* 414–419 (1981).

6 Samii, M.; Moringlane, J.R.: Thermocoagulation of the dorsal root entry zone for the treatment of intractable pain. Neurosurgery *15:* 953–955 (1984).

7 Schvarcz, J.R.: Postherpetic craniofacial dysaesthesiae: their management by stereotaxic trigeminal nucleotomy. Acta neurochir. *38:* 65–72 (1977).

8 Schvarcz, J.R.: Spinal cord stereotactic techniques re trigeminal nucleotomy and extralemniscal myelotomy. Appl. Neurophysiol. *41:* 99–112 (1978).

J.M. Siqueira, MD, Av. do Contorno, 9530, Hospital Felicio Rocho,
Belo Horizonte, MG (Brazil)

Proc. 9th Meeting World Soc. Stereotactic and Functional
Neurosurgery, Toronto 1985
Appl. Neurophysiol. *48:* 281–282 (1985)

A Quantitative Determination of Stimulation Parameters of Transcutaneous Electrical Nerve Stimulation for Pain Relief

B.H. Sjölund

Educational Branch, Medical Board of the Armed Forces, Karolinen, Karlstad, Sweden

Key Words. Transcutaneous electrical nerve stimulation · Parameters · Nocifensive reflex · Rat

Transcutaneous electrical nerve stimulation (TENS) is now a well-established technique to alleviate chronic pain [1, 2]. We have previously found that when conventional, high frequency TENS does not produce pain relief, short impulse trains at a low repetition rate and at an intensity evoking muscle twitches may produce analgesia (acupuncture-like TENS [3]. This analgesia is probably mediated via an endorphinergic link [4].

It is thus important to systematically investigate which afferent inputs should be activated at which parameters to most effectively suppress transmission of nociceptive information. To avoid subjective pain ratings from patients, the size of a C-fiber evoked nocifensive flexion reflex in the lightly anesthetized rat has been utilized as a measure of such transmission in the present study. This reflex activity parallels the impulse pattern in important parts of the spinothalamic pathways [5]. In a previous study [6], I reported the results of conditioning high frequency continuous stimulation in this model. I have now extended the study to include conditioning stimulation with short trains at a low repetition rate.

Briefly, Wistar rats, anesthetized with N_2O–O_2–halothane, had their plantar (Pl), sural (Sur) and gastrocnemius (Gastr) nerves dissected for stimulation and their common peroneal (Per) and sciatic (Sci) nerves dissected for bipolar recording on one side. Conditioning stimulation of a skin (Sur) or a muscle (Gastr) nerve for 30 min with trains of 8 or 16 pulses at 100 Hz, given at repetition rates of 1 or 5 Hz, was delivered at strengths recruiting coarse myelinated (2 T) or fine myelinated (10 T) afferents. Test stimulation was given at 100 T to the Pl nerve and the nocifensive reflex was recorded in the Per nerve, rectified and integrated for quantification.

Only one combination of parameters produced a significant inhibition with skin nerve stimulation, namely trains of 8 pulses at 1 Hz repetition rate with a high stimulus intensity. On the other hand, all parameters tested produced inhibition with muscle nerve stimulation. It thus seems important to put electrodes over muscle nerves when treating with low frequency, acupuncture-like ('burst') TENS.

Acknowledgement

Supported by Medtronic Inc. and the Swedish MRC (project No. 05658).

References

1 Eriksson, M.; Sjölund, B.; Nielzén, S.: Pain, *6:* 335-347 (1979).
2 Eriksson, M.; Sjölund, B.; Sundbärg, G.: J. Neurosurg. *61:* 149-155 (1984).
3 Eriksson, M.; Sjölund, B.: In Zotterman, Sensory functions of the skin, pp. 575-581. (Pergamon, Oxford 1976).
4 Sjölund, B.; Eriksson, M.: Brain Res. *173:* 295-301 (1979).
5 Schoenborg, J.; Sjölund, B.: J. Neurophysiol. *50:* 1108-1121 (1983).
6 Sjölund, B.: J. Neurosurg. (in press, 1985).

B.H. Sjölund, MD, Educational Branch, Medical Board of the Armed Forces, Karolinen, S-65180 Karlstad (Sweden)

Proc. 9th Meeting World Soc. Stereotactic and Functional
Neurosurgery, Toronto 1985
Appl. Neurophysiol. *48:* 283–287 (1985)

Stereotactic Pallidotomy in Extrapyramidal Disorders

J. Burzaco

Servicio de Neurocirurgia, Fundación Jimenez Diaz, Madrid, Spain

Key Words. Pallidotomy · Extrapyramidal disorders · Spatial representation · Stereotactic surgery · Surgical indication

Abstract. The results of stereotactic pallidotomy in 37 patients with extrapyramidal disorders are presented. All patients had the same RF lesions and target coordinates. The patients are classified into 5 groups according to the clinical picture. These results are compared with those obtained by thalamotomy in a similar group of patients. The main indications for pallidotomy are given. The spatial representation of globus pallidus medialis according to Andrews and Watkins, Talairach and the author are shown and their differences discussed.

Stereotactic pallidotomy was used for the first time in 1947 by *Spiegel and Wycis* [4] to receive hyperkinesia in an athetotic patient. In the fifties the globus pallidus medialis was a frequently used target for the stereotactic treatment of Parkinson's disease, but its use later declined in favor of thalamic lesions.

Patients

During the period 1962–1984, we operated on 82 patients with extrapyramidal disorders. Pallidotomy was performed in 37 patients; in 24 it was a unilateral lesion, and in 12 it was combined with a contralateral thalamotomy. Only in 1 case did we do a bilateral pallidotomy.

The patients have been classified into 5 groups according to the clinical symptomatology:

Group I – bilateral dystonic-hyperkinetic syndromes (21 patients/10 pallidotomies): A history of birth injury is the common etiological factor in all the patients of this group. Most patients were severely disabled by a combination of dystonic symptoms, choreoathetotic movements and a variable degree of spasticity and motor palsy. The operation was performed in order to relieve some of the most severe symptoms that made the daily attendance of the patient very troublesome.

Group II – focal dystonic-hyperkinetic syndrome (21 patients/8 pallidotomies): The symptoms mainly affect one limb or one side of the body. The etiology is diverse: vascular, traumatic, injury at birth, etc.

Group III – bilateral hyperkinetic syndromes (12 patients/3 pallidotomies): Patients in this group suffered from Huntington's chorea, multiple sclerosis, tremor. Three of the patients have had a contralateral thalamotomy before.

Group IV – bilateral dystonic syndromes (16 patients/10 pallidotomies): Most of these patients suffered from dystonia muscularum deformans. Five also had contralateral thalamotomy.

Group V – torticollis (12 patients/7 pallidotomies): Patients with purely neck symptoms and patients showing slight extrapyramidal disturbances limited to the face or to one limb. If the extrapyramidal symptoms were more relevant the patient was included in one of the other groups. The only case of bilateral pallidotomy was performed in a patient with torticollis.

Pallidotomy was selected as the surgical target (1) when hypertonic or dystonic symptoms predominated, (2) to avoid bilateral symmetrical thalamic lesions, (3) in the dominant hemisphere when there was concern about speech disturbances.

All patients were operated using Leksell's technique, bipolar RF thermolesion, 8 mm long × 6 mm wide, at 65–67 °C. Target coordinates: X = 4 mm in front of the mid-intercommissural plane; Y = 1 mm above the bicommissural line; Z = 19 mm lateral to the midline. Local anesthesia was used routinely.

Results

The evaluation of the results obtained after pallidotomy is based on the five-grade standard scale: R-1, symptoms abolished or greatly reduced with good functional capacity. R-2, great improvement of the dystonic or hyperkinetic symptoms but functional capacity is reduced. R-3, slight improvement or unsatisfactory functional recovery. R-4, no significant change in the patient's status. R-5, some sort of deterioration occurs after the operation.

The results of pallidotomy for the 5 clinical groups are shown in table I. In table II, the results R-1 and R-2 of pallidotomy can be compared with those of thalamotomy in the 5 groups of patients. The good results of pallidotomy in the dystonic syndromes, both focal and bilateral, and the satisfactory effects of thalamotomy in the bilateral hyperkinetic group as well as in the dystonic group are noteworthy. The results are rather poor for both types of lesions in group I, as should be expected in cerebral palsy patients.

Table I. Extrapyramidal syndromes

Group	Syndrome	Pallidotomy					Total
		R-1	R-2	R-3	R-4	R-5	
I	Bilateral D-H	–	5	5	–	–	10
II	Focal D-H	2	4	2	–	–	8
III	Bilateral H	–	1	2	–	–	3
IV	Bilateral D	5	3	2	–	–	10
V	Torticollis	1	3	3	–	–	7
	Total	8	16	14			38

D = dystonic; H = hyperkinetic

Table II. Extrapyramidal syndromes, percent satisfactory results

Group	Syndrome	Pallidotomy		Thalamotomy	
		%	n	%	n
I	Bilateral D-H	50	5/10	46	7/15
II	Focal D-H	75	6/8	81	9/11
III	Bilateral H	33	1/3	57	8/14
IV	Bilateral D	80	8/10	69	9/13
V	Torticollis	57	4/7	57	4/7
	Total	63		61	

Discussion

The purpose of the classification of extrapyramidal disorder patients into 5 groups is to gather the few objective items that one can find in these various cases to analyze the results on a more objective basis.

Torticollis should, from the standpoint of surgical treatment, be considered as a different entity from dystonia, although as a rule is classified as a localized form of a dystonic syndrome. The 12 patients with torticollis exhibited marked differences in the age of onset, clinical picture and evolution as compared with those patients with focal or

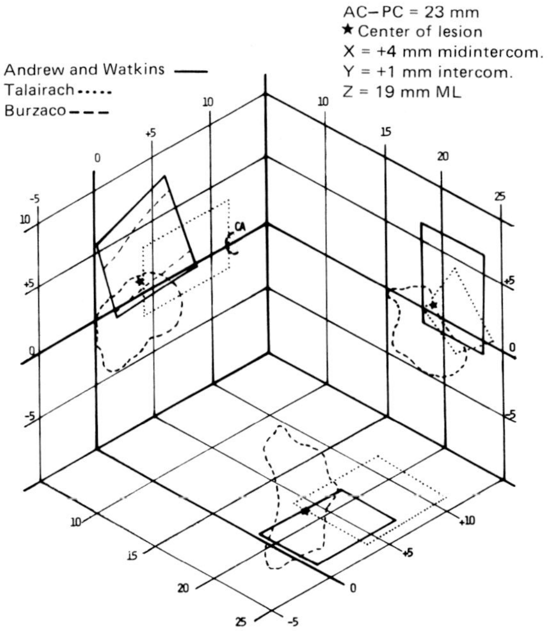

Fig. 1. A three-plane representation of the globus pallidus medialis in three different locations.

bilateral syndromes. On the other hand, torticollis responds to pallidal and thalamic lesions quite differently than do the dystonic syndromes.

There is no significant difference in the overall results between pallidotomy and thalamotomy, although it seems evident that the response of hyperkinetic symptoms to thalamotomy is much better than that of pallidotomy, but the reverse is true in dystonic symptoms.

Speech disturbances are among the most distressing side effects in stereotactic surgery. Out of 47 dominant hemisphere lesions, the incidence of immediate transitory speech disturbances has been 14% in 16 pallidotomies, and 17% in 31 thalamotomies. We find that recovery is better for pallidal complications. The only 3 cases with serious permanent dysphasia were patients with bilateral thalamotomy.

In general, it can be said that the immediate results of pallidotomy may look less dramatic than those of thalamotomy, but in the long term, pallidotomy patients get a better functional result.

Figure 1 is a three-plane representation of the globus pallidus medialis in three different locations: *Talairach's* demarcation area, *Andrews and Watkins'* [1] medial statistical value, and the 'safety area' elaborated by us [2] from *Shaltenbrand and Bailey's* [3] 'Atlas of the Human Brain'. There are some significant variations in the GPM location: Talairach's demarcation is more frontal than Andrews and Watkins' medial statistical value, or our safety area. On the other hand, Talairach and Andrews and Watkins locate the GPM mainly above the AC-PC plane, while we locate it mainly below that plane. The values of Talairach's and Andrews and Watkins' representation of GPM have been corrected to fit with a AC-PC distance of 23 mm.

These differences justify new studies in order to clarify more precisely the anatomical location of the globus pallidus medialis, if this structure is to continue to be used as a stereotactic target.

References

1 Andrews, J.; Watkins, E.S.: A stereotaxic atlas of the human thalamus and adjacent structures (Williams & Wilkins, Baltimore 1969).
2 Burzaco, J.A.: Sistema de representación tridimensión de los nucleos mesodiencefalicos para uso en cirugia estereotactica; tesis Madrid (1972).
3 Shaltenbrand, G.; Bailey, P.: Introduction to stereotaxis with an atlas of the human brain, vol. 3 (Thieme, Stuttgart 1959).
4 Spiegel, E.A.; Wycis, H.T.: Development of stereoencephalotomy for extrapyramidal diseases. J. Neurosurg. *24:* 433–439 (1966).
5 Talairach, J.; David, M.; Tournoux, P.; Corredor, H.; Kvasina, T.: Atlas d'anatomie stéréotaxique (Masson, Paris 1957).

Dr. J.A. Burzaco, Servicio de Neurocirurgia, Fundación Jimenez Diaz,
Av. Reyes Catolicos 2, E-28003 Madrid (Spain)

Proc. 9th Meeting World Soc. Stereotactic and Functional
Neurosurgery, Toronto 1985
Appl. Neurophysiol. *48:* 288–292 (1985)

Plastic Change of Thalamic Organization in Patients with Tremor after Stroke

C. Ohye, T. Shibazaki, T. Hirai, Y. Kawashima, M. Hirato, M. Matsumura

Department of Neurosurgery, Gunma University School of Medicine, Maebashi, Gunma, Japan

Key Words. Human thalamus · Microrecording · Stereotactic thalamotomy · Tremor after stroke · Reorganization

Abstract. Thirteen patients with tremor after stroke were treated by stereotactic thalamotomy. Prior to making therapeutic lesions, microrecordings were tried and the findings were compared with our own results obtained in Parkinson's disease. Several characteristic features were revealed in terms of changes in electrical activity in and around the thalamic Vim nucleus. These findings support the idea that reorganization of the thalamic sensory nuclei might take place.

Selective stereotactic Vim (ventralis intermedius) thalamotomy using a microelectrode has been shown to be quite reliable and satisfactory for ameliorating various kinds of tremor [1,4]. In a previous study, however, we have shown that the coagulation volume necessary for arresting tremor after stroke is often much more (200–300 mm^3) than that for parkinsonian (PA) tremor (40–60 mm^3).

To elucidate the neural basis underlying the possible thalamic disorganization in stroke cases, an electrophysiological study was conducted in 13 operated cases with tremor after stroke.

Using Leksell's stereotactic apparatus, a pair of semimicroelectrodes (bipolar concentric type, outer diameter 0.3 mm, tip about 10–20 μm, interpolar distance about 0.3 mm, electrical resistance 100 $k\Omega$) were introduced from the prefrontal area to the lower border of the Vim nucleus. Basic neural activity and unitary and multiunitary spike discharges were analyzed. Observations were made in awake patients under local anesthesia.

Table I. Post-CVD tremor (1982–1985/6)

No.	Case	Sex	Age	Central damage	Ope.	Tracking	Background activity	Kinesth. neuron	Effect
I	K.T.	m	51	(pons)	1	4	low	(eye mov.)	B
II	K.F.	f	63	cerebell.	1	2	low	4 (face:4)	A
III	S.W.	f	64	(thal.)	1	4	low	(eye mov.)	A
IV	T.S.	m	22	cerebell.	1	6	low	1+2 tactile }	B
								(face: 8)	↓
	T.S.	m	22	cerebell.	2	4	low	6+3 tactile }	A→B
V	H.M.	m	42	pons	1	4	high	(eye mov.)	A
VI	Y.S	f	61	thal.	1	2	high	3 (face: 1)	A
VII	K.A.	f	47	midbrain	1	2	low	rhythm × 2	A

Among 13 cases, 6 were treated before 1980 and 7 after 1981. In the early series, using the same tentative target point as in cases with PA, kinesthetic neurons were recorded from Vim in only 2 cases with general low background activity. Consequently, the results of thalamic surgery were not satisfactory: complete tremor arrest in 3 cases, slight residual in 1 and considerable residual in 2. Therefore, since 1981, we changed the strategy slightly, and in the next 7 cases (1 was operated twice) electrical activity in and around the Vim nucleus was extensively explored (table I). Thus, several characteristic features in terms of changes in electrical activity compared with that in PA were found. In summary: (1) The general basic activity was much lower than that in PA. In a total of 8 explorations, reduced activity was found in 6 and high activity in 2. This might be relevant to the fact that in the latter 2 cases with thalamic high basic activity, severe paresthesia was noticed clinically together with the tremulous involuntary movement [2]. (2) Sensory neurons, including kinesthetic neurons, were less frequently encountered. In cases with tremor after stroke, a total of 21 sensory neurons were found in 28 trackings (21/28 = 0.75), while in PA, for example, 48 sensory neurons in 40 trackings (48/40 = 1.2). (3) Among 21 sensory neurons, adequate natural peripheral stimuli were determined. Five (24%) responded to tactile (surface, light touch) and 16 (76%) to

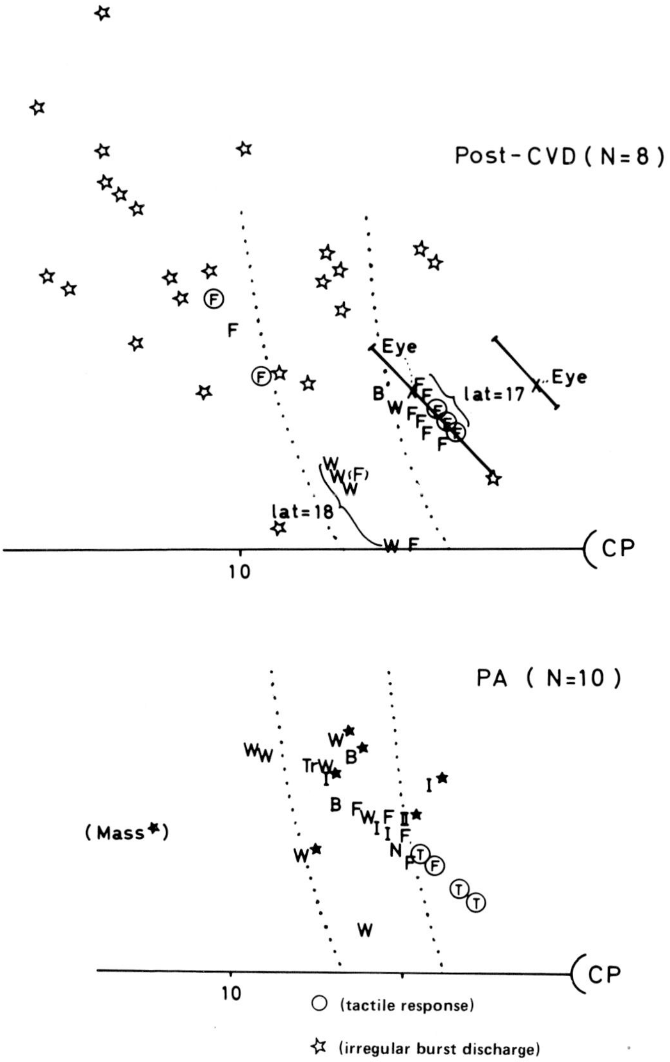

Fig. 1. Profile of thalamic distribution of the identified sensory neurons and burst discharge during the course of stereotactic thalamotomy for tremor after stroke (upper) and Parkinson's disease (lower). Recorded points are represented by a capital letter related to each peripheral receptive field (B = biceps; Eye = ocular movement; F = face; I = thumb; II = index finger; N = neck; Tr = triceps; W = wrist). Area between dotted lines is standard Vim area. These points were reconstructed from X-ray film referring to commissure posterior (cp) and intercommissural line (horizontal line).

deep or kinesthetic stimuli (compression of the muscle, passive and active movement of joint, or tapping). This proportion was contrasted to 8% (tactile) and 92% (deep), respectively in PA's thalamus. (4) These tactile and kinesthetic neurons were distributed in and around the Vim nucleus, intermingling with each other (fig. 1). In cases with PA, there was clear-cut separation; kinesthetic neurons were found rostrally and tactile neurons caudally. (5) Sensory neurons representing the face area were encountered in an extremely high percentage, 8 among 16 kinesthetic neurons (50%). In PA, this ratio was about 15% in our experience. (6) In general, in our systematic tracking in the Vim area in PA, kinesthetic neurons representing the contralateral upper limb were the most frequent (64%). However, in this series, upper limb neurons were found only in 7%. (7) Slow rhythmic discharge synchronous with abnormal ocular movement was recorded in 3 cases. In one particular case with pontine hemorrhage, this kind of slow rhythmic discharge was encountered in a wide area in the rostral part of the ventralis caudalis (VC) nucleus, (referring to the standard atlas of the human thalamus) (fig. 1). In the thalamus of PA, neurons related to the ocular movement were never recorded. (8) Many irregular burst activities were encountered in the dorsal part of the Vim nucleus and its rostral part (fig. 1), which was reminiscent of the findings in the thalamus of cases with writing tremor [5]. In cases with PA, rhythmic activity time-locked with tremor were easily found but irregular burst activities were rare.

All these findings are quite different from those in PA, in which basic activity is very high in the Vim area and, within it, kinesthetic neurons were topographically organized, and separately distributed from tactile neurons [3]. The difference might be attributed to the possible reorganization that took place after the vascular accident in the area connected, more or less, to this particular thalamic nucleus. The results of operation in the 7 patients in the later series are much better; complete arrest in 5 and slight residual in 2.

References

1 Hirai, T.; Miyazaki, M; Nakajima, H.; Shibazaki, T.; Ohye, C.: The correlation between tremor characteristics and predicted volume of effective lesions in stereotaxic Vim thalamotomy. Brain *106:* 1001–1018 (1983).

2 Hirato, M.; Kawashima, Y.; Wada, H.; Nagaseki, Y.; Hirai, T.; Shibazaki, T.; Denda, Y.; Ohye, C.: Quantitative analysis of neural activity of the thalamic Vim nucleus in patients with thalamic pain. Appl. Neurophysiol. *47:* 85–86 (1984).
3 Ohye, C.: Depth microelectrode studies; in Schaltenbrand, Walker, Stereotaxy of the human brain, pp. 372–389 (Thieme, Stuttgart 1982).
4 Ohye, C.; Hirai, T.; Miyazaki, M.; Shibazaki, T.; Nakajima, H.: Vim thalamotomy for the treatment of various kinds of tremor. Appl. Neurophysiol. *45:* 275–280 (1982).
5 Ohye, C.; Miyazaki, M.; Hirai, T.; Shibazaki, T.; Nakajima, H.; Nagaseki, Y.: Primary writing tremor treated by stereotactic selective thalamotomy. J. Neurol. Neurosurg. Psychiat. *45:* 988–997 (1982).

C. Ohye, MD, Department of Neurosurgery, Gunma University School of Medicine, 3-39 Showa-machi, Maebashi, Gunma (Japan)

Proc. 9th Meeting World Soc. Stereotactic and Functional
Neurosurgery, Toronto 1985
Appl. Neurophysiol. *48:* 293 (1985)

Postoperative and Long-Term Results of 1,561 Stereotactic Operations in Parkinsonism

F. Mundinger

Neurochirurgische Universitätsklinik, Freiburg i. Br., FRG

Key Words. Parkinson's disease · Stereotactic surgery

Abstract. Out of a series of 3,808 (31.5.84) Parkinson operations the postoperative and long-term results of 1,561 stereotactic procedures are evaluated. The results are compared, especially in respect to the focus of therapeutic lesion (internal pallidum, oral ventral nuclei, subthalamic zona incerta and radiatio prelemniscalis). In the long range, tremor and rigidity are abolished or markedly improved in more than 80%, the associated Parkinson symptoms in between one and two thirds of cases. In the further development of the diseases the progression of the positive symptoms is blocked as well as the medically induced dyskinesia. The ability for work and better living are achieved in 60% and amelioration of the psychic situation in 30% of the cases. Operative mortality is 0.4% and morbidity is less than 2%.

Prof. Dr. F. Mundinger, Neurochirurgische Universitätsklinik,
Hugstetter Strasse 55, D-7800 Freiburg i.Br. (FRG)

Proc. 9th Meeting World Soc. Stereotactic and Functional
Neurosurgery, Toronto 1985
Appl. Neurophysiol. *48:* 294–304 (1985)

Present Role of Stereotactic Thalamotomy for Parkinsonism

Retrospective Analysis of Operative Results and Thalamic Lesions in Computed Tomograms

T. Miyamoto, H. Bekku, E. Moriyama, S. Tsuchida

Department of Neurosurgery, Fukuyama National Hospital, Fukuyama City, Hiroshima, Japan

Key Words. Parkinson's disease · Stereotactic surgery · Thalamus · Tomography · CT scanning

Abstract. 14 cases of unilateral and 5 cases of bilateral thalamotomy for parkinsonism were reviewed, with 32–144 months' (mean 67.8) and 54–212 months' (mean 110) follow-up, respectively, after the initial operation. Rigidity and tremor disappeared in approximately 80% of cases and was reduced in the remaining 20%. 68% improved by one or two grades in the Hoehn-Yahr scale after operation. Thalamotomy abolished dyskinesias and on-off phenomena on the operated sides. 36% of cases discontinued levodopa therapy after operation. CT study of the lesions suggested that destruction of a large part of basal Vop was most important to obtain the best results.

Materials and Methods

19 parkinsonian patients who underwent ventrolateral (VL) thalamotomy were reviewed. There were 15 women and 5 men, with ages ranging from 33 to 70 (mean 56.9) years at the time of the first operation. The 14 cases operated on unilaterally were followed-up 1–70 months (mean 18.2) preoperatively and for 33–144 months (mean 67.8) postoperatively. The 5 cases with bilateral surgery were followed up for 1–62 months (mean 24.8) before the first operation, 2–9 years (25–35 months in 4 cases) before the second operation. These patients were divided into subgroups according to the Hoehn-Yahr scale [2] as shown in figure 1.

Thalamotomy was used to treat rigidity and/or tremor in normal patients or those with slightly abnormal EEG and CT examinations whose disabilities were mainly caused by tremor and rigidity predominantly on one side either as an initial treatment or following levodopa. Background EEG α averaged 9–10 Hz in 8, and 8.0–8.5 Hz in 7 of the 18

Grade	First exam.	First op. preop.	First op. postop.	Second op. preop.	Second op. postop.	Final state
N			●			○ ▲
I	○○ ●	○ ●	○○ △△△△ □ ▲	●	●▲	○ △△△ ●
II	△△△ △△ ▲▲	○ △△△ ◎ ▲	△□□□ ◎◎ ◇ ▲■◉	▲		△ □□□□ ◎◎ ■
III	□□ □□ ■	△△ □□□□ ■			▲■◉	◇ ▲◉
IV	◎◎ ◉	◎ ◇ ▲◉		▲■◉		
V	◇					
death						△

Fig. 1. Clinical courses of the disabilities according to Hoehn-Yahr's grading of patients with unilateral and bilateral thalamotomy. An open figure shows a patient destined for unilateral surgery, and a closed figure shows a patient destined for bilateral surgery. Symbols: single circle = grade 1 at first examination; triangle = grade II; square = grade III; double circle = grade IV; diamond = grade V.

cases examined. Cerebral atrophy as shown by CT was minimal in 11 and slight in 8 out of the 19 cases.

Using the Sugita stereotactic apparatus, electrothermal coagulation was carried out at 65 or 70 °C for 1–2 min with electrodes whose exposed tips measured 3–4.5 mm in length and 1.8 mm in diameter in the Vop nucleus so that the electrode tip was located 2 mm above the inferior border of the thalamus.

For retrospective analysis of the lesions, CT scans were made within a few days and 2 months to a few years after surgery, the lesions being plotted on a horizontal section of the brain from *Schaltenbrand and Bailey's* [12] atlas.

Daily drug dosages were as follows: 750–2,500 mg levodopa, 200–750 mg levodopa/20–75 mg carbidopa as a combined preparation, 100–300 mg amantadine, 6 mg trihexyphenidyl-HCl, 6 mg piroheptine-HCl, and 3 mg biperiden.

Table I. Effects of VL thalamotomy on major signs and symptoms of parkinsonism

		First operation		Second operation	
		discharge	follow-up	discharge	follow-up
Rigidity	disappeared	14	14	4	4
	reduced	3	3	1	1
Tremor	disappeared	9	10	2	2
	reduced	3	2		
Gait disturbances	disappeared	10	7	1	1
	reduced	7	8	4	4
	worsened		2		
Incoordination	disappeared	16	13	3	3
	reduced	1	4	2	2
Progression in nonoperated side or of axial signs	yes		11		2
	no		6		3

Results

Table I presents the effects of surgery on the presenting parkinsonian features in the 19 cases.

Contralateral rigidity disappeared in 78% (11/14) after the first operation and 80% (4/5) after the second-sided operation. In the remaining cases, reduction of rigidity was observed. Surgical benefits were maintained throughout the follow-up periods.

Tremor disappeared in 75% (9/12) at discharge from the hospital after the first operation and 80% at the last follow-up. In all bilateral cases, tremor disappeared completely. Gait disturbances improved contralaterally in all cases early after discharge following the first operation, but the effects declined so that the incidence of gait disturbances fell from the initial 59% (10/17) to 47% (7/17) at later follow-up. Although definite improvement of gait was also observed in all patients operated upon bilaterally, only 20% (1/5) were free of impairment, because of increased akinesia. Incoordination of upper limbs initially improved in all cases, but it later got worse – 76% (13/17) after

Table II. Effects of VL thalamotomy on medical treatment for parkinsonism

	Cases n	Stop or no need	Main-tained	In-creased	Changed to LD	CD	CA
Unilateral operation							
Levodopa (LD)	6	1[1]	3			1	1[1]
Levodopa Carbidopa (CD)	6	1[1]	1	1	2		1[1]
Anticholinergics (C) Amantadine (A)	2		1[1]		1		
Bilateral operation							
LD 1st op.	4		1			3	
2nd op.	1			1			
CD 2nd op.	3		2	1			
CA 1st op.	1		1[1]				
2nd op.	1		1[1]				

[1] Patients with no levodopa or levodopa/carbidopa treatment.

the first operation and 60% (3/5) after the second operation. Progression of neurological signs and symptoms on the nonoperated side or axial signs were seen in 65% (11/17) after the first operation, but the remaining 35% escaped from progression of major parkinsonian signs. In 40% of bilateral cases, no progression of symptoms was observed.

Table II shows the various drugs used before and after operation. Levodopa alone or combined levodopa/carbidopa was primarily used. Amantadine and anticholinergics were also used as an adjunct. Of 14 cases with unilateral thalamotomy, no levodopa was necessary in 5 cases (36%) and preoperative doses of levodopa were enough in 4 cases (29%) for the entire follow-up period. An increase of levodopa dose or an addition of levodopa was necessary in only 2 cases. Out of 5 cases with bilateral surgery, progression of contralateral symptoms after the first operation necessitated combined levodopa/carbidopa in 3 cases (60%) and readministration of amantadine and anticholinergics following temporary postoperative withdrawal in 1 case. After the second operation, 4 cases were maintained under levodopa therapy (including a combined carbidopa preparation) with an increase of dose in 2 cases.

One case with bilateral surgery was well controlled with 200 mg amantadine and 3 mg biperiden until 3 years after the second operation. In all, 32% (6/9) of the patients became free of levodopa treatment.

Figure 1 shows the clinical courses of 19 operated patients according to Hoehn-Yahr's scale. Postoperative progression of the disease was classified by impairment of activities of daily living (ADL) due to contralateral signs and akinesia as follows: grade I, unilateral signs or subnormal; II, slight akinesia; III, moderate akinesia, and IV, marked akinesia or on-off signs but still semi-selfsufficient in ADL.

The first operation was carried out because of progression by one or two grades in 3 cases, and because of an increase of unilateral signs with no change of grade in 6 cases, even under drug therapy. The other 8 patients were operated on 1 or 2 months after minimal medication. Postoperatively, 53% (10/19) remained in grade II, 42% (8/9) in grade I, and 1% remained normal. In bilateral cases, the disability became worse in all cases before the second operation, especially in 3 cases which progressed to grade IV. After the second surgery, the status improved by one grade in 80% at the time of discharge, whereas 40% of the patients improved two grades during the follow-up period, 1 case to normal. The overall follow-up showed that 11% (2/19) of the patients were normal, 26% grade I, 42% grade II, 16% grade III and 5% died from other causes.

Levodopa-induced dyskinesias were observed in 1 case with unilateral operation and 3 cases with bilateral operation. Dyskinesias were seen only on the nonoperated side and disappeared completely after bilateral operation.

On-off phenomena were observed in 1 case with unilateral operation and 2 with bilateral operation. The on-off phenomena disappeared after the second operation in bilateral cases, but the phenomenon recurred in 1 case with progression of akinesia 3 years after the second surgery, showing sudden association of movements even though rigidity was completely abolished.

There were no operative complications after the first surgery except transient mental confusion in 2 cases. After the second operation, mild dysarthria was observed, but was tolerable in daily verbal communication.

Figure 2 shows the localization of the thalamic lesions plotted on the *Schaltenbrand and Bailey's* atlas from available CT of 19 sides. Early postoperative CT showed much broader areas of low density in

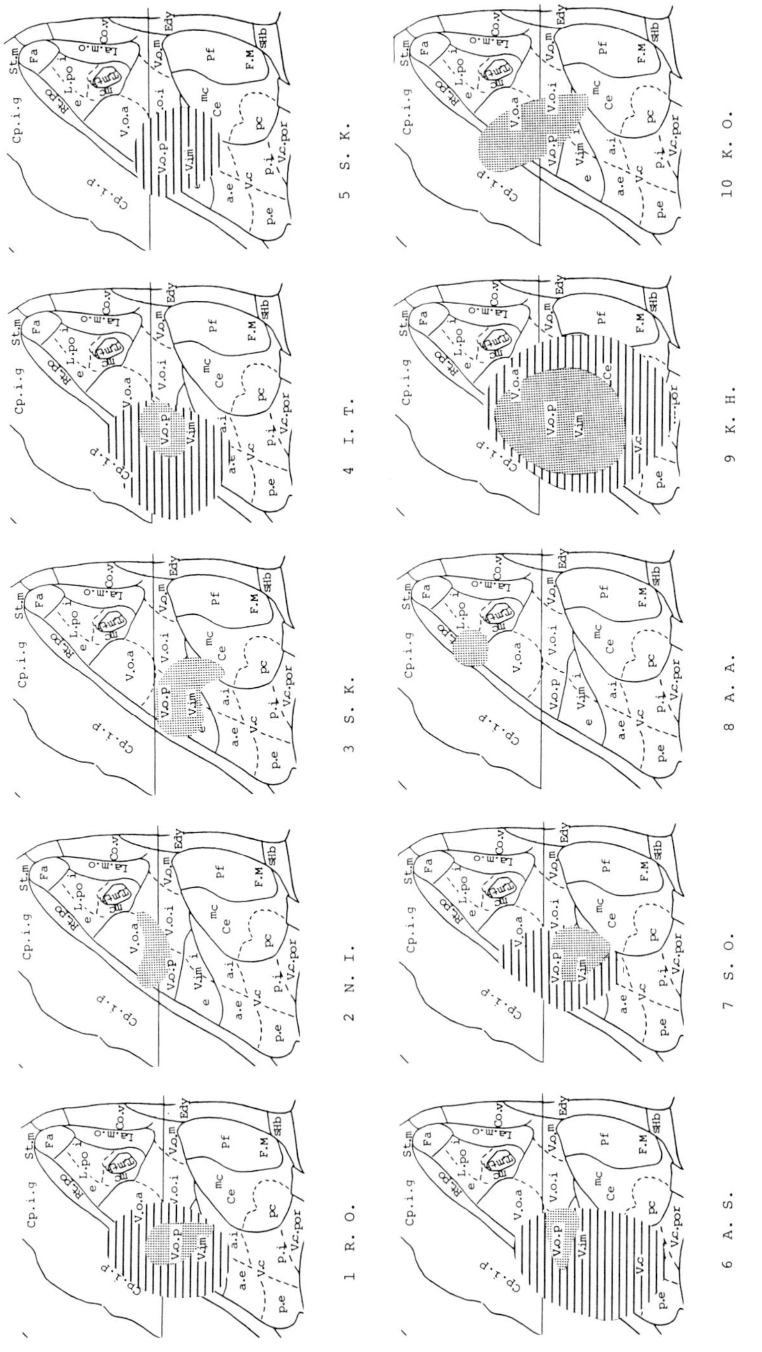
1 R. O.
2 N. I.
3 S. K.
4 I. T.
5 S. K.
6 A. S.
7 S. O.
8 A. A.
9 K. H.
10 K. O.

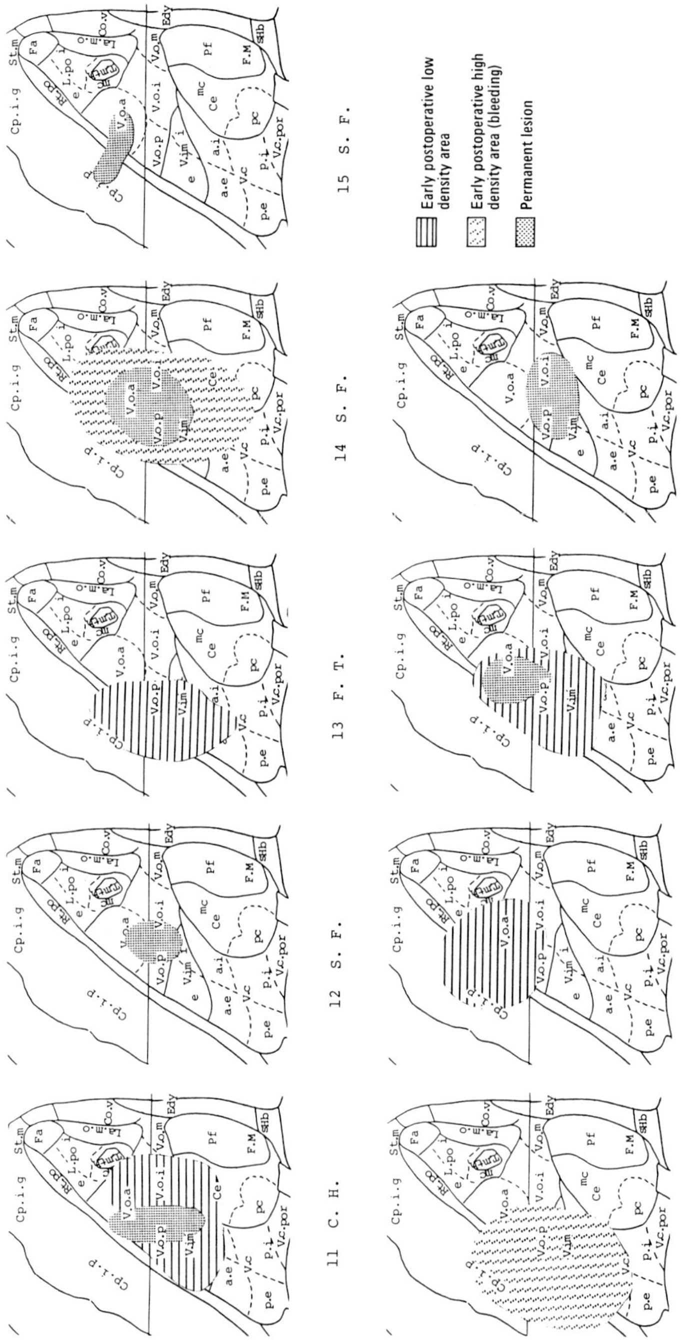
11 C. H.
12 S. F.
13 F. T.
14 S. F.
15 S. F.
16 K. O.
17 I. Y.
18 F. S.
19 S. K.
Early postoperative low density area
Early postoperative high density area (bleeding)
Permanent lesion

the ventrolateral thalamus and the adjacent structures. Some lesions displaced anteriorly and some others displaced posteriorly. The whole Vop nucleus was involved in 11 out of 12 sides of CT. However, clinical results of operation did not reflect any precise correlation with the location of the lesions, because some showed remaining rigidity or tremor after operation. High density areas indicating hemorrhage were seen in 2 cases. Two months to a few years after surgery, small lesions were observed in only one or two slices of CT images. No permanent subthalamic lesions were identified, as we intended to restrict lesions only to the thalamus.

In 6 cases with completely abolished rigidity and tremor (fig. 2, cases 1-6), 4 out of 5 permanent lesions presented as mediolaterally directed small lesions. Vop was involved fairly extensively in cases 1-4, and 6. The anterior part of Vim was also involved with transverse extension in cases 3, 4, and 6. Voa was involved only a little in case 2. In 7 cases, 7-9 and 13-16, whose rigidity was completely abolished, permanent lesions of the entire Vop nucleus were seen in 40% (2/5) of cases with permanent lesions, and others were seen in the medial half of Vop and Voa in 1 (fig. 2, case 7) in the posterior half of Voa and Cp.i.p. in 1 (case 15), and in Lpo.e. and partial Voa in the remaining case (fig. 2, case 8). Out of 3 cases with remaining tremor (cases 7-9), 1 showed a lesion of the medial half of Vop and Voa, and another showed no Vop or Vim lesion; case 9 was exceptional in that he still demonstrated a tremor, even with a total Vop and Vim lesion. In 6 cases (10-12 and 16-18) with remaining rigidity, permanent lesions extended anteroposteriorly but not mediolaterally in 80% (4/5) of cases with permanent lesions. The lateral half of Vop was not destroyed in all 5 cases. Partial posterior destruction of Voa and nearly half or more destruction of Voa was seen in 40% (2/5) respectively.

Fig. 2. CT thalamograms plotted on the atlas of *Schaltenbrand and Bailey* [12]. 1-12 show cases with both rigidity and tremor, and 13-19 show cases with rigidity alone. Both rigidity and tremor were completely abolished in 1-6. Tremor persisted in 7-9 and rigidity persisted in 10-12 and 17-19. Rigidity was abolished in 13-16. Thalamic lesions were shown on the same side of the atlas for convenience. Cases in which either early or late CT was not available show either lesion in each atlas.

Discussion

The medical treatment of Parkinson's disease, once so promising after the introduction of levodopa, is now facing many problems [3, 4, 8]. Drugs are unable to delay progression of the disease [8]. Drug effects subside with the passage of time; *Marsden and Parkes* [8] stressed that a third of 85% of patients with good initial response to treatment lost all benefit over 5 years of therapy. Oscillations in motor performances (akinetic periods and dyskinesias) and psychiatric disturbances have been very troublesome [3, 4].

Stereotactic thalamotomy until recently was regarded as an unfavorable procedure [3, 7, 13] except for a limited group of patients with tremor. On the other hand, some authors still regard thalamotomy as a useful procedure [5, 9, 10, 15, 16]. Our results show that unilateral or bilateral VL thalamotomy contributed to long-lasting relief from rigidity and/or tremor in approximately 80% of patients where these symptoms were responsible for disabilities. Thalamotomy also benefitted gait and coordination of the limbs on the operated side, even though some exacerbation or progression of akinesia was unavoidable.

In our series, thalamotomy was performed as an initial treatment of choice following failure of short-term medical therapy in 42% of our cases, or after treatment with levodopa or other drugs for 1–6 years (mean 20 months) in 48%, indicating that a period of levodopa treatment does not interfere with the operative results [5, 6, 15].

Drug therapy was continued even after operation. VL thalamotomy allowed reduced doses or discontinuation of drugs in many cases until akinesia or symptoms on the nonoperated side progressed, in contrast to Vim thalamotomy, which was reported to bring less striking improvement of rigidity and no improvement of locomotion and other skillful movements [14]. In 36% (5/14) of unilateral cases, levodopa became unnecessary and in another 29% no increase of levodopa was necessary. 20% (1/5) of bilateral cases did well only with amantadine and an anticholinergic drug, and 40% of bilaterally operated cases needed no increase of levodopa after the second operation.

These results strongly suggest that thalamotomy may delay or stop progression of the symptoms to a significant degree, as *Matsumoto* et al. stressed [9]. VL thalamotomy prevented or abolished dyskinesias and on-off phenomena with increased rigidity on the operated side, because combined surgical and medical treatment allowed significant reduction in doses of the drugs. In a recent report, drug-induced dyskinesia was abolished by a Vop and Voa lesion but not by a Vim lesion [11]. Other authors also reported VL thalamotomy abolished dyskinesias on the operated limbs [5, 9, 15]. In our series no psychiatric complications were encountered.

There are still controversies concerning bilateral thalamotomy. *Matsumoto* et al. [9] stress the beneficial effects of bilateral surgery, while other authors oppose bilateral surgery because of severe morbidity and complications [15, 16]. Our results indicate that bilateral thalamotomy can effectively alleviate parkinsonian disability and major levodopa-induced side effects. Mild but tolerable dysarthria was the only unavoidable complication [9]. Key factors for better results were an interval of more than 2 years between the first and the second operation and complete abolishment of bilateral rigidity.

Reviewing these results, the natural history of the disease [2, 8] might have been hopefully changed into slower progression by the surgical intervention [9], because most of the patients were doing better by one or two grades throughout the follow-up periods than would have been anticipated comparing with the status prior to the first operation, either in unilateral or bilateral operation. *Kelly and Gillingham's* [5] strategy of thalamotomy is to delay the start of levodopa treatment until akinesia progresses.

Finally, CT analysis of the lesions indicated that permanent thalamic lesions should be produced in the VL nucleus. Especially the lesion should be produced in Vop and Voa for rigidity, and in Vop with partial Voa and anterior part of Vim for both rigidity and tremor, although Lpo.e. or Voa lesions also abolished rigidity. Destruction of a large part of Vop as a central target at the base of the VL nucleus seemed to be critically important, as other authors reported [1, 5, 16].

References

1 Hassler, R.; Mundinger, F.; Riechert, T.: Stereotaxis in Parkinson's syndrome, pp. 236–248 (Springer, Berlin 1979).
2 Hoehn, M.M.; Yahr, M.D.: Parkinsonism: onset, progression, and mortality. Neurology *17:* 427–442 (1967).
3 Horstink, M.W.I.M.: Problems of levodopa treatment. Clin. Neurol. Neurosurg. *86:* 196–206 (1984).

4 Kase, M. Atarashi, J.; Ando, K.; Ito, K.; Ohomoto, T.: Ten years' treatment of Parkinson's disease with levodopa - observations of 239 patients in 27 institutions. Adv. neurol. Sci. *25:* 737–747 (1981).
5 Kelly, P.J.; Gillingham, F.J.: The long-term results of stereotaxic surgery and *L*-dopa therapy in patients with Parkinson's disease. A 10-year follow-up study. J. Neurosurg. *53:* 332–337 (1980).
6 Knutsson, E.; Martensson, A.; Meyerson, B.A.; Risberg, A.M.: The influence of a previous thalamotomy on the *L*-dopa effects on mono-manual dexterity in parkinsonism. Scand. J. rehabil. Med. *5:* 130–133 (1973).
7 Marsden, C.D.; Fahn, S.: Surgical approaches to dyskinesias - After-word; in Marsden, Fahn, Movement disorders, pp. 345–347 (Butterworth Scientific, London 1982).
8 Marsden, C.D.; Parkes, J.D.: Success and problems of long-term levodopa therapy in Parkinson's disease. Lancet *i:* 345–349 (1977).
9 Matsumoto, K.; Shichijo, F.; Fukami, T.: Long-term follow-up review of cases of Parkinson's disease after unilateral and bilateral thalamotomy. J. Neurosurg. *60:* 1033–1044 (1984).
10 Meyer, C.H.A.: Parkinsonism: If surgery is necessary, can it help spontaneous movement and motor fatiguing? Acta Neurochir. *54:* 149–155 (1980).
11 Narabayashi, H.; Yokochi, F.; Nakajima, Y.: Levodopa-induced dyskinesia and thalamotomy. J. Neurol. Neurosurg. Psychiat. *47:* 831–839 (1984).
12 Schaltenbrand, G.; Bailey, P.: Introduction to stereotaxis with an atlas of the human brain (Thieme, Stuttgart 1959).
13 Siegfried, J.: Neurosurgical treatments of Parkinson's disease. Present indications and value; in Rinne, Klinger, Stamm, Parkinson's disease, pp. 369–376 (Elsevier/North-Holland, Amsterdam 1980).
14 Tasker, R.R.; Organ, L.W.; Hawrylyshyn, P.: Investigation of the surgical target for alleviation of involuntary movement disorders. Appl. Neurophysiol. *45:* 261–274 (1982).
15 Van Buren, J.M.; Li, Choh-luh; Sapiro, D.Y.; Henderson, W.G.; Sadwsky, D.A.: A qualitative and quantitative evaluation of parkinsonians three to six years following thalamotomy. Confinia neurol. *35:* 202–235 (1973).
16 Van Manen, J.; Spleeman, J.D.; Tans, R.J.J.: Indications for surgical treatment of Parkinson's disease after levodopa therapy. Clin. Neurol. Neurosurg. *86:* 207–212 (1984).

T. Miyamoto, Department of Neurosurgery, Fukuyama National Hospital,
4-14-17 Okinokami-cho, Fukuyama City, Hiroshima 720 (Japan)

Proc. 9th Meeting World Soc. Stereotactic and Functional
Neurosurgery, Toronto 1985
Appl. Neurophysiol. *48:* 305–308 (1985)

Cross-Correlation Analysis of Thalamic Neurons and EMG Activity in Parkinsonian Tremor[1]

F.A. Lenz, R.R. Tasker, H.C. Kwan, S. Schnider, R. Kwong, J.T. Murphy

Departments of Neurosurgery, Physiology and Electrical Engineering, University of Toronto and Toronto General Hospital, Toronto, Canada

Key Words. Cross-correlation analysis · Parkinson's disease · Stereotactic surgery · Thalamus · Tremor

Abstract. Bursting activity in cells cross-correlated with electromyographic (EMG) activity during parkinsonian tremor. Statistically significant evidence of cross-correlation was found for 49% of cells located at the lesion target for relief of tremor. Statistically significant correlation was found for 90% of cells having tremor frequency power greater than twice 'average power' at nontremor frequencies. This population of cells may be involved in the generation of parkinsonian tremor.

Introduction

Neurons which fire at about the frequency of tremor have often been described at the thalamic lesion site for relief of parkinsonian tremor [reviewed in 3]. It has been hypothesized that these cells, called 'tremor cells', drive parkinsonian tremor, and that tremor is driven by direct or linear transmission of tremor cells activity to muscles in the periphery. An initial step in testing that hypothesis was to examine the correlation between EMG, as a measure of peripheral tremor, and thalamic tremor cell activity.

[1] Supported by PSI Foundation (Toronto, Canada) and MRC (Canada).

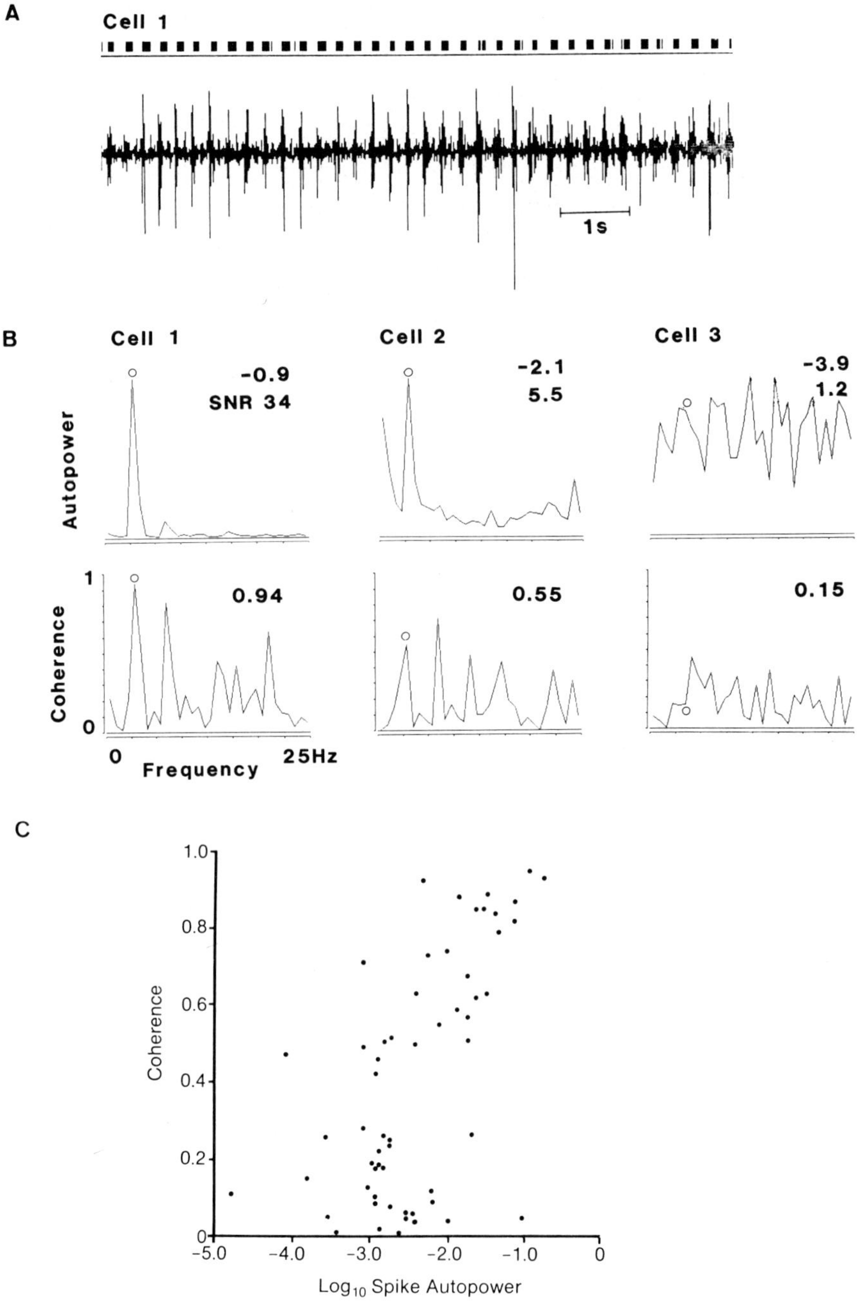
A
Cell 1
1s
B
Cell 1
Cell 2
Cell 3
-0.9
SNR 34
-2.1
5.5
-3.9
1.2
Autopower
Coherence
1
0
0.94
0.55
0.15
0
25Hz
Frequency
C
Coherence
1.0
0.8
0.6
0.4
0.2
0
-5.0
-4.0
-3.0
-2.0
-1.0
0
Log10 Spike Autopower

Materials and Methods

Thalamic neuronal spike trains were recorded by high impedance microelectrodes during stereotactic surgery for relief of parkinsonian tremor. EMG activity was recorded simultaneously and all data were subsequently digitized and subjected to spectral cross-correlation analysis [1, 2]. The autopower and coherence spectra were used to indicate, respectively, the intensity of tremor frequency, neuronal activity and the likelihood of statistically significant correlation between the two processes. The coherence function has a value of 1 if the two processes are perfectly correlated and a value 0 if they are completely uncorrelated. By the technique employed in these computations, a coherence of greater than 0.42 indicates correlation between thalamic EMG activity with $p < 0.05$ [1]. All cells described in the present report were located at the lesion site for relief of parkinsonian tremor.

Results

The upper panel of figure 1A shows the spike train of a thalamic cell (cell 1) firing at about the frequency of tremor as seen by comparison with simultaneous EMG of wrist flexors displayed in the lower panel of figure 1A. The spike autopower spectra and coherence for this cell are displayed in figure 1B with the log autopower and signal-to-noise ratio (SNR) at tremor frequency as listed. Log autopower is calculated from the autopower spectrum whereas the SNR is the ratio of the autopower at tremor frequency to the average value of all other frequencies in the autopower spectrum. Thus, the log autopower and SNR indicate the intensity of tremor frequency activity in absolute terms and in relation to other components of the spectrum, respectively. For cell 1, the coherence is greater than 0.42 at the peak of the spike autopower spectrum which occurs at tremor frequency (indicated

---

Fig. 1. Spectral cross-correlation analysis of tremor cells in parkinsonian patients. **A** Thalamic spike train (upper trace) and EMG activity (lower trace) for cell 1. Each vertical line in the spike train indicates the occurrence of an action potential. **B** Autopower and coherence spectra for cell 1 (left panel) and two other cells. The vertical axis of the autopower spectrum is different for each cell. To the upper right of the autopower spectra are tremor frequency values for log autopower (upper number) and SNR (lower number). Coherence spectra have a uniform vertical axis from 0 to 1. The number listed to the upper right of the coherence spectra is the coherence at tremor frequency. Circles indicate tremor frequency as measured from the EMG spectra (not shown). **C** Coherence and log autopower are plotted against each other for 59 cells.

by the circle). Hence, thalamic and EMG activity are significantly correlated at this frequency. The autopower and coherence spectra of two other cells are shown in figure 1B. In these three cells, the log autopower varies from -0.9 to -3.9, while the SNR varies from 34 to 1.2. Cells with a tremor frequency component of twice the average for other frequency components (SNR >2) were arbitrarily defined as tremor cells. Similar calculations have been performed on 59 cells and coherence and autopower values are plotted against each other in figure 1C. 49% of cells were correlated with EMG activity to a statistically significant level. 49% of cells were classified as tremor cells (SNR >2) of which 90% were significantly correlated with tremor, 64% of these cells were unresponsive to somatosensory stimulation.

Discussion

These results demonstrate that 90% of tremor cells located at the lesion site were correlated with parkinsonian tremor to a statistically significant level. Hence, the activity of these cells is consistent with the hypothesis that parkinsonian tremor is driven by transmission of tremor cell activity to the periphery. Exploration of other properties of these cells may be important in elucidating the mechanism of parkinsonian tremor.

References

1 Glaser, E.M.; Rushkin, D.S.: Principles of neurobiological signal analysis (Academic Press, New York 1976).
2 Lenz, F.A.; Tasker, R.R.; Kwan, H.C.; Murphy, J.T.; Nguyen-Huu, H.H.: Techniques for the analysis of spike trains in the human central nervous system. Acta neurochir. *33:* suppl., pp. 57–61 (1984).
3 Tasker, R.R.; Organ, L.W.; Hawrylyshyn, P.A.: The thalamus and midbrain of man: a physiologic atlas using electrical stimulation (Thomas, Springfield 1982).

Dr. R.R. Tasker, Division of Neurosurgery, Room 14–215, Eaton N. Wing, Toronto General Hospital, 200 Elizabeth St., Toronto, Ont. M4Y 2C4 (Canada)

Proc. 9th Meeting World Soc. Stereotactic and Functional
Neurosurgery, Toronto 1985
Appl. Neurophysiol. *48:* 309–314 (1985)

Idiopathic Oromandibular Dyskinesia Treated by Vo Complex Microstereotactic Thalamotomy

H. Narabayashi, F. Yokochi, Y. Nakajima

Department of Neurology, Juntendo University School of Medicine,
Hongo, Bunkyo-ku, Tokyo, Japan

Key Words. Striato-pallido-thalamic projection · Vo complex · Stereotactic surgery · Dyskinesia

Abstract. Two cases of oromandibular or buccolingual dyskinesia, which did not respond to medical therapy, had lesions produced in the Vo complex of the thalamus by microstereotactic surgery with almost complete relief of symptoms. It was assumed the symptom, as well as levodopa-induced dyskinesia, may depend on the striato-pallido-thalamic projection.

Introduction

Idiopathic oromandibular or buccolingual dyskinesia is a peculiar involuntary movement around the face, jaw, tongue and neck, often observed after the age of 50 [1, 3]. This condition has become of interest after the experiences of levodopa-induced dyskinesia of similar distribution in elderly parkinsonian patients. As in levodopa-induced dyskinesia, it is postulated that dopamine is involved in this condition.

The cases of oromandibular dyskinesia which did not respond to medical treatment underwent microstereotactic Vo complex[1] thalamotomy with satisfactory results, as will be described.

[1] Vo complex is the term used for both the ventralis oralis anterior, Voa, and posterior, Vop, nuclei of the thalamus by *Hassler* [2], which is almost synonymous to the ventrolateral nucleus, VL, in American terminology.

A B

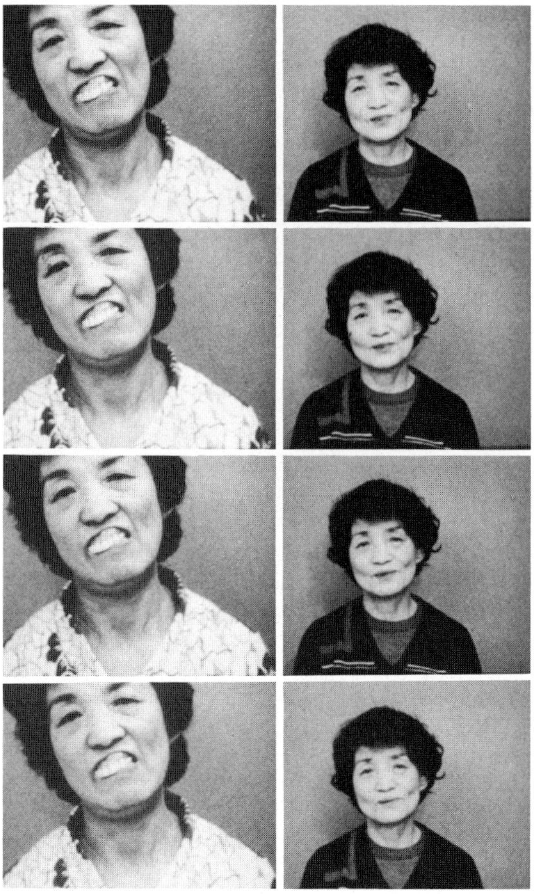

Fig. 1. Oromandibular dyskinesia in case 1, dislocation of jaw pushing out the artificial teeth. **A** Preoperative. **B** Postoperative improvement.

Case Reports

Case 1 – 60-year-old female. Without any preceding history of illness, the patient started to complain of stiffness of the right shoulder at the age of 45. Within several months, abnormal contraction of facial muscles, deviation of the jaw to the left or to the right (a little more severely to the left side), facial grimacing (more on the right side), and involuntary tonic contraction of the right shoulder muscles became apparent and gradually worse. Trials with almost all medicines, including muscle relaxants, tranquilizers and dopaminergic or antidopaminergic agents at about ten neurological centers failed to improve the symptoms even slightly.

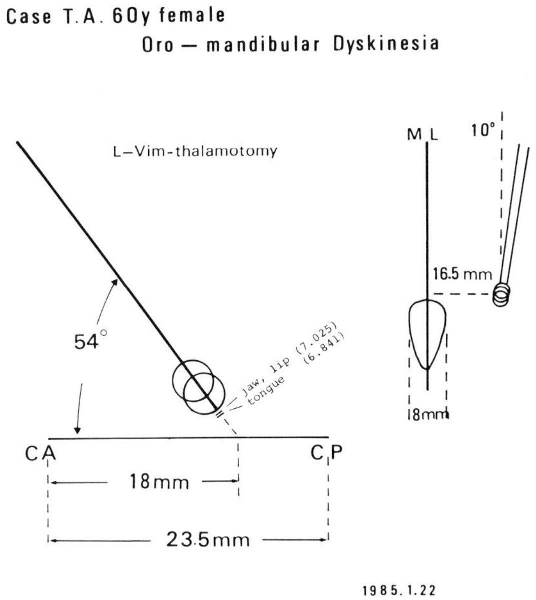

Fig. 2. In case 1 the location of the thermocoagulation lesion (open circle) was decided after confirming the proprioceptive neurons in Vim. Jaw, lip and tongue indicate the place of the neuron presenting evoked spike discharges as pressing or movement of each part. The number is the distance in microns above the tentative target (4,000) measured radiologically. Lateral distance in AP view includes 10% parallax.

On admission the patient presented with marked difficulty in biting and in speech because of these abnormal movements. Involuntary movements in the facial, oral area and tongue were so severe that dislocation of the jaw resulted in pushing her artificial teeth out of her mouth (fig. 1). Functions of the distal part of the right arm were normal and the left extremities were not affected. There were no pyramidal, cerebellar or other extrapyramidal signs.

The side of surgery was decided by the coexisting symptom of the right shoulder, although the facial and jaw dyskinetic movements were almost symmetrical. On January 22, 1983, the microstereotactic procedure on the left Vo complex of the thalamus was carried out, which resulted in about 70–80% diminution of the involuntary movements. Involuntary tonic contraction of the right shoulder muscles was completely abolished. Facial and jaw dyskinesia became much less, as seen in figure 1A and B, and involuntary tongue protrusion was also almost diminished. Speech and biting became much easier.

The target structure for the lesion was decided by a microelectrode recording technique. Neurons responding to passive or active jaw movement and pressing on the jaw, lip, or tongue (proprioceptive neurons) were identified within the thalamus in the ventral part of the ventralis intermedius nuclei, Vim. The needle tip was pulled back for 1.8 mm

A B

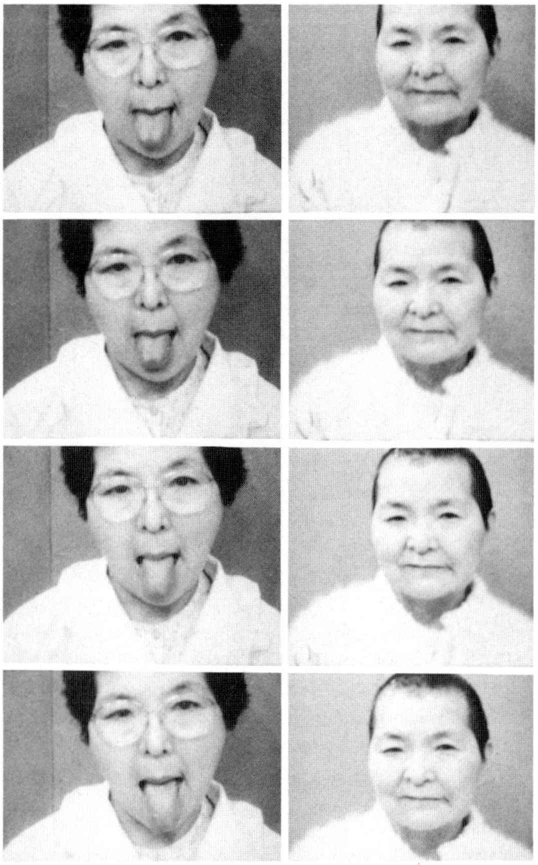

Fig. 3. Oromandibular dyskinesia in case 2. **A** Preoperative. **B** Postoperative improvement.

and two successive lesions, each being about 4 mm in diameter, were produced, as shown in figure 2 [4, 5, 7]. These two medium-sized lesions were assumed to be located selectively in the ventral base of the Vo complex.

Case 2 – 63-year-old female. About a year ago, slight involuntary movement of the jaw to the left or right started, and 6 months ago forced involuntary protrusion of the tongue started, which became quickly worse.

Whenever the patient was awake, the severe continuous maximum protrusion of the tongue was present, which was impossible to manipulate or draw back voluntarily (fig. 3). Because of this, speech and biting were almost impossible and only fluid meals were possible. There were no other neurological manifestations in other cranial nerves or extremities.

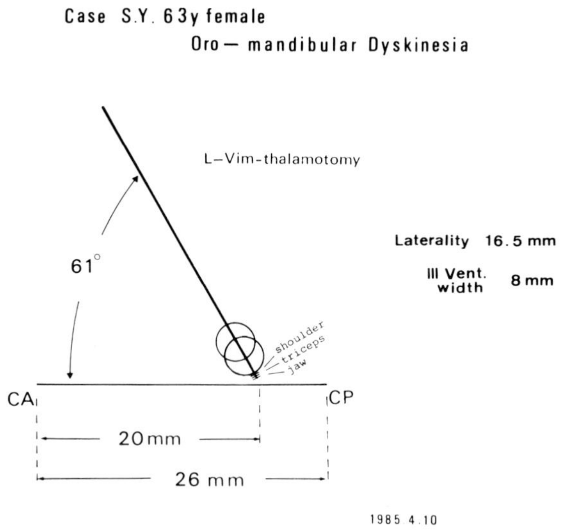

Fig. 4. In case 2 the location of the thermocoagulation lesion (open circle) was decided after confirming the proprioceptive neurons in Vim. Explanations are the same as in figure 2.

Left Vo complex thalamotomy on October 31, 1984, and the right thalamotomy on April 10, 1985, were performed. Almost complete alleviation of forced tongue protrusion was obtained, as shown in figure 3A and B. No side effects in speech or psychological functions occurred. Chewing, swallowing and speech were almost normalized.

The target structure was decided similarly to case 1, after confirming the proprioceptive neurons for shoulder muscles, triceps brachii muscle and jaw movement, as demonstrated in figure 4.

Discussion

These observations suggest that the idiopathic oromandibular dyskinesia is a symptom presumably depending on the pallido-thalamic projection, similar to levodopa-induced dyskinesia, which was described in detail by the author [6]. These presumed striato-pallido-thalamic disorders are usually modified by changing the level of striatal dopamine by pharmacological agents. However, when such medicine does not influence these symptoms, a small lesion exactly placed stereotactically within the Vo complex by using the microelectrode technique is an effective and perhaps the only way to alleviate the symptoms.

References

1 Delwaide, P.J.; Desseilles, M.: Spontaneous buccolinguofacial dyskinesia in the elderly. Acta neurol. scand. *56:* 256–262 (1977).
2 Hassler, R.: Anatomy of the thalamus; in Schaltenbrand, Bailey, Introduction to stereotaxis with atlas of the human brain, pp. 230–290 (Thieme, Stuttgart 1959).
3 Marsden, C.D.: The problem of adult-onset idiopathic torsion dystonia and other isolated dyskinesia in adult life (including blepharospasm, oromandibular dystonia, dystonic writer's cramp, and torticollis, or axial dystonia); in Eldridge, Fahn, Advances in neurology, vol. 14, pp. 259–276 (Raven Press, New York 1976).
4 Narabayashi, H.; Ohye, C.: Importance of microstereoencephalotomy for tremor alleviation. Appl. Neurophysiol. *43:* 222–227 (1980).
5 Narabayashi, H.: Recent status of stereotaxic surgery. Surg. Neurol. *19:* 493–496 (1983).
6 Narabayashi, H.; Yokochi, F.; Nakajima, Y.: Levodopa-induced dyskinesia and thalamotomy. J. Neurol. Neurosurg. Psychiat. *471:* 831–839 (1984).
7 Ohye, C.; Saito, Y.; Fukamachi, A.; Narabayashi, H.: An analysis of the spontaneous rhythmic and non-rhythmic burst discharges in the human thalamus. J. neurol. Sci. *22:* 245–259 (1974).

H. Narabayashi, MD, Department of Neurology, Juntendo University
School of Medicine, Hongo, Bunkyo-ku, Tokyo 113 (Japan)

Proc. 9th Meeting World Soc. Stereotactic and Functional Neurosurgery, Toronto 1985
Appl. Neurophysiol. *48:* 315 (1985)

Evaluation of Thalamotomy by Positron Emission Tomography and Magnetic Resonance Imaging

T.W. Hood, S.S. Gebarski

Section of Neurosurgery and Neuroradiology, University of Michigan Medical Center, Ann Arbor, Mich., USA

Key Words. Stereotactic surgery · Magnetic resonance imaging · Positron emission tomography · Thalamotomy

Abstract. Positron emission tomography (PET) and magnetic resonance imaging (MRI) can be used to evaluate patients with movement disorders at the previously unavailable levels of metabolism and proton environment. The abnormalities seen in these studies, which do not appear in conventional X-ray computed tomography (CT), may contribute to the understanding of the pathophysiology of these disorders. Postoperative PET and MRI in conjunction with the postoperative functional result can further elucidate the effect of thalamotomy at these levels.

Since January 1984, patients with Parkinson's disease, spasmodic torticollis, and dystonia who were candidates for VL thalamotomy have had preoperative PET, MRI and CT. Follow-up PET, MRI and CT were obtained at least 3 months postoperatively to permit resolution of edema. Postoperative CT demonstrated the accuracy of lesion localization.

The pre- and postoperative PET, MRI, and CT. PET employed 18-fluorodeoxyglucose as the isotopic metabolic substrate. MRI used a superconducting system with spin-echo sequences to image hydrogen nuclei. Both T_1 and T_2 weighted MRI was carried out to best define the range of aberrant proton behavior in these lesions. All imaging was acquired in axial planes comparable to those employed by the Leksell frame. MRI images were also acquired in various orthogonal planes to further define the lesion and predict electrode path.

T.W. Hood, MD, Section of Neurosurgery, University of Michigan Medical Center, 1405 East Ann Street, Ann Arbor, MI 48109 (USA)

Proc. 9th Meeting World Soc. Stereotactic and Functional Neurosurgery, Toronto 1985
Appl. Neurophysiol. *48:* 316–323 (1985)

Cell Sparse Zones in the Ventrolateral Thalamic Mass in Humans, Monkeys and Cats: Their Special Reference to Kinesthetic Neurons

T. Hirai, Y. Nagaseki, H. Wada, T. Shibazaki, M. Matsumura, C. Ohye

Department of Neurosurgery, Gunma University School of Medicine, Maebashi, Gunma, Japan

Key Words. Cell sparse zone · Vim nucleus · VPLo nucleus · VLs nucleus · Kinesthetic neuron · Tremor

Abstract. The Vim nucleus of the human thalamus is the cell sparse zone. The neurons in this zone respond to peripheral stimuli of kinesthetic modality with a short latency. In the cytometrical study, the cell sparse zone is identifiable in both the monkey and cat thalamus. The cell dimension and density in a 1 mm^2 area in the cell sparse zone of each species are as follows: humans – large neuron 500–900 μm^2, medium neuron 200–400 μm^2, cell density 60–90/mm^2/50 μm thickness; monkeys – large neuron 400–800 μm^2, medium neuron 200–400 μm^2, cell density 120–250/mm^2/50 μm thickness; cats – large neuron 400–800 μm^2, medium neuron 200–400 μm^2, cell density 120–250/mm^2/50 μm thickness. In this zone, there are large and medium thalamocortical relay neurons defined by the Golgi impregnated and HRP studies. It is still obscure which neurons respond to kinesthetic stimulation and which neurons or afferent fibers play important roles in the tremor mechanism.

The Vim nucleus of the human thalamus [4,5,9,15] is the cell sparse zone. The neurons in this zone respond to peripheral stimuli of kinesthetic modality [10,11] with a short latency, and a small coagulative lesion within the Vim nucleus of the human thalamus ameliorates various kinds of tremor including Parkinson's tremor. To compare anatomically these findings of the Vim nucleus of humans to those of other species, a cytometrical study was conducted on the ventrolateral thalamic mass of monkeys and cats by the same method reported previously [5].

Six brains of neurologically normal humans, 3 Macaca brains and 3 cat brains were used for measuring the cell density and dimension of each thalamic nucleus [2, 3, 4, 7, 9, 12, 14, 15] by the same method reported previously using a microscopic image analyzer (Olympus VIP-21CH). Three human brains, 2 Macaca brains and 2 cat brains were used for examining the shape of individual neurons in the cell sparse zone by the Golgi impregnated method. Two cats and a Macaca were used to examine the dimension and shape of the thalamocortical relay neurons in the cell sparse zone by the retrograde labelling of HRP after injection of a large amount of HRP in the sensory motor cortex.

The cell sparse zone of the thalamus of humans, monkeys and cats is most easily distinguished [1,13] in horizontal section and each is very similar to the other in terms of location in the thalamus and cytoarchitecture (fig. 1). The anterior border between the cell sparse zone and the VL complex was clearly distinguished in humans and monkeys. In the cat thalamus, this border was obscure in the VL complex, but the anterior part of the VL complex was more densely packed with more smaller cells than the posterior part of the VL complex (the cell sparse zone). The posterior border between the cell sparse zone and the VB complex could be distinguished in terms of the difference of cell density, cell variety and the diminution of large cells.

The cell dimension and density in 1 mm^2 areas in the cell sparse zone of each species are as follows: humans - dimension of large cell 500–900 μm^2, medium cell 200–400 μm^2 and cell density 60–90/mm^2/50 μm thickness; monkeys - dimension of large cell 400–800 μm^2, medium cell 200–400 μm^2 and cell density 120–250/mm^2/50 μm thickness; cats - dimension of large cell 400–800 μm^2, medium

Fig. 1. The histogram of cell dimension and density in 1 mm^2 area (humans) and 0.25 mm^2 area (monkeys and cats) in various thalamic nuclei about 1.9 mm (humans) 0.6 mm (monkeys) and 0.2 mm (cats) above the intercommissure line in the horizontal section. The horizontal line is drawn at the level of the posterior commissure. The three vertical lines indicate midline, 10 mm, 20 mm (humans) or midline, 5 mm, 10 mm (monkeys and cats) from the midline. The histograms are so distributed as occupying the corresponding position shown in the black squares on the right upper drawing. In each histogram, the abscissa represents cell dimensions (μm^2) and the ordinate the number of cells per 1 mm^2 (humans), or 0.25 mm^2 (monkeys and cats). The ventrolateral thalamic nuclei were classified based on the dimension and density of each neuron group referring to Hassler's (in humans), Olszewski's (in monkeys) and Berman and Jones's (in cats) classification and terminology. Note that the cell sparse zone is rich in large neurons but that they are less densely arranged.

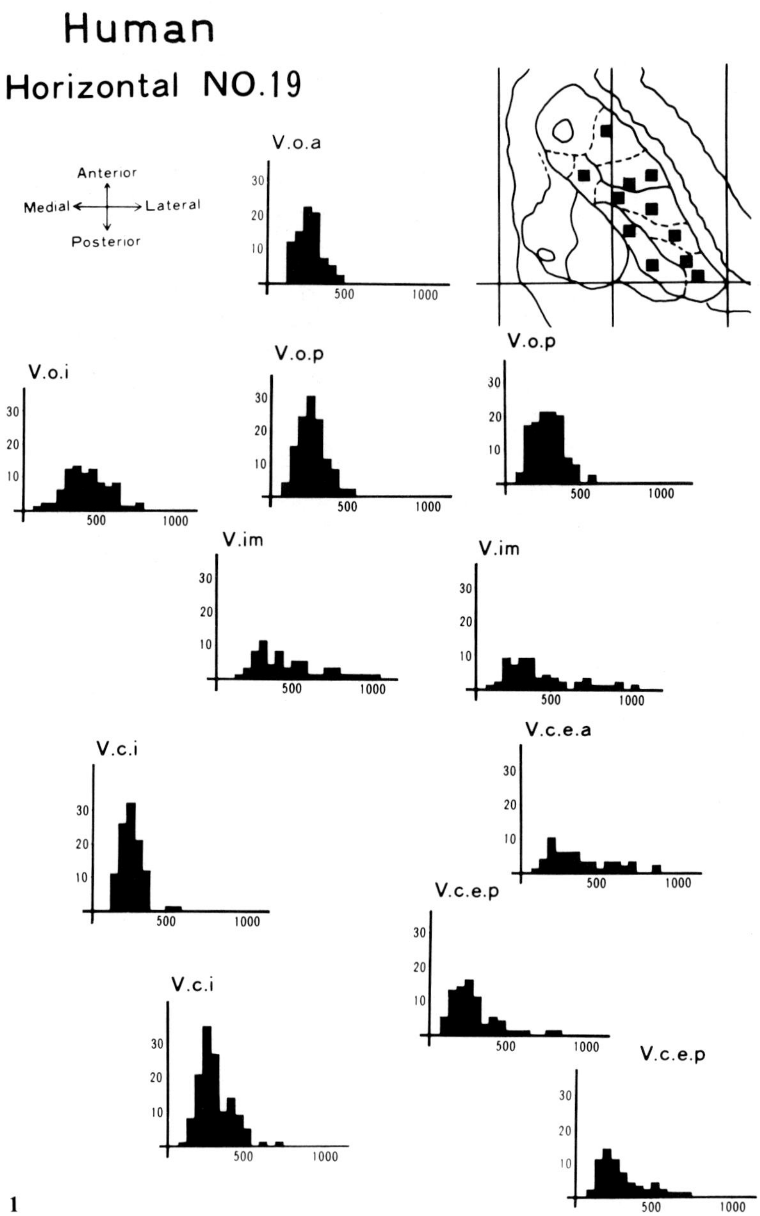
Human
Horizontal NO.19
Anterior
Medial
Lateral
Posterior
V.o.a
V.o.i
V.o.p
V.o.p
V.im
V.im
V.c.i
V.c.e.a
V.c.e.p
V.c.i
V.c.e.p
30
20
10
500
1000

1

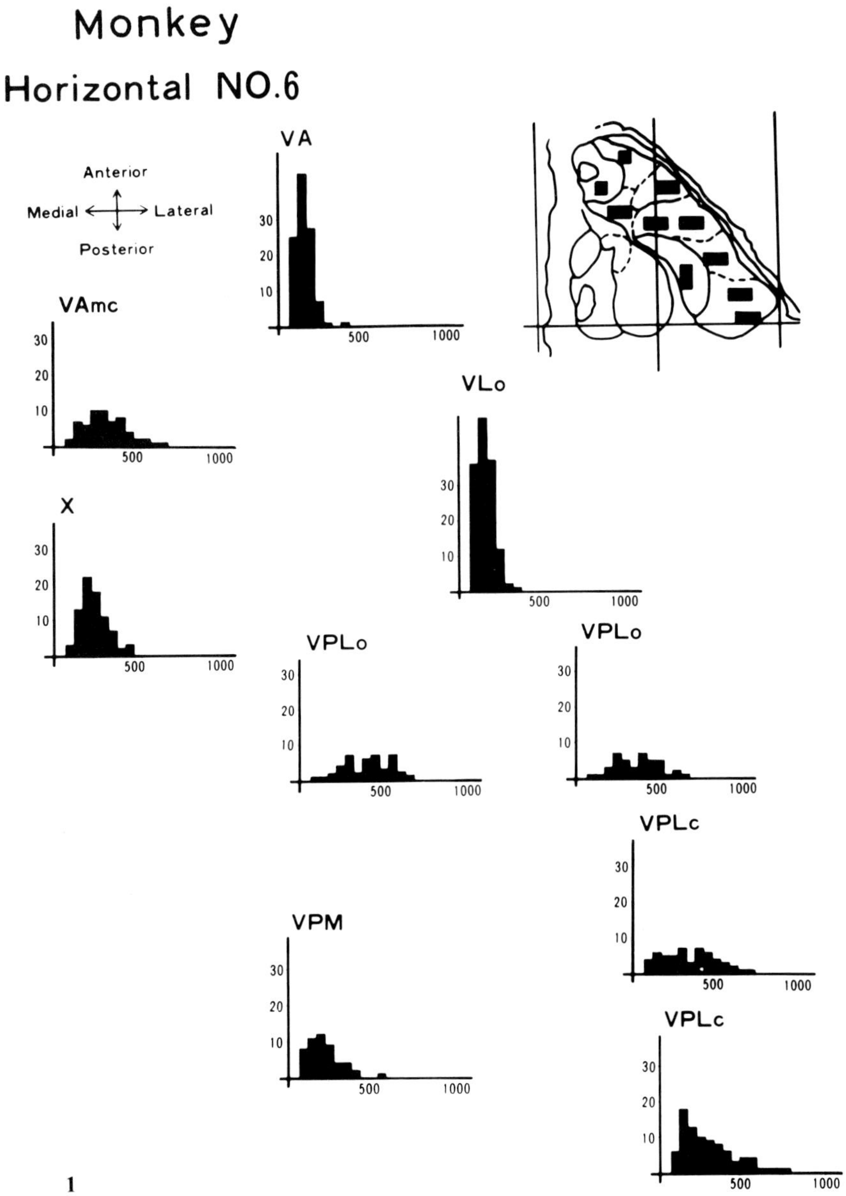
Monkey
Horizontal NO.6
Anterior
Medial
Lateral
Posterior
VA
VAmc
X
VLo
VPLo
VPLo
VPLc
VPM
VPLc
30
20
10
500
1000

1

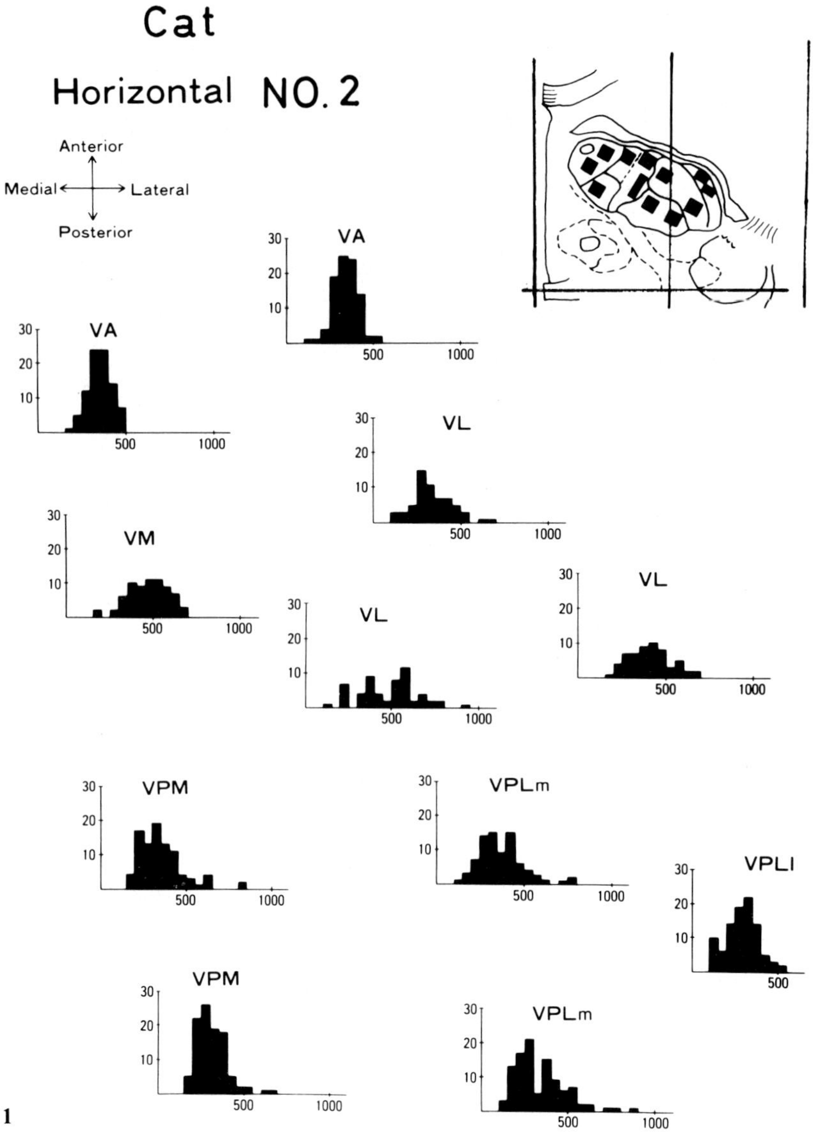
Cat
Horizontal NO. 2
Anterior
Medial
Lateral
Posterior
VA
VA
VL
VM
VL
VL
VPM
VPLm
VPLl
VPM
VPLm
10
20
30
500
1000

1

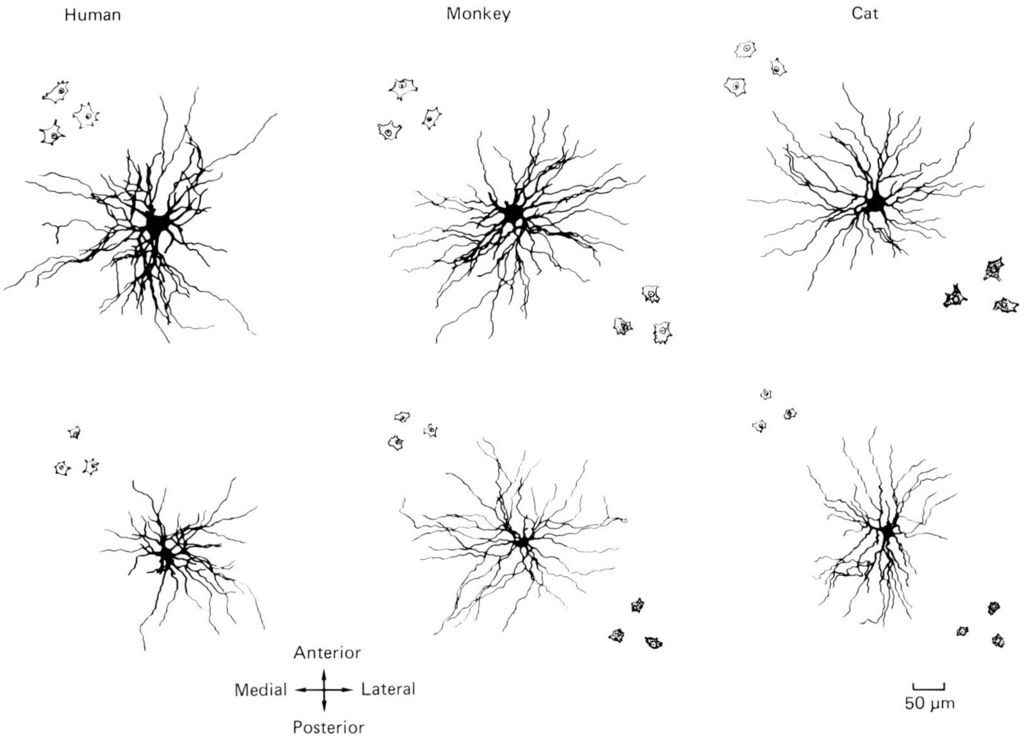

Fig. 2. The camera lucida drawing of large and medium thalamocortical relay neurons found in the cell sparse zone of the thalamus in humans, monkeys and cats. Large and medium neurons stained by the Golgi-impregnated method (humans) and labelled by HRP (monkeys and cats) are shown. Three neurons, drawn on the upper left side, indicate the neurons in the cell sparse zone stained with cresyl violet. Three neurons, drawn on the lower right side, indicate the neurons in the cell sparse zone labelled by HRP after injection of a large amount of HRP in the sensory motor cortex. Both neurons are typical thalamocortical relay neurons and have 6–8 proximal dendrites which arborize in almost all directions extending at least 500–600 μm.

cell 200–400 μm^2 and cell density 120–250/mm^2/50 μm thickness. The cell sparse zone of monkeys and cats was more densely packed than that of humans and the cells in this zone were relatively smaller than that of humans.

We identified the large and the medium thalamocortical relay neurons in the cell sparse zone (fig. 2). The large neurons are generally multiangular and usually have 6–8 proximal dendrites. Each of the proximal dendrites branches into 2–3 short secondary dendrites. One secondary branch, shortly after the origin, branches into 2–3 distal dendrites which become progressively thinner up to the termination. These dendrites arborize in almost all directions at least 500–600 μm in length. Medium neurons have relatively round and cubic cell soma, and usually have 6–8 proximal dendrites. The dendritic ramification as a whole is similar to, but generally less extensive and sparser than that of the large cells.

The cell sparse zone named hitherto by the anatomists is the following: Vim nucleus of humans [4, 9, 15], VPLo nucleus of monkeys [8, 12], VLs part in VL nucleus of cats [2, 3, 7, 14].

The Vim nucleus of the human thalamus is the cell sparse zone [4, 5, 9, 15] which contains large and medium thalamocortical relay neurons. We have not as yet been able to identify which neurons respond to kinesthetic stimulation and which neurons or afferent fibers play important roles in the tremor mechanism. The functional property and the precise fiber connections of this nucleus are still obscure.

References

1 Berkley, K.J.: Spatial relationships between the terminations of somatic sensory and motor pathways in the rostral brainstem of cats and monkeys. II. Cerebellar projections compared with those of the ascending somatic sensory pathways in lateral diencephalon. J. comp. Neurol. *220:* 229–251 (1983).

2 Berman, A.L.; Jones, E.G.: The thalamus and basal telencephalon of the cat (University of Wisconsin Press, Madison 1982).

3 Boivie, J.: The termination of the spinothalamic tract in the cat. An experimental study with silver impregnation methods. Exp. Brain Res. *12:* 331–353 (1971).

4 Hassler, R.: Architectonic organization of the thalamic nuiclei; in Schaltenbrand, Wahren, Atlas for stereotaxy of the human brain; 2nd rev. ed. (Thieme, Stuttgart 1977).

5 Hirai, T.; Nagaseki, Y.; Kawashima, Y.; Wada, H.; Tsukahara, Y.; Imai, S.; Ohye, C.: Large neurons in the thalamic ventrolateral mass in humans and monkeys. Appl. Neurophysiol. *45:* 245–250 (1982).

6 Hirai, T.; Miyazaki, M.; Nakajima, H.; Shibazaki, T.; Ohye, C.: The correlation between tremor characteristics and the predicted volume of effective lesions in stereotactic nucleus ventralis intermedius thalamotomy. Brain *106:* 1001–1018 (1983).

7 Jones, E.G.; Burton, H.: Cytoarchitecture and somatic sensory connectivity of the thalamic nuclei other than the ventrobasal complex in the cat. J. comp. Neurol. *154:* 395–432 (1974).

8 Jones, E.G.; Friedman, D.P.; Hendry, S.H.C.: Thalamic basis of place and modality specific columns in monkey somatosensory cortex: a correlative anatomical and physiological study. J. Neurophysiol. *48:* 545–568 (1982).
9 Mehler, W.R.: The posterior thalamic region in man. Confinia neurol. *26:* 18–29 (1966).
10 Ohye, C.; Fukamachi, A.; Miyazaki, M.; Isobe, I.; Nakajima, H.; Shibazaki, T.: Physiologically controlled selective thalamotomy for the treatment of abnormal movement by Leksell's open system. Acta neurochir. *37:* 93–104 (1977).
11 Ohye, C.; Narabayashi, H.: Physiological study of presumed ventralis intermedius neurons in the human thalamus. J. Neurosurg. *50:* 290–297 (1979).
12 Olszewski, J.: The thalamus of the *Macaca mulatta*. An atlas for use with the stereotaxic instrument (Karger, Basel 1952).
13 Pearson, J.C.; Haines, D.E.: On the question of the ventral intermediate nucleus in primate thalamus: a study of the lesser bushbaby, *Galago senegalensis*. Brain Behav. Evol. *19:* 108–125 (1981).
14 Rinvik, E.: A re-evaluation of the cytoarchitecture of the ventral nuclear complex of the cat's thalamus on the basis of corticothalamic connections. Brain Res. *8:* 237–254 (1968).
15 Van Buren, J.M.; Borke, R.C.: The nuclei and cerebral connections of the human thalamus (Springer, Berlin 1972).

T. Hirai, MD, Department of Neurosurgery, Gunma University School of Medicine, 3-39 Showa-machi, Maebashi, Gunma (Japan)

Proc. 9th Meeting World Soc. Stereotactic and Functional Neurosurgery, Toronto 1985
Appl. Neurophysiol. *48:* 324–338 (1985)

Spinal Cord Stimulation in the Treatment of Spasmodic Torticollis[1]

Joseph M. Waltz, Carmen A. Scozzari, David P. Hunt

Department of Neurological Surgery, St. Barnabas Hospital, New York, N.Y., USA

Key Words. Spinal cord stimulation · Four-electrode system · Spasmodic torticollis · Sensory input modulation

Abstract. This report presents our observations in 63 patients undergoing chronic spinal cord stimulation for treatment of spasmodic torticollis. In this series there were 23 patients (36.5%) who demonstrated marked improvement, characterized by no evidence of torticollis, full range of motility of the head and neck and no pain. Moderate improvement was found in 20 patients (31.8%) who showed minimal residual torticollis, but had full motility and no pain. There were 5 patients (7.9%) considered mildly improved who demonstrated decrease in their torticollic position, spasms and pain, but retained some element of torticollis and/or some limitation of motility. Correlations were made demonstrating the effect on the results of age, sex, electrode array, the configuration of the applied field and the parameters of stimulation.

The aberrant neuronal mechanisms underlying the involuntary movement of the head and neck in spasmodic torticollis has been the focus of extensive experimental research. Direction-specific rotary movement of the head can be achieved by stimulation of numerous extrapyramidal structures located within the mesodiencephalon. Contraversive rotary movements are effected via the influence of the pallidum

[1] This study was supported in part by grants from Lawrence S. Rockefeller and Dr. Lucy R. Waletzky.

internum and its thalamic and other descending connections [6]. Rotary movements are also produced by the interstitial nucleus of Cajal and its connections, particularly those contributions emanating from the nucleus ventralis oralis internus of the thalamus [4].

Rotary movement of the head can be induced through stimulation of the midline cerebellar nuclei and sites within the cerebellar peduncle [5]. With lesions placed within the medial reticular formation, brachium conjunctivum and mesancephalic tegmentum in monkeys, *Foltz* et al. [2] have produced a condition in the primate remarkably similar to human torticollis.

These observations have added support to the theory that torticollis and retrocollis are at least partly a result of an abnormality of sensory motor communication from the cerebellum to the motor and premotor cortex via the thalamus.

The introduction of spinal cord stimulation has offered a less destructive and hazardous avenue than ablative procedures to achieve sensory input modulation.

In 1975, we began investigating this concept of therapeutic neuromodulation in disorders of the motor system. During the past 10 years, in over 650 cases, we have demonstrated, along with other investigators, that selectively stimulating the cervical spinal cord can reverse and improve disabling motor symptoms regardless of etiology, including spasticity, athetosis, ataxia, pseudobulbar dysfunction and dystonic spasms and posture, including spasmodic torticollis [10–15]. Crucial to the therapeutic effectiveness of spinal cord stimulation has been the evolution of its technique and instrumentation. In 1978, we reported in our initial 130 cases the significance of the cord level stimulated in relation to the results [10]. These observations led us that time to the design of a system which would allow stimulation at selected cord levels and at various frequencies. The result was a four-electrode system which subsequently was shown to improve the results of spinal cord stimulation in motor disorders [12]. These results were further improved by introduction of a computerized system [15], which eliminated percutaneous leads and a second stage operation for receiver implantation, has resulted in a reduced risk of infection, and allows an indefinite period for selection of the stimulation parameters which in the case of torticollis is extremely important. This report presents observations in 63 patients undergoing spinal cord stimulation for the treatment of axial cervical dystonia (torticollis).

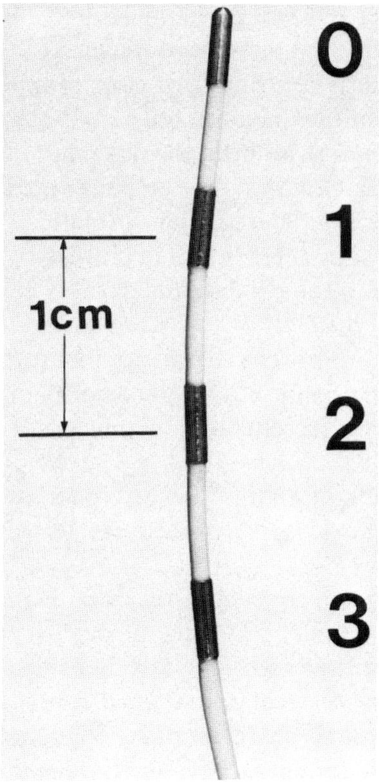

Fig. 1. The multilevel four-electrode catheter assembly with platinum electrodes 1.2 mm in diameter and spaced 1 cm apart from center to center.

Technique

Two electrode systems were used in this series: the earlier two-electrode system and the newer four-electrode system. Both of these systems were implanted by percutaneous and open techniques.

Two-Electrode Percutaneous Implantation

This technique was employed during the period of 1975–1978. The procedure was carried out under local anesthetic, when possible; a general anesthetic, if necessary. The patient was placed in the prone position with the cervical-dorsal junction flexed. The needles were introduced over the superior lip of the lamina at a shallow angle to enter the epidural space with hustead epidural needles at the upper or midthoracic level. The two epidural electrodes were introduced Neuromed, Fort Lauderdale, Florida cephalad in the epidural space, their course being monitored by fluoroscopy. The electrodes were po-

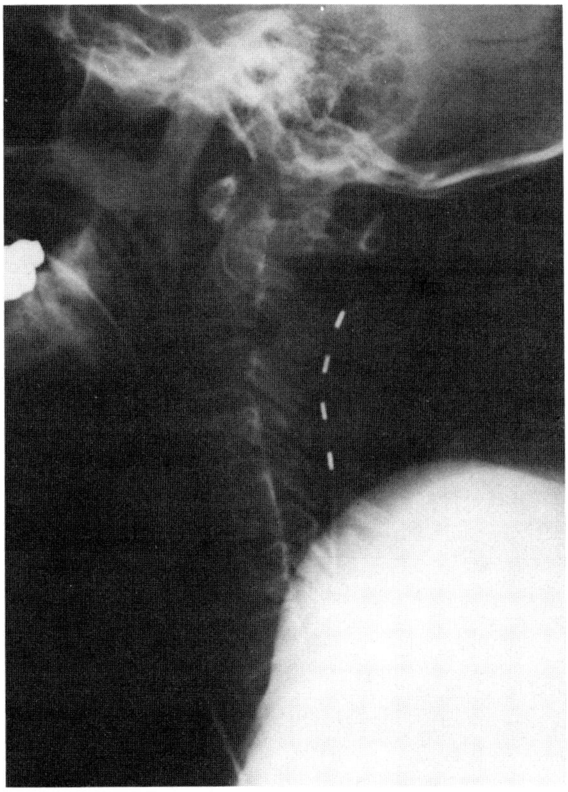

Fig. 2. Lateral cervical X-ray showing the four-electrode system in place.

sitioned in the midline, separated by a distance of approximately 1-2.5 cm. The connecting leads were externalized for a period of test stimulation of 7-10 days. If no improvement was noted, the system was removed. If sufficient improvement was noted, the system was interiorized by connecting the epidural electrodes to a subcutaneously placed receiver for chronic stimulation.

Two-Electrode Open Implantation

In certain cases, because of broken wires, displaced electrodes or inability to achieve satisfactory electrode placement, it was necessary to place the electrode in position by a laminectomy. The electrodes used in this case were a pair of platinum buttons mounted in a dacron mesh, coated with silicone rubber. A laminectomy over 2 levels was carried out and the electrode plate was sutured in place to the dura in the midline. Electrodes were connected to the subcutaneously placed receiver. No test period was possible with this system.

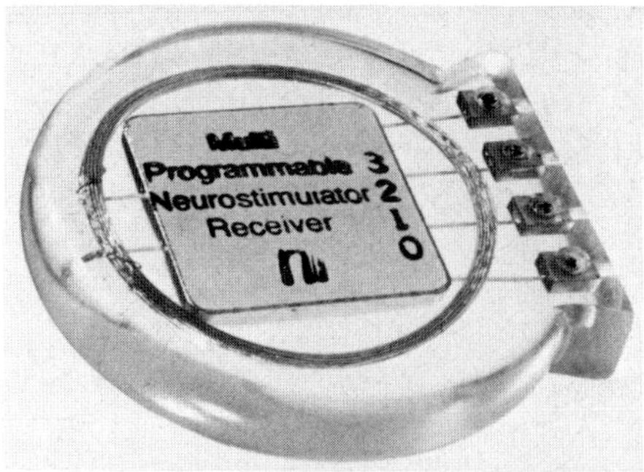

Fig. 3. The computerized receiver which is internalized subcutaneously and permits external adjustment of multiple stimulation parameters through a control panel in the transmitter.

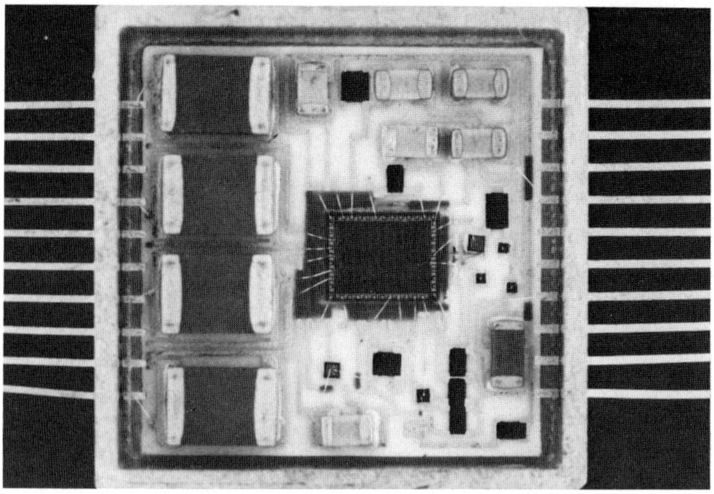

Fig. 4. The hermetically sealed electronic hybrid circuit, contained in the receiver, which decodes the programming signals from the external transmitter.

Four-Electrode Implantation Technique

From 1978 to 1979 the four-electrode system was implanted in the cervical area through a simple laminectomy placed in the epidural space in the midline under direct vision [9]. Since, we have used a percutaneous technique (9, 12) in which four electrodes are incorporated into a thin catheter system which can be inserted through a single 16-gauge epidural needle. The multielectrode assembly consists of four platinum electrodes, 4 mm in length, 1.2 mm in diameter and spaced 6 mm apart (1 cm center to cen-

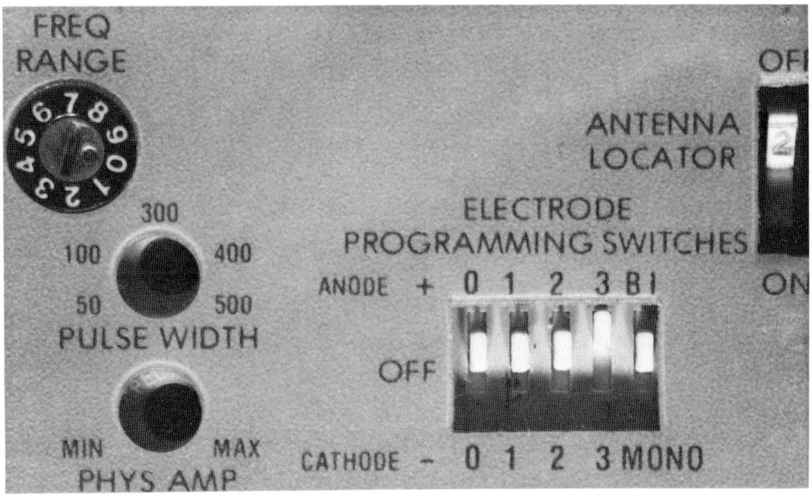

Fig. 5. The control panel located in the transmitter which permits selection of any combination of the four electrodes, polarity and either monophasic or biphasic stimulation within a frequency range of 25–1,500 Hz.

Table I. Spinal cord stimulation electrode combinations

	Neg–Pos		Neg–Pos
1.	0–1	2.	1–0
3.	0–2	4.	2–0
5.	0–3	6.	3–0
7.	1–2	8.	2–1
9.	1–3	10.	3–1
11.	2–3	12.	3–2
13.	0–1 2–3	14.	1–0 3–2
15.	0–2 1–3	16.	2–0 3–1
17.	0–1 3–2	18.	1–0 2–3

The four-electrode configuration allows 18 combinations of settings, 9 in each cathode polarity orientation, one series being oriented cephalad and the other caudad. In each series, there are six single bipolar and three double bipolar settings.

ter) (fig. 1). The needle is placed in the epidural space in the middorsal area and the electrode assembly is passed through the needle and under fluoroscopic control is advanced to the C2 level in the epidural space (fig. 2). Initially, four temporary extensions were externalized for testing various levels of stimulation on the patient. The development of the computerized receiver and transmitter allows the receiver to be implanted initially, requiring no percutaneous extensions (fig. 3). The receiver (fig. 4) decodes the radiofrequency programming signals from the external computerized transmitter. The transmitter contains within it a control panel (fig. 5) which permits selection of any combination of four electrodes, polarity, and either monophasic or biphasic stimulation at a frequency range of 10–1,500 Hz[2].

We find that patients respond to specific electrode combinations. Parameters of stimulation must be established in each case. A set protocol is followed in which 18 electrode settings are tried in sequence (table I). Observations are made on each to establish the best electrode combination. This is then followed by a frequency analysis with observations made at 100-Hz increments from 100 to 1,500 Hz. The period of analysis usually requires 4–6 weeks before the proper parameters are established.

Population

We have treated 63 patients suffering from spasmodic torticollis with high cervical cord stimulation (table II). There were 36 females and 27 males, ranging in age from 30 to 61 years, with a mean age of 44.5 years. The duration of symptoms ranged from 8 months to 27 years, with a mean duration of 5.3 years. Follow-up time ranged from 1 to 10 years with a mean follow-up time of 4.3 years.

Results

Two-Eletrode System (table III)

The two-electrode system was employed in 17 patients suffering from spasmodic torticollis, including 5 males and 12 females. There were 5 cases (29%) which were not internalized because no effect was noted during the trial stimulation of 7–10 days. These cases were stimulated at multiple levels and at various stimulation parameters. 12 cases of this series were internalized because of satisfactory response to the stimulation. Of these 12 patients, 5 (29.4%) showed marked improvement, 4 (23.5%) showed moderate improvement, with a combined moderate to marked improvement of 52.9%, 1 case showed mild improvement (5.9%), and 2 cases showed no improvement after internali-

[2] This system has eliminated the need for a second surgical procedure, reduced the length of hospitalization and decreased the risk of infection. The system allows an indefinite period for electrode analysis, which becomes of great importance in evaluating the dystonic and spasmodic torticollis patient.

Table II. The composition of the group of 63 patients with spasmodic torticollis submitted to spinal cord stimulation

Females	36
Males	27
Age	30–61 years (mean 44.5 years)
Duration of s/s	8 months to 27 years (mean 5.3 years)
Follow-up	1–10 years (mean 4.3 years)

Table III. The results observed in the 17 patients who were submitted to two-electrode spinal cord stimulation

Improvement	Female, n = 12		Male, n = 5		Total, n = 17	
	n	%	n	%	n	%
Marked	4	33.3	1	20.0	5	29.4
Moderate	3	25.0	1	20.0	4	23.5
Mild	1	8.4	0	0.0	1	5.9
Unimproved	4	33.3	3	60.0	7	41.2

zation with a failure rate of 11.7%. The 5 cases which showed marked improvement were implanted in the C2, C3 area. There was a rather significant correlation in this group of age and gender, with all patients being in their third decade and 4 of the 5 being female. The moderately improved group, which consisted of 4 cases, were implanted in the C2, C3 level. Three of the 4 cases were female. One remaining case of mild improvement was a 46-year-old female, with the level of stimulation being at C2.

Four-Electrode System (table IV)

Forty-six patients with spasmodic torticollis underwent implantation of the quadrapolar system. In this series, marked improvement was noted in 18 patients (39.1%). Moderate improvement was found in 16 patients (34.8%) with marked to moderate improvement being noted in 34 patients (73.9%). Mild improvement was demonstrated in 4 patients (8.7%). Significantly increased improvement was demonstrated with the four-electrode system when compared with the two-

Table IV. The results observed in the 46 patients who had four-electrode spinal cord stimulation

Improvement	Female, n = 24		Male, n = 22		Total, n = 46	
	n	%	n	%	n	%
Marked	13	54.2	5	22.7	18	39.1
Moderate	5	20.8	11	50.0	16	34.8
Mild	1	4.2	3	13.6	4	8.7
Unimproved	5	20.8	3	13.6	8	17.4

Table V. The results observed in the 63 patients who had spinal cord stimulation for their spasmodic torticollis

Improvement	Female, n = 36		Male, n = 27		Total, n = 63	
	n	%	n	%	n	%
Marked	17	47.2	6	22.2	23	36.5
Moderate	8	22.2	12	44.4	20	31.8
Mild	2	5.6	3	11.1	5	7.9
Unimproved	9	25.0	6	22.2	15	23.8

electrode system. Marked to moderate improved cases increased from 52.9 to 73.9% and unimproved cases fell from 41.2 to 17.4%.

Combined Series (table V)

In the total series, there were 23 patients (36.5%) who demonstrated marked improvement. Moderate improvement was observed in 20 patients (31.8%) who showed minimal residual torticollis, but had full motility without pain. There were 5 patients (7.9%) who were considered mildly improved, demonstrated decrease in their spasms, pain and torticollic neck position, but retained some element of torticollis and/or some limitation of motility. 15 patients (23.8%) were not helped. None of the patients were made worse by the procedure. There was no correlation of gender bias with both male and female showing similar overall response.

Table VI. The incidence of the optimal frequency observed in the 46 patients undergoing four-electrode spinal cord stimulation

Hz	%	Hz	%
100	5.6	800	2.8
200	8.3	900	5.6
300	8.3	1,000	11.1
400	5.6	1,100	13.9
500	8.3	1,200	5.6
600	8.3	1,300	–
700	8.3	1,400	8.3

Table VII. Complications observed in 63 cases undergoing spinal cord stimulation

Complication	n	%
Infection	1	1.5
Insulation defect	2	3.1
Electrode fracture	5	7.9

No specific electrode setting combination was found to be uniformly superior for this condition with relatively equal dispersion of the settings among the group. Some combinations occurred slightly more often than others, which was of no predictive value. The more frequent occurrence of electrode combinations appears to correlate with the size of the applied field. The polaritiy of the applied field was noted to be important with the cathode orientation being cephalad in 72.2% of the cases and caudad in 27.8% of the cases. In general, as noted by *Gildenberg* [3], the torticollic patient shows a tendency to respond to the higher frequency range of stimulation with 55.5% of the patients responding to frequencies of 700 Hz or higher and 72.2% responding to 500 Hz or higher (table VI).

This procedure entails little or no risk to the patient (table VII). Infections occurred in 1.5% of the cases. The system must be temporarily removed and reimplanted in 4–6 months. Fractured electrodes occurred in 7.9% and the insulation defects occurred in 3.1%. Revision of the stimulator system, when these problems occur, is accomplished eas-

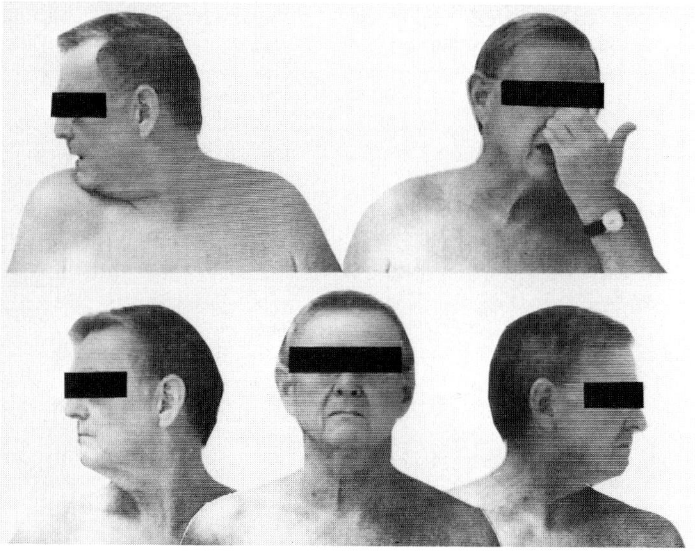

Fig. 6. A 62-year-old man with severe painful spasmodic torticollis. The patient demonstrates the use of sensory input to overcome his nuchal posturing to the right. The patient is shown 1 year postoperatively with relief of his spasmodic torticollis and full motility of the neck.

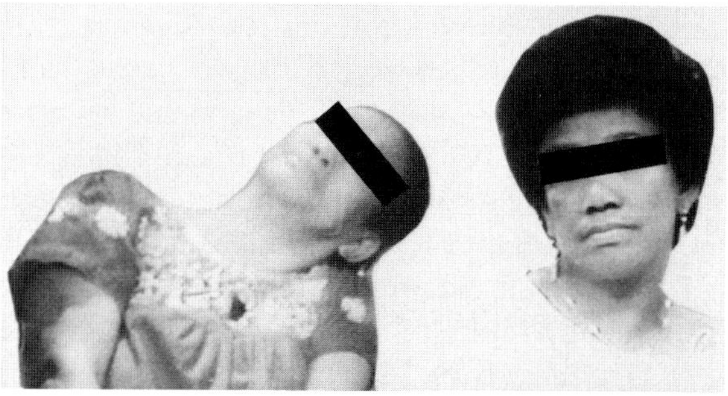

Fig. 7. Severe uncontrolled painful spasms had incapacitated this 31-year-old woman for over 3 years. Preoperative photos show the patient's ability to temporarily overcome the constant spasms by exerting pressure over her face and forehead. Postoperatively, the patient demonstrates complete relief of torticollis. The patient now has complete range of motion of her neck and has been without painful cervical spasms for the past 5 years.

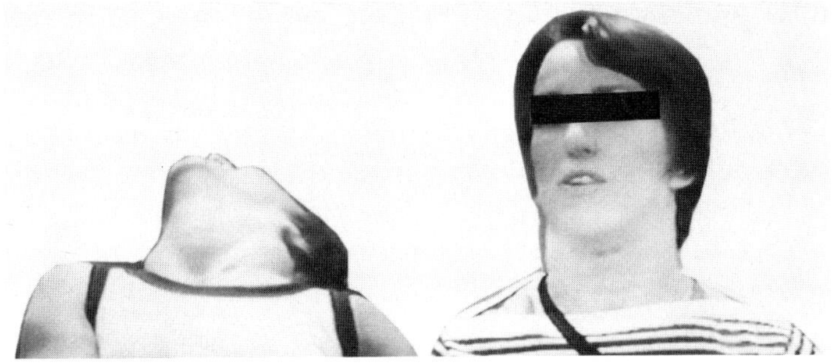

Fig. 8. The patient is a 29-year-old female, with a 20-year history of progressive axial dystonia. The patient had been refractory to all medication and had undergone bilateral thalamectomies at another institution, which proved ineffective in relieving her problem. The patient is shown 2 years postoperatively, having undergone implantation of the spinal cord stimulator system with marked improvement in the dystonia.

ily. In our experience, there has been no mortality and no worsening of any patient's neurologic status.

No correlation was evident between the type or severity of the torticollis with the degree of clinical response noted. The degree of clinical improvement was found to be equal when comparison among the specific types of theses dystonic states were made. Those patients afflicted with lateralcollis (fig. 6), who manifest sensory input correction, responded quite as well as those patients with fixed posturing (fig. 7). No disparity in the level of improvement was noted between the group of patients suffering from anterocollis and those with retrocollis (fig. 8). Even patients with severe intermittent titubation of the head, i.e., Woodpecker dystonia, manifested an equally positive degree of improvement.

Discussion

Both voluntary motor function and postural maintenance represents the product of an intricate balance and elegant mosaic of the harmonious integration of sensory and motor impulses at both central and segmental levels. This sensory motor performance is a closed-loop type of interraction with continuity of a sensory feedback control and multisensory integration [8]. Part of the postural mechanisms of the neck, mediated through the reticular formation, are the tonic neck reflexes, which are modulated by a multitude of sensory input information and servomechanisms. The integrity of such a closed-loop type of sensory motor interaction is essential for voluntary and postural motor control. Any sizeable defect in the flow or organization of afferent sensory information will result in disturbance of the motor function. In its abnormal state, such as spasmodic torticollis, the mosaic has now become a chaotic collage devoid of form and structure, totally lacking in integration.

One of the factors underlying hyperkinesis of nuchal musculature in torticollis is a failure of servomechanisms that modulate somatic motor pathways and tonic neck reflexes which maintain the head and neck in its normal position. The spasmodic jerks often accompanying torticollis appear to be attempts to correct this forced abnormal position. More specifically, this may be due to an imbalance of the tonic neck reflexes where there has been a physiologic resetting of the reflexes due to an abnormal sensory input causing the neck to be rotated, tilted or twisted in position. This resetting of the tonic neck reflexes is obvious in the titubation-like movements. Many patients find that substitute sensory input servomechanisms temporarily overcome the tonic neck reflex and return the head to its normal position. This sensory input modulation can be achieved by placing the hand on the chin, face, forehead or neck on the side ipsilateral to the head deviation. This requires little force, but the head returns to its previous reset tonic neck reflex state as soon as the stimulation is removed. *Brundy* et al. [1] have supplied further evidence of the ability of sensory input modulation to modify tonic neck reflexes in the nuchal dystonic patient. They demonstrated biofeedback suppression of motor activity in the torticollic patient, which they felt indicated that an overriding servomechanism had been established. The response of the dystonic patient to the sensory input modulation by thalamic lesions added further credence to these observations and the conclusion that these abnormal states of sensory communication could be altered by changing the reflex arch by prosthetic input modulation. This theory prompted *Gildenberg* [3] to use spinal cord stimulation in torticollis patients to alter the abnormal pattern of the tonic neck reflexes. The effect of spinal cord stimulation on tonicity was shown graphically by Siegfried et al. [7]. In patients with hypertonicity; stimulating the spinal cord at the C2, C3 level, they showed modification of tonicity with objective measurements, as well as H reflex amplitude diminution up to 86% and, in some cases, totally inhibited.

The level at which the reticular formation is stimulated, the polarity of the electrical field and the frequency of stimulation are all crucial factors in achieving maximal therapeutic results and must be established on an individualized basis. This determination of the optimal stimulation parameters for the individual patient is conveniently and definitively accomplished with the computerized version of the four-electrode multilevel system. Ongoing efforts to maximize therapeutic results have resulted in the computerized version of the multilevel spinal cord stimulation system currently in use. This system was evolved with the intended purpose of refining our surgical intervention by precluding the necessity of a second stage procedure and affording the opportunity for an unrestricted trial period in which to establish optimal stimulation parameters best suited to the individual requirements of the patient so crucial to outcome.

To further improve the therapeutic response in torticollis, the clinical results must be correlated and analyzed with various stimulation criteria, including frequency, polarity, pulse width, impedance, site of stimulation and evoked potentials. In consideration of the refractory nature of the axial dystonias to conventional therapeutic modalities, with their attendant risks, it appears that spinal cord stimulation provides a safer alternative with enhanced efficacy.

References

1 Brundy, J.; Grynbaum, B.B.; Korein, J.: Spasmodic torticollis: treatment by feedback display of the EMG. Archs. phys. Med. Rehabil. *55:* 403–408 (1974).

2 Foltz, E.L.; Knopp, L.M.; Ward, A.A.: Experimental spasmodic torticollis. J. Neurosurg. *16:* 55–72 (1959).

3 Gildenberg, P.L.: Treatment of spasmodic torticollis by dorsal column stimulation. Appl. Neurophysiol. *41:* 113–121 (1978).

4 Hassler, R.; Hess, W.R.: Experimentelle und anatomische Befunde über die Drehbewegungen und ihre nervösen Apparate. Arch. Psychiat. NervKrankh. *192:* 488–526 (1954).

5 Koella, W.P.: Motor effects from electrical stimulation of the basal cerebellum in the unrestrained cat. J. Neurophysiol. *18:* 558–573 (1955).

6 Montanelli, R.P.; Hassler, R.: Motor effects elicited by stimulation of the pallido-thalamic system in the cat; in Bargmann, Schade, Lectures on the diencephalon, pp. 56–66 (Elsevier, Amsterdam 1964).

7 Siegfried, J.; Krainick, J.U.; Hass, H.; Adorjani, C.; Meyer, M.; Thoden, U.: Electrical spinal cord stimulation for spastic movement disorders. Appl. Neurophysiol. *41:* 134-141 (1978).
8 Smith, K.U.; Henry, J.P.: Cybernetic foundations for rehabilitation. Am. J. phys. Med. *46:* 379-467 (1967).
9 Waltz, J.M.; Andreesen, W.H.: Multiple lead spinal cord stimulation: technique. Appl. Neurophysiol. *44:* 30-36 (1981).
10 Waltz, J.M.; Davis, J.A.: Cervical cord stimulation in the treatment of athetosis and dystonia; in Fahn, Calne, Shoulson, Advances in neurology, vol. 37: Experimental therapeutics of movement disorders, pp. 225-237 (Raven Press, New York 1983).
11 Waltz, J.M.; Pani, K.C.: Spinal cord stimulation in disorders of the motor system. Proc. VIth Int. Symp. External Control of Human Extremities, 1978, pp. 545-556.
12 Waltz, J.M.; Reynolds, L.O.; Riklan, M.: Multi-lead spinal cord stimulation for control of motor disorders. Appl. Neurophysiol. *44:* 244-257 (1981).
13 Waltz, J.M.: Spinal cord stimulation for palsies. Patient Care *13:* 118-206 (1979).
14 Waltz, J.M.: Surgical approach to dystonia; in Marsden, Fahn, Neurology, vol. 2: Movement disorders, pp. 300-307 (Butterworths, London 1981).
15 Waltz, J.M.: Computerized percutaneous multi-level spinal cord stimulation in motor disorders. Appl. Neurophysiol. *45:* 73-92 (1982).

J.M. Waltz, Department of Neurological Surgery, St. Barnabas Hospital, New York, NY 10457 (USA)

Proc. 9th Meeting World Soc. Stereotactic and Functional Neurosurgery, Toronto 1985
Appl. Neurophysiol. *48:* 339–346 (1985)

Bipolar Spinal Cord Stimulation for Spasmodic Torticollis

G. Dieckmann, G. Veras

Division of Functional Neurosurgery, Georg August University Medical Center, Göttingen, FRG

Key Words. Spasmodic torticollis · Dorsal cord stimulation · Spinal cord stimulation

Abstract. Four years' experience with electrical stimulation of the cervical cord is reported for 18 patients suffering from spasmodic torticollis. Permanent 1,100-Hz stimulation of the C2–C4 level resulted in a marked improvement in 50% of the patients, in a satisfactory result in 27.8% and in an unsatisfactory result in 22.2%. Muscular tension and related pain were reduced within 8 days to 4 months postoperatively. A measurable improvement of head posture rendered objective by a mechanoelectrical measuring device could only be observed after a continuous stimulation over 8–12 months. The procedure is nondestructive and reversible, complications consisted only in those related to the stimulation system itself.

Introduction

For improvement of the posture of the head in spasmodic torticollis, stereotactic thalamotomy or subthalamotomy has proved to be highly effective [1, 2, 4, 8]. There are long-lasting improvements, especially in connection with a specific postoperative physiotherapy [3], and in some cases even total elimination of the false posture of the head. The long-term results are often very much better than the frequently disappointing early results [4]. However, this is an ablative technique in the depth of the brain in a neuronal system which is in itself already damaged. Side effects, especially motor impediments contralateral to the central site of elimination from motor neglect [8] to

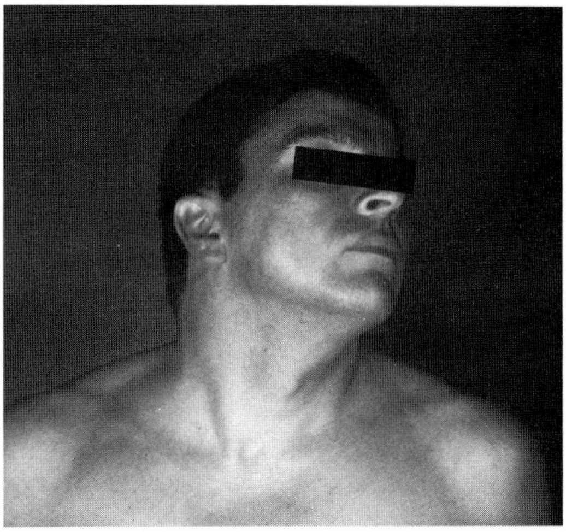

Fig. 1. Head movements around a craniocaudal as well as an anterior-posterior axis in a torticollis patient.

hemiparesis and pseudobulbar disorders [10], detract from the result of surgery, which is actually good. It was hence of interest to obtain a nondestructive technique for interruption of transmission of the disinhibited subcortical impulses to the throat and neck musculature as described by *Gildenberg* [5, 6] and *Waltz* [11]. Accordingly, we have performed a cervical high frequency stimulation for spasmodic torticollis with a permanent implanted electrode since 1980.

Materials and Methods

From 1980 to 1983, we treated 30 patients surgically for spasmodic torticollis. In 12 of these patients, a stereotactic subthalamotomy was performed, and in 18 patients there was a cervical high frequency stimulation. These 18 patients were investigated in the present study. They comprised 12 women and 6 men. The men developed the disease at an average age of 35.2 years, and the women at an average age of 43.7 years.

The following investigations were carried out preoperatively: (a) specific neurological examination for torticollis patients; (b) EMG investigation; (c) Akineton test; (d) radiological examination (cervical spine, head, chest); (e) cerebral computer tomography; (f) ENT examination; (g) neuro-ophthalmological examination; (h) psychological evaluation test (MMPI); (i) mechanoelectrical measurement of head mobility, and (j) stereophotography (only in a portion of the patients).

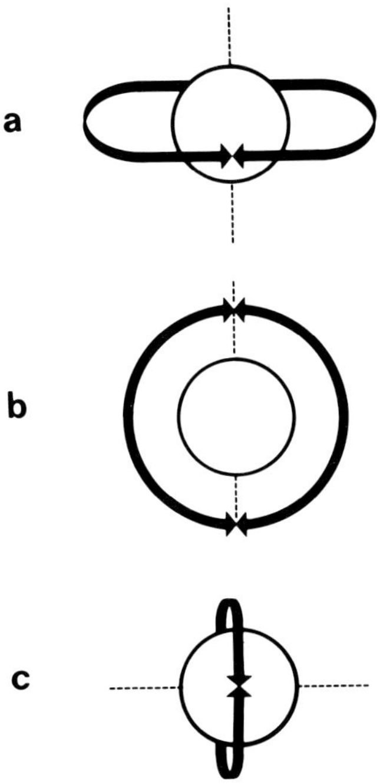

Fig. 2. Angular movements of the head in its three main axes in torticollis patients: **a** rotatory movements in the horizontal; **b** rotatory movement to the side; **c** backwards or forwards movements.

The follow-up examinations were carried out on discharge of the patients, 6 months, 1 or 2 years after the operation. They comprised the positions a, b and c. Both the preoperative and the postoperative examination were carried out under inpatient conditions. The diagnosis of spasmodic torticollis was made on the basis of the clinical picture (fig. 1) and the electromyographic result.

The mechanoelectronic measurement of the head mobility angle allows an objective quantitative evaluation of the improvement of angular movements of the head. The method is inexpensive and reliable. The necessary instruments were developed in collaboration with the Department of Medical Physics and Biophysics at the Georg August University in Göttingen.

The instrument allows head mobility to be measured in its three main movements axes. These are movements around (fig. 2) (1) a craniocaudal axis, i.e. rotatory movements in the horizontal; (2) an anterior-posterior axis, i.e. rotatory movements to the side, in which the ear becomes closer to the shoulder, and (3) a binauricular axis, in order to move the head backwards or forwards in the sense of a retrocollis or anterocollis.

The head movements around these three spatial axes were registered by means of a basal ring applied on the head with a vertical target bow similar to the stereotactic device of Riechert, but of Plexiglas, and transmitted to an electronic system for recording and further processing of the mechanical impulses coming from the basal ring. The electronic impulses were read off on a digital display and simultaneously made graphically visible as movement deflections on a paper strip.

Surgical Technique

In 10 of the cervically implanted patients, a four-pole platelet electrode was implanted by means of partial laminectomy under general anesthesia. The upper platelet came to rest at the level of C2, and the lower platelet at the level of C4. The bipolar stimulation by means of platelet electrodes comprised the segment regions between C2 and C4. This does not correspond to the data of *Gildenberg* [5], who originally recommended the stimulation of the C1/C2 segment. It corresponds to the communication of *Waltz and Pani* [13] who saw the best results in involuntary movements when the electrodes were situated between the segments C2 and C4, as was confirmed in our investigations. In the other 8 patients, we inserted two monopolar epidural spinal electrodes percutaneously from high-thoracic levels under local anesthesia. The level of placing the active surface of the electrodes at the segments C2 and C4 was retained. The rest of the equipment such as electrode extension, receiver and antenna is the same as with the four-polar platelet electrode; it depends on the manufacturing company.

Four days after the implantation, stimulation was commenced. Stimulation was initially carried out with frequencies between 800 and 1,500 Hz, and then only with 1,100 Hz. This stimulation is also only possible bipolarly, and hence we punctated two stimulus electrodes into the spinal canal. The duration of stimulation was 8–12 h on average, during the day or, if desired by the patient, also during the night. The patients were instructed to maintain the stimulation continuously. They were informed that a positive effect of stimulation is only to be reckoned with after a long period of time.

Results

Only muscular contractures and the accompanying pain improved immediately after the operation within the first days up to 2 months after the beginning of stimulation. An objective improvement of the torticollis could not be detected at this time. This only commences between the 8th and 12th months after the beginning of stimulation, and occasionally even only up to 2 years afterwards (fig. 3).

The result of stimulation was evaluated according to the following classification:

Very good: Patients who did not have any torticollis under the stimulation, who had returned to work completely and in whom the symptoms are not triggered even by special circumstances.

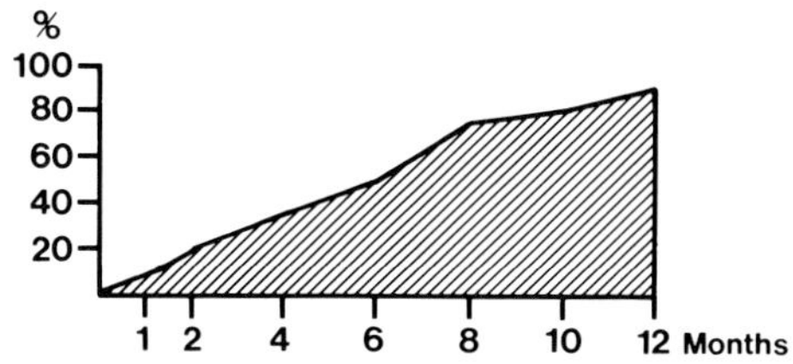

Fig. 3. Results of epidural cervical stimulation in patients with torticollis. The improvement of the involuntary head movement increases by time. Stimulation parameters: 1,100 Hz, 4–5.5 V, 12 h/day continuous.

Good: Patients who notice a motor improvement, do not have any torticollis at rest, no longer complain of contractures of the shoulder and neck musculature, but in whom symptoms of torticollis occur under special circumstances (physical and/or emotional strain).

Satisfactory: The patients report on a subjective improvement in which a moderate improvement of the torticollis is also shown objectively. These also include patients with a short period of follow-up observation or secondary treatment (1 patient died of myocardia infarction after implantation, and a second patient did not present for follow-up examination).

Unsatisfactory: Patients who do not sense any efficacy of this stimulation subjectively or in whom no motor improvement could be rendered objective in the course of the follow-up examination.

On the basis of these criteria, a very good result of treatment was found in 7 patients (38.9%), a good result in 2 patients (11.1%), a satisfactory result in 5 (27.8%) patients and an unsatisfactory result in 4 (22.2%) patients. Table I shows the results of permanent cervical epidural stimulation with regard to the effect of the involuntary head movement in 18 consecutive patients with torticollis. No patient had deteriorated.

The unsatisfactory or unchanged results include 3 patients in whom the stimulation device had to be totally removed because of disturbance of wound healing with subsequent infection. There were no complications regarding the neurological finding in any case. Five patients showed disorders of wound healing several weeks after the implantation with consecutive ascending infections, which necessitated seven revisions. In 3 patients, the system then had to be removed and remained removed. Until very recently, we did not carry out implanta-

Table I. Results of permanent cervical epidural stimulation with regard to the effect on the involuntary head movements in 18 consecutive patients with torticollis

Classification	Patients	Percentage	
Very good	7	38.9	50.0
Good	2	11.1	
Satisfactory	5	27.8	
Unsatisfactory	4	22.2	
Worse	0	0.0	

tions under the antibiotic protection which is usual elsewhere; this may be the reason for the striking frequency of infection in the implants. Another complication, or more precisely a side effect, was a hyperperistalsis with diarrhea under stimulation with higher voltage in 2 patients; this subsided immediately after reduction of the stimulus intensity. There were no other complications in any patient.

Discussion

With 50% very good or good improvement of the torticollis, our results obtained with electrical stimulation of the cervical cord are not as good as those of *Gildenberg* [7], 11 out of 14 of whose patients were improved in this classification. They are also not as favorable as the improvements of 83% in dystonia patients communicated by *Waltz and Davis* [12]. It is possible that the reason may be a different indication. Just as in stereotactic subthalamotomy for improvement of a torticollis, the purely horizontal forms of torticollis also correspond better in stimulation treatment than the rotatory forms or the combined horizontal-rotatory forms. For the stimulation treatment, we have deliberately made no restriction of the indications on the basis of the clinical neurological picture. It is also conceivable that there was a worsening of our statistics by the 3 patients in whom the implantation device had to be explanted because of infections and in whom a fresh implantation was not carried out.

Our study cannot make any contribution to the discussion on the mechanism of action of neuroaugmentative treatment of torticollis. We must refer here to the speculative interpretation made by *Gildenberg* [6] according to which the cervical stimulation blocks or depolarizes afferent propriospinal fibers which were involved in the regulation of tonic reflexes of the neck, so that the asymmetrical tonic neck reflex pattern is interrupted. On the other hand, *Waltz and Davis* [12] see the mechanism of action of high frequency stimulation in an action on the reticular activating system.

The late onset of the therapeutic effect only after months or even after years of continuous stimulation is striking. Although an explanation of this is not known and has also not been discussed so far, it is in agreement with other reports in the literature regarding subthalamotomy [4, 9].

However, the side effects known so far and to be expected from neuroaugmentative treatment of torticollis are very much less than the side effects after stereotactic lesioning. These have been known for years and cause some surgeons to dispense completely with stereotactic therapy for treatment of spasmodic torticollis. In view of the side effects of neurodestructive treatment by means of stereotactic subthalamotomy, epidural stimulation proves to be a welcome alternative in treatment of spasmodic torticollis. Permanent side effects do not occur with this treatment. However, the question remains open as to what consequences may result from a continuous stimulation in the vicinity of the reticular activating system for 8–12 h practiced over years. Incidentally, as suggested by first observations, it appears to be the case that the duration and frequency of stimulation can be reduced or the entire stimulation may be discontinued after stimulation for several years, when the false posture of the head has normalized.

References

1 Augustinsson, L.E.; Essen, C. von; Lindqvist, G.: VOI thalamotomy in spasmodic torticollis. Third Meeting of the European Society of Stereotactic and Functional Neurosurgery, Freiburg 1977, abstr. 5.9.

2 Bertrand, C.; Molina-Negro, P.; Martinez, S.N.: Combined stereotactic and peripheral surgical approach for spasmodic torticollis. Appl. Neurophysiol. *41:* 122–133 (1978).

3 Bold, R.M.; Grossmann, A.: Stemmführung nach R. Brunkow (Enke, Stuttgart 1978).

4 Essen, C. von; Augustinsson, L.E.; Lindqvist, G.: VOI thalamotomy in spasmodic torticollis. Appl. Neurophysiol. *43:* 159–163 (1980).

5 Gildenberg, P.L.: Treatment of spasmodic torticollis by dorsal column stimulation. Rev. Inst. Nal. Neurologia *10:* 11–15 (1976).

6 Gildenberg, P.L.: Treatment of spasmodic torticollis by dorsal column stimulation. Appl. Neurophysiol. *41:* 113–121 (1978).

7 Gildenberg, P.L.: Comprehensive management of spasmodic torticollis. Appl. Neurophysiol. *44:* 233–243 (1981).

8 Hassler, R.; Dieckmann, G.: Die stereotaktische Behandlung des Torticollis aufgrund tierexperimenteller Erfahrungen über die richtungsbestimmten Bewegungen. Nervenarzt *41:* 473–487 (1970).

9 Hernesniemi, J.; Laitinen, L.: Résultats tardifs de la chirurgie dans le torticolis spasmodique. Neuro-Chirurgie *23:* 123–131 (1977).

10 Molina-Negro, P.: Functional surgery of abnormal movements; in Rasmussen, Marino, Functional neurosurgery, pp. 89–121 (Raven Press, New York 1979).

11 Waltz, J.M.: Spinal cord stimulation for palsies? Patient Care *13:* 188–206 (1979).

12 Waltz, J.M.; Davis, J.A.: Cervical cord stimulation in the treatment of athetosis and dystonia; in Fahn, Calne, Shoulson, Advances in neurology; experimental therapeutics of movement disorders, pp. 225–237 (Raven Press, New York 1983).

13 Waltz, J.M.; Pani, K.C.: Spinal cord stimulation in disorders of the motor system. Proc. VIth Int. Symp. External Control of Human Extremities, 1978, pp. 545–556.

Gert Dieckmann, MD, Division of Functional Neurosurgery,
Georg August University Medical Center, D-3400 Göttingen (FRG)

Proc. 9th Meeting World Soc. Stereotactic and Functional
Neurosurgery, Toronto 1985
Appl. Neurophysiol. *48:* 347–350 (1985)

Spasmodic Head Movements Produced by Destruction of Unilateral Ventromedial Tegmentum in Cats

Kazuo Mori, Haruhiro Shimabukuro, Katsumi Yamashiro, Hitoshi Miyake, Teruaki Kawano

Department of Neurosurgery, Nagasaki University, Nagasaki, Japan

Key Words. Torticollis · Ventral tegmental area · Serotonin · Brain dialysis

Abstract. In cats, unilateral electrolytic destruction in the dorsomedial parts of the ventral tegmental area (VTA) (Tsai) led to the appearance of torticollic rotatory head postures associated with a marked drop of the corresponding caudate serotonin. Results obtained from fluorescence histochemistry and brain dialysis also revealed that decrease in serotonin shared the leading role. However, since a chemical lesion produced by neurotoxic agents failed to induce such abnormal postures, concomitant interruption of nonaminergic fibers at VMT might also be the essential factor. Among them the interstitial nucleus (Cajal) and its descending tract were the most suspicious.

Cats with Ventral Tegmental Area Lesions

Torticollic rotatory head postures (the chin rotated to the destroyed side) could be produced in cats by making unilateral electrolytic destruction at the dorsomedial parts of the ventral tegmental area (VTA) of Tsai [3]. The lesion commonly was impinging upon the medial longitudinal fasciculus, interstitial nucleus of Cajal and its descending tract, crossing components of the medial tectospinal tract, and invaded a part of the red nucleus and VTA. Abnormal postures became remarkable within 2–3 days following destruction and lasted usually 7–10 days. In addition, animals were frequently ataxic and showed ocular signs due to third nerve paresis [6].

Contrariwise, sustained bending of the head to the contralateral side was a prominent feature, if the lesion extended more laterally and widely, including the central tegmental tract, the adjoining reticular substance and so on (lateroflexional type).

Changes in Monoamine Concentrations

As the ascending serotonergic fibers are located mainly in the dorsomedial parts of VTA [2], electrolytic destruction inevitably produced a decline in the concentration of serotonin on the lesioned side. Especially, the corresponding caudate serotonin decreased to 40% of the concentration of the nonlesioned side. On the contrary, in the lateroflexion type, a lesion involving the nigrostriatal pathways and decrease in the ipsilateral caudate dopamine and norepinephrine were the most conspicuous findings [3].

Fluorescence Histochemical Study

In the rotatory type, disturbed serotonergic pathways were also demonstrated with the fluorescence histochemical method. In these animals, strongly fluorescent serotonergic axons were clearly evident ventral to the lesion. Swollen varicose fibers were observed running ventromedial to VTA, indicating retrograde accumulation of serotonin caused by the interruption of axonal flow. On the contrary, the dopaminergic outflow from the pars compacta of the substantia nigra and paranigral nucleus appeared normal [2].

An intraperitoneal injection of *L*-5-HTP (100 mg/kg) induced marked exaggeration of the rotatory movements. Contrariwise, *L*-dopa (100 mg/kg) did not significantly alter the postures that were already present [3].

Intracerebral Dialysis

Correspondence, if any, between the animals' head postures and endogenous extracellular levels of amine metabolites were studied in vivo by using an intracerebral dialysis technique. In all of the 4 animals which showed rotatory head postures, the ratio of HVA to 5-HIAA in perfusates obtained from the ipsilateral caudate nucleus was significantly high compared to the intact (control) cats throughout the course of dialysis. On the contrary, in 2 animals in which rotatory head movements had disappeared at the time of dialysis, an increase in the ratio was less prominent or within the control range (fig. 1). This result also

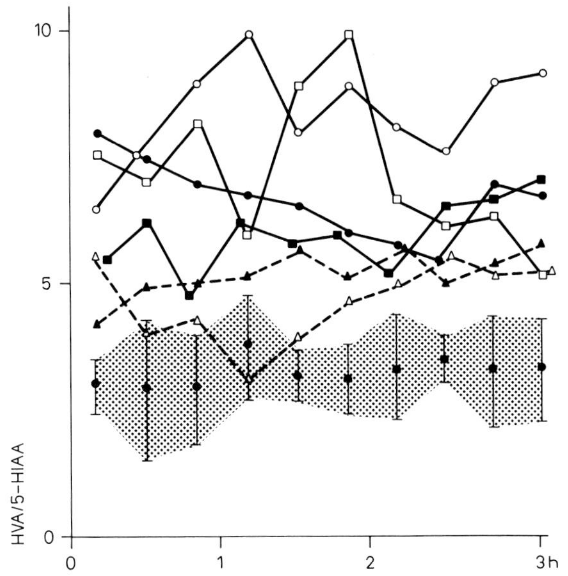

Fig. 1. In vivo measurement of the ratio of HVA to 5-HIAA, studied by intracerebral dialysis. After making an electrolytic lesion in the dorsomedial parts of VTA (Tsai), dialysis tubing was implanted into both sides of the caudate nucleus. Subsequently, dialysis was continued for about 5 h with Ringer's solution at a flow rate of 20 μl/min. Perfusates were collected at 20-min intervals and assayed for extracellular levels of HVA and 5-HIAA. In 4 cats with rotatory head posturs (solid lines), the HVA/5-HIAA ratio from the ipsilateral caudate nucleus was increased significantly. In 2 cats in which rotatory movements had disappeared at the time of dialysis (dotted lines), this ratio was less prominent, and in 1 cat it showed partly within the control values.

indicates, although indirectly, that a decrease in ipsilateral caudate serotonin might play an important role in the manifestation of rotatory torticollic postures in this animal model.

Chemical Lesioning

Since an electrical current destroys both aminergic and nonaminergic pathways, observation was made in chemically denervated cats with 6-hydroxydopamine, 5,6- or 5,7-dihydroxytryptamine by which a marked difference in concentrations of bioamines between the two sides could be produced. Mechanical (nonspecific) tissue destruction caused by injection was so slight that it could be negligible. In neurotoxic lesions, however, abnormal movements were not produced, except 1 cat which had an associated large hemorrhage produced at the time of injection [4].

In the light of these findings and the findings of other workers [1, 5], it is appealing to assume that for the manifestation of torticollic rotatory head posture, destruction of the nonaminergic pathways at VMT (especially the descending tract from the Cajal nucleus) is essential. Imbalance in the concentration of serotonin could act to enhance the rotatory head movements.

References

1 Hassler, R.; Dieckmann, G.: Die stereotaktische Behandlung des Torticollis aufgrund tierexperimenteller Erfahrungen über die richtungsbestimmten Bewegungen. Nervenarzt *41:* 473–487 (1970).
2 Ishikawa, M.: Fluorescence histochemical study of the central monoaminergic neuron system on experimental torticollis in the cat. Arch. jap. Chir. *45:* 457–470 (1976).
3 Mori, K.; Fujita, Y.; Shimabukuro, H.; Ito, M.; Handa, H.: Some considerations for treatment of spasmodic torticollis. Clinical and experimental studies. Confinia Neurol. *37:* 265–269 (1975).
4 Mori, K.; Kawano, T.; Tsujimura, M.; Iwayama, K.: Spasmodic torticollis-like posture by chemical denervation of the ventromedial tegmentum (VMT) in cats. Appl. Neurophysiol. *42:* 302–321 (1979).
5 Poirier, L.J.; Sourkes, T.L.; Bouvier, G.; Boucher, R.; Carabin, S.: Striatal amines, experimental tremor and the effect of harmaline in the monkey. Brain *89:* 37–55 (1966).
6 Shimabukuro, H.; Mori, K.: The role of the mesencephalic tegmentum upon manifestation of the spasmodic torticollis-like posture and ocular symptoms in cats. Arch. jap. Chir. *38:* 626–632 (1969).

Kazuo Mori, MD, Department of Neurosurgery, Nagasaki University School of Medicine, 7-1 Sakamoto-machi, Nagasaki 852 (Japan)

Proc. 9th Meeting World Soc. Stereotactic and Functional
Neurosurgery, Toronto 1985
Appl. Neurophysiol. *48:* 351–357 (1985)

Phrenic Nerve Stimulation (Diaphragm Pacing) in Respiratory Paralysis

H. Fodstad[a], *G. Andersson*[b], *S. Blom*[c], *H. Linderholm*[d]

Departments of [a] Neurosurgery and [d] Clinical Physiology, University of Umeå;
[b] Department of Anaesthesiology, Danderyd Hospital, Stockholm, and
[c] Department of Clinical Neurophysiology, University of Uppsala, Sweden

Key Words. Cervical cord lesion · Diaphragm pacer · Phrenic nerve stimulation · Respiratory insufficiency

Abstract. Phrenic nerve stimulators (diaphragm pacers) were implanted in 16 patients with partial or total respiratory insufficiency due to high cervical medullary lesions and brain stem lesions (14 cases) or central hypoventilation syndrome (2 cases). At 5–72 months' follow-up (M=35) 12 patients are entirely independent of conventional respirator, 2 of them after 8 years of total respirator dependency. Two patients are dead and the final 2 cases had limited help from diaphragm pacing.

Introduction

Artificial respiration by electrostimulation of the phrenic nerve is a well-known technique in the history of medicine [2, 10, 13]. The modern diaphragm pacemaker was developed by *Sarnoff* et al. [12, 14] and *Glenn* et al. [7, 8]. The main indications for electrophrenic stimulation are respiratory paralysis after cervical-medullary injury above the origin of the phrenic motor neurons and the chronic central hypoventilation syndrome (sleep apnea or Ondine's curse) [4, 7–9]. The method has also been tried in chronic obstructive pulmonary disease [6] and chronic hiccup [3, 5]. Since 1979 we have implanted diaphragm pacers in 16 patients with respiratory insufficiency of central nervous origin.

Material and Method

Sixteen patients [10 males and 6 females, age 6–63 years (M=24)] with partial or total respiratory insufficiency due to high cervical cord lesions, brain stem lesions or cen-

Table I.

Case No.	Year of birth (age) sex	CNS lesion	Preop. respirator dependency	Pacer implantation date	Follow-up months	Late result
1	1969 (10 y) male	abscess C:1–C:3 tetraplegia	fully dependent for 8 years	left side June 1979 right side Sept. 1979	72	independent of respirator with full-time pacing some spontaneous respiration
2	1958 (22 y) female	congenital exostosis C:2 tetraplegia	partially dependent for 4 years	left side March 1980, revised Febr. 1982 right side June 1980, revised Dec. 1981 and Aug. 1982	63	independent of respirator with full-time pacing some spontaneous respiration
3	1970 (10 y) male	central hypoventilation sy. (M. Morquio) tetraparesis	continuous manual ventilation for 1 year	left side Oct. 1980	-	died of pneumonia 3 weeks after operation
4	1961 (19 y) male	trauma C:4–C:5 tetraplegia	fully dependent for 8 months	right side Oct. 1980 left phrenic nerve without function	56	dependent on respirator at night; autonomous spontaneous respiration during daytime pacing stopped 1983
5	1965 (16 y) male	trauma foramen magnum – C:1 tetraplegia	fully dependent for 18 months	left side June 1981, revised Sept. 1981 right side Sept. 1981	48	independent of respirator with full-time pacing some spontaneous respiration

Table I. (continued)

Case No.	Year of birth (age) sex	CNS lesion	Preop. respirator dependency	Pacer implantation date	Follow-up months	Late result
6	1956 (25 y) male	trauma C:3 tetraplegia	fully dependent for 8 years	left side June 1981, revised Oct. 1981, July 1983 and June 1985 right side June 1981	48	independent of respirator with full-time pacing some spontaneous respiration
7	1967 (14 y) male	central hypoventilation sy. (sleep apnea)	partially dependent for 4 months	right side Nov. 1981 left side Dec. 1981, revised Sept. 1984	43	independent of respirator with pacing at night and spontaneous respiration during daytime
8	1965 (17 y) female	foramen magnum herniation (suprasellar tumor) tetraplegia	fully dependent for 5 years, partially for 2 years	left side July 1982 right side July 1982	35	independent of respirator with full-time pacing some spontaneous respiration
9	1972 (10 y) male	brain stem (foramen magnum/ post. fossa tumor) tetraplegia	fully dependent for 2 months	left side Oct. 1982 right side Oct. 1982	32	independent of respirator with full-time pacing some spontaneous respiration
10	1920 (62 y) male	brain stem (Wallenberg's syndrome) tetraparesis	fully dependent for 6 months	left side Nov. 1982, revised Nov. 1982 right side Nov. 1982	31	independent of respirator with full-time pacing some spontaneous respiration

Table I. (continued)

Case No.	Year of birth (age) sex	CNS lesion	Preop. respirator dependency	Pacer implantation date	Follow-up months	Late result
11	1920 (63 y) female	infarction C:2–C:3 (art. spinalis ant. thromb.) tetraparesis	fully dependent for 8 months	left side March 1983 right side March 1983 (malfunctioning left phrenic nerve)	21	dependent on respirator at night; pacing during daytime; died of cardiac/respiratory arrest Jan. 1985
12	1963 (20 y) male	trauma C:3–C:4 tetraplegia	fully dependent for 11 months	right side May 1983	25	independent of respirator with pacing at night and spontaneous respiration during daytime
13	1921 (62 y) female	brain stem (acoustic neurinoma)	partially dependent for 6 months	left side July 1983	23	independent of respirator with pacing at night and spontaneous respiration during daytime
14	1962 (21 y) male	trauma C:4 tetraplegia	fully dependent for 2½ years, partially for 9 months	left side July 1984 right phrenic nerve without function	11	dependent on respirator occasionally pacing during daytime
15	1978 (6 y) female	tumor C:2–C:3 (Recklinghausen's disease) tetraplegia	fully dependent for 5 months	left side Sept. 1984 right side April 1985	9	independent of respirator with full-time pacing
16	1973 (11 y) female	trauma C:1 tetraplegia	fully dependent for 14 months	left side Jan. 1985 right side Jan. 1985	5	independent of respirator with full-time pacing

tral hypoventilation syndrome received phrenic nerve stimulators (table I). Fourteen patients were tetraplegic/tetraparetic and had been fully or partially dependent on respiratory assistance in hospitals for 2 months to 8 years. The pacemaker (Avery model S 202 unilateral/pocket) was implanted bilaterally in 11 patients and unilaterally in 5 patients. The technical description and operative procedure have been reported elsewhere [4, 8, 9].

Preoperatively, both phrenic nerves were transcutaneously stimulated under fluoroscopy of the diaphragm and ventilation and blood gas studies were undertaken.

Results

At 5–72 months' follow-up (M=35) 12 patients are entirely independent of conventional respirators (table I). Nine are pacing full time, each phrenic nerve being stimulated for 12 hours at a time. Three patients can breathe spontaneously during the daytime and use their pacers at night. One patient stopped using the pacer after 2 years when he developed an autonomous spontaneous respiration that interfered with the stimulator. One additional patient uses the pacer only occasionally and is dependent on the respirator most of the time. Two patients are dead – 1 died 3 weeks postoperatively of pneumonia and the other died in her sleep 21 months after surgery. Five patients went through altogether 9 reoperations because of receiver failure, electrode failure due to fibrosis around the phrenic nerve or skin necrosis over the implanted receiver. Postoperative studies of ventilation and blood gases while using the pacer have shown normal values after a diaphragm-conditioning period of 1–3 months in all patients who had become independent of their respirator. Interestingly, 6 of the patients with cervical-medullary lesions have developed some spontaneous respiration after the first weeks of diaphragm pacing – 2 of them after 8 years of total respirator dependency. The tracheostomy has been removed in 3 patients, whereas 6 patients can talk with the aid of a tracheal speaking valve. Eleven patients have left the hospital and stay in their homes, 5 attend school 2–7 h/day and 1 is working 4 h/day.

Discussion

The implantation of electrophrenic stimulators has been of significant benefit to the majority of our patients. The reason for this is probably careful patient selection as well as adequate preoperative investigations and postoperative controls. Problems which occasionally will arise are fibrosis around the phrenic nerve at the site of the electrode cuff [4, 11], diaphragm fatigue [1, 7] and failure of the radioreceiver [4]. Other difficulties are related to the energy source, the lack of an alarm system in case of pacemaker failure and the high cost of the equipment. With regard to the technical problems, the risk of complications and the limited number of patients suitable for this operation,we think that implantation of phrenic nerve stimulators should be concentrated in a few centers and units with the necessary resources and experience. International cooperation, improvement of the technique involved and less expensive devices would undoubtedly trigger the interest in this method and prevent the 'best means of imitating natural respiration' [2] fading into the shadows.

References

1 Ciesielski, T.E.; Fukuda, Y.; Glenn, W.W.L.; Gorfien, J.; Jeffery, K.; Hogan, J.F.: Response of the diaphragm muscle to electrical stimulation of the phrenic nerve. A histochemical and ultrastructural study. J. Neurosurg. *58:* 92–100 (1983).

2 Duchenne, G.: De l'électrisation localisée et de son application à la pathologie et à la thérapeutique; 3rd ed. (Baillière, Paris 1972).

3 Fodstad, H.; Blom, S.: Phrenic nerve stimulation (diaphragm pacing) in chronic singultus. Neurochirurgia *27:* 115–116 (1984).

4 Fodstad, H.; Blom, S.; Linderholm, H.: Artifical respiration ba phrenic nerve stimulation (diaphragm pacing) in patients with cervical cord and brain stem lesions. Scand. J. Rehabil. Med *15:* 173–181 (1983).

5 Glenn, W.W.L.: The diaphragm. Hiccup (singultus); in Glenn, Thorac. Cardiovasc, Surg.; 4th ed., pp. 359–360 (Appleton Century Crofts, Publishing Division Prentice-Hall, East Norwalk 1983).

6 Glenn, W.W.L.; Gee, J.B.L.; Schachter, E.N.: Diaphragm pacing. Application to a patient with chronic obstuctive pulmonary disease. J. thorac. cardiovasc. Surg. *75:* 273–281 (1978).

7 Glenn, W.W.L.; Hogan, J.F.; Loke, J.S.O.; Ciesielski, T.E.; Phelps, M.L.; Rowedder, R.: Ventilatory support by pacing of the conditioned diaphragm in quadriplegia. New Engl. J. Med. *310:* 1150–1155 (1984).

8 Glenn, W.W.L.; Holcomb, W.G.; Gee, J.B.L.; Rath, R.: Central hypoventilation. Long-term ventilatory assistance by radiofrequency electrophrenic respiration. Ann. Surg. *172:* 755–773 (1970).

9 Glenn, W.W.L.; Phelps, M.; Gersten, L.M.: Diaphragm pacing in the management of central alveolar hypoventilation; in Guilleminault, Dement, Sleep apnea syndromes, pp. 333–345 (Liss, New York 1978).

10 Israel, F.: Über die Wiederbelebung scheintoter Neugeborener mit Hilfe des elektrischen Stromes. Z. Geburtsh. Gynäk. *91:* 602–622 (1927).
11 Kim, J.H.; Manuelidis, E.E.; Glenn, W.W.L.: Diaphragm pacing, Histopathological changes in the phrenic nerve following long-term electrical stimulation. J. thorac. cardiovasc. Surg. *72:* 602–608 (1976).
12 Sarnoff, S.J.; Hardenbergh, E.; Whittenberger, J.L.: Electrophrenic respiration. Am. J. Physiol. *155:* 1–9 (1948).
13 Ure, A.: An account of some experiments made on the body of a criminal immediately after execution, with physiological and practical observations. Sci. Arts, Lond. *6:* 283–294 (1819).
14 Whittenberger, J.L.; Sarnoff, S.J.; Hardenbergh, E.: Electrophrenic respiration. II. Its use in man. J. clin. Invest. *28:* 124–128 (1949).

H. Fodstad, PhD, Department of Neurosurgery, University of Umeå,
Umeå (Sweden)

Proc. 9th Meeting World Soc. Stereotactic and Functional
Neurosurgery, Toronto 1985
Appl. Neurophysiol. *48:* 358–361 (1985)

Preliminary Report on the Use of Fetal Tissue Transplantation to Correct MPTP-Induced Parkinson-Like Syndrome in Primates

Roy A.E. Bakay, Massimo S. Fiandaca, Daniel L. Barrow, Arthur Schiff, Delwood C. Collins

Emory University Clinic, Atlanta, Ga., USA

Key Words. Parkinson's disease · Primates · Tissue transplant · N-methyl-4-phenyl-1,2,3,6-tetrahydropyridine · Fetal tissue

Abstract. A Parkinson-like syndrome was produced in nonhuman primates and successfully reversed through transplantation of heterologous fetal mesencephalic brain tissue. Rigidity and bradykinesia were induced by the chronic administration of N-methyl-4-phenyl-1,2,3,6-tetrahydropyridine. Once the deficits were fixed, *Macaca mulatta* with well-developed Parkinson-like behavior received fetal mesencephalic cell preparations stereotactically implanted into multiple sites of the head of the caudate bilaterally. Both animals demonstrated a normalization of CSF *L*-dopa and significant improvement in observed activity. The neuropathological studies performed 2 months following transplantation demonstrated successful integration of fetal cells in the caudate.

Introduction

The transplantation of fetal tissue into adult animals to correct behavioral abnormalities is well established in the rat [1]. Lesions to the substantia nigra in the rat which lead to abnormal circling behavior can be successfully reversed by transplantation of fetal tissue provided that it is performed within a 'critical' developmental age of the donor [2]. This appears to be at the time of the final mitosis before migration and differentiation into dopaminergic neurons. Experience with transplantation of fetal tissue in nonhuman primates is extremely limited [7] and was reported to be unsuccessful, probably because of incorrect fetal donor age [6].

The drug N-methyl-4-phenyl-1,2,3,6-tetrahydropyridine (MPTP) is a selective neurotoxin that destroys dopaminergic cells in the nigrostriatal pathway resulting in a movement disorder with many of the characteristics of parkinsonism [3]. The purpose of this study was to see whether or not the movement disorder induced by MPTP could be reversed through the transplantation of fetal mesencephalic tissue.

Methods

Baseline behavioral data was obtained by videotaping normal *Macaca mulatta* caged activity and scoring the observed movements. Multiple hours of recording on each animal were broken down into 15-second segments and the dominant activity in that segment recorded. CSF was obtained from the cisterna magna and catecholamine activity determined by radioenzymatic assay [5]. Drug was administered as previously described by *Burns* et al. [3]. An additional two sets of doses were required to obtain the degree of movement abnormality desired.

Postdrug biochemical and behavioral data were obtained 3 months following the initial administration of MPTP. Fetal tissue was obtained at the 35th and 37th postgestational days as determined by timed breeding. The fetus was carefully dissected under the operating microscope and the mesencephalon removed. Gentle tissue disruption was performed using a 0.01% trypsin and gentle agitation [2]. The cell suspension was then stereotactically implanted into the head of the caudate of the recipient animal, bilaterally along a 1-cm tract in three separate areas 5 mm apart.

At 1 and 2 months postoperatively, behavior and biochemical data were obtained. The right caudate was then surgically removed, sectioned and immediately frozen over dry ice for flourescence histochemistry [4]. The animal was then perfused with 10% formalin for histopathological study.

Results and Discussion

Following the administration of MPTP, both animals demonstrated a significant tendency to spend more time in a stationary position. This increase in sedentary behavior was at the expense of 'active' behavior (circling, acrobatics, etc.). The degree of movement deficits corresponded to a decrease in CSF *L*-dopa levels with a reduction of 76 and 78%. Two months following fetal transplantation, both animals demonstrated an increase in activity and a decrease in time sitting. The time spent in 'active behavior' increased but never reached the same degree of activity as prior to MPTP treatment. CSF *L*-dopa similarly increased to baseline concentrations.

mal. All graft sites were extremely small, with the largest being only 1 mm in diameter. Catecholamine-flourescent cells were observed along transplantation tracts and in grafts.

Catecholamine-flourescent fibers extend into the host tissue with bouton-like enlargements suggestive of normal synaptic contacts. The animals' behavioral and biochemical improvement strongly suggest a functional interaction between graft and host. This type of improvement was not seen spontaneously except in inadequate MPTP preparations.

Discussion

The primate brain is many orders of magnitude larger than the rodent brain and therefore techniques successful in the rodent may have to be dramatically altered in order to achieve succes, in the primate. Using multiple stereotactically implanted injection sites, bilaterally in the caudate nucleus, appears to be a promising tactic. Not all of these implantation sites were successful and despite the overal improvement in movement, there still appears to be a persistent deficit in terms of overall motor repertoire. Additional techniques for transplantation will need to be explored.

Although this work represents a promise for future transplantation in Parkinson disease, a number of cautions are in order. The succes of this procedure needs to be repeated and long-term studies performed. The transplant must be able to continue to survive and function on a chronic basis without host injury. Studies to investigate this are underway.

Acknowledgements

From the Neurosurgery and Medical Research Service Veterans Administration and the Division of Neurosurgery, Emory University School of Medicine and Yerkes Regional Primate Center (NIH Co-Grant RROO-165) Emory University.

We wish to thank the outstanding staff at Yerkes Primate Center for their support without which this project would be impossible. We also wish to thank *Joyce Klemm*, BS, MT (ASCP) and *Mary Alice Smith*, MS, for their technical assistance.

References

1 Bjorklund, A.; Stenevi, U.: Reconstruction of the nigrostriatal dopamine pathway by intracerebral nigral transplant. Brain Res. *177:* 555–560 (1979).

2 Bjorklund, A.; Stenevi, U.; Schmidt, R.H.; Dunnett, S.B.; Gage, F.H.: Intracerebral grafting of neuronal cell suspensions. 1. Introduction and general methods of preparation. Acta physiol. scand., suppl. 522, pp. 1–7 (1984).

3 Burns, R.S.; Chiueh, C.C.; Markey, S.P.; Ebert, M.H.; Jacobowitz, D.M.; Kopin, I.J.: A primate model of parkinsonism: selective destruction of dopaminergic neurons in the pars compacta of the substantia nigra by N-methyl-4-phenyl-1,2,3,6-tetrahydropyridine. Proc. natn. Acad. Sci. USA *80:* 4546–4550 (1983).

4 De la Torre, J.C.: An improved approach to histoflourescence using the SPG method for tissue monoamines. J. neurosci. Meth. *3:* 1–5 (1980).

5 Johnson, G.A.; Gren, J.M.; Kupiecki, R.: Radioenzymatic assay of dopa (3,4-dihydroxyphenylalanine). Clin. Chem. *24:* 1927–1930 (1978).

6 Levitt, P.; Rakic, P.: The time of genesis, embryonic origin and differentiation of the brain stem monoamine neurons in the rhesus monkey. Devl. Brain Res. *4:*35–57 (1982).

7 Morihisa, J.M.; Nakamura, R.K.; Freed, W.J.; Mishkin, M.; Wyatt, R.J.: Adrenal medulla grafts survive and exhibit catecholamine flourescence in the primate brain. Expl. Neurol. *84:* 643–653 (1984).

R.A.E. Bakay, MD, Emory University Clinic, 1365 Clifton Road, N.E., Atlanta, GA 30322 (USA)

Proc. 9th Meeting World Soc. Stereotactic and Functional
Neurosurgery, Toronto 1985
Appl. Neurophysiol. *48:* 362–366 (1985)

Changes in Cerebral Blood Flow after Stereotactic Thalamotomy[1]

Gunvor Kullberg[a], *Jarl Risberg*[b]

Departments of [a] Neurosurgery and of [b] Psychiatry, University Hospital, Lund, Sweden

Key Words. Cerebral blood flow · Thalamotomy · Stereotactic surgery · Blood flow measurements · Xenon

Abstract. Regional cerebral blood flow (rCBF), a parameter of neuronal activity in the brain, was measured by the ^{133}Xe inhalation method in 43 patients undergoing stereotactic thalamotomy. A postoperative flow reduction of about 2% in the operated hemisphere was found, persisting in further measurements performed after a year. There was no consistent change in the pattern of regional flow distribution. The results indicate a diminished level of activity in the hemisphere subjected to thalamotomy, but the change could not be linked to any specific area or function.

Due to the coupling between blood flow, metabolism and neuronal activity of the brain, measurement of the regional cerebral blood flow (rCBF) can be used for mapping of cerebral function. The aim of the present investigation was to study changes of rCBF following stereotactic thalamotomy, performed as a treatment for tremor.

Material and Methods

The study is based on 43 operations, 25 on the left side and 18 on the right side, in 37 patients. Five of the patients had bilateral operations, left side preceding right side, 1 patient had two operations on the right side because of recurrent tremor. The mean age of the patients was 60 years, range 36–74 years. The diagnosis was Parkinson's disease in 32 patients and other types of tremor in 5.

[1] Supported by the Swedish Medical Research Council (project No. 4969).

Table I. Mean hemisphere flow

	n	Hemisphere flow			pCO_2
		mean and standard deviation		difference between sides	
		op. side	contralateral		
Preoperation	43	41.7 (6.0)	41.5 (6.0)	+0.2[a]	39.3
Postoperation (1–2 weeks)	43	39.1 (5.9)	39.8 (5.9)	−0.8[c]	37.5
		Change from preop. to postop.:		−1.0[c]	
Preoperation	25	42.4 (7.2)	42.1 (7.1)	+0.3[a]	40.5
Follow-up (½–2 years)	25	39.9 (6.5)	40.6 (6.2)	−0.7[b]	39.4
		Change from preop. to follow-up:		−1.0[c]	

[a] Not significant; [b] $0.01 < p < 0.025$; [c] $p < 0.001$ (Wilcoxon test for pair differences).

Table II.

	n	Hemisphere flow adjusted to $pCO_2 = 40$	
		op. side	contralat.
Preoperation	25	42.2	42.0
Postoperation	25	41.0	41.7
	Difference:	-1.2[a]	-0.3[b]

[a] $p = 0.05$; [b] not significant (Wilcoxon test for pair differences).

The operative procedure included ventricular puncture through a burr hole just behind the coronal suture with injection of air for pneumoencephalography, followed by stereotactic placement of a coagulation lesion in the ventrolateral thalamus.

The rCBF was determined by the ^{133}Xe inhalation technique [1] with simultaneous measurements in 16 regions of each hemisphere. The ISI (initial slope index [2]) was used as a measure of mainly cortical blood flow. The mean flow of the 16 regions will be referred to as hemisphere flow. The measurements were made with the patients resting with closed eyes.

The patients were studied before the operation, during the 2nd postoperative week, and in 25 cases also after ½–2 years.

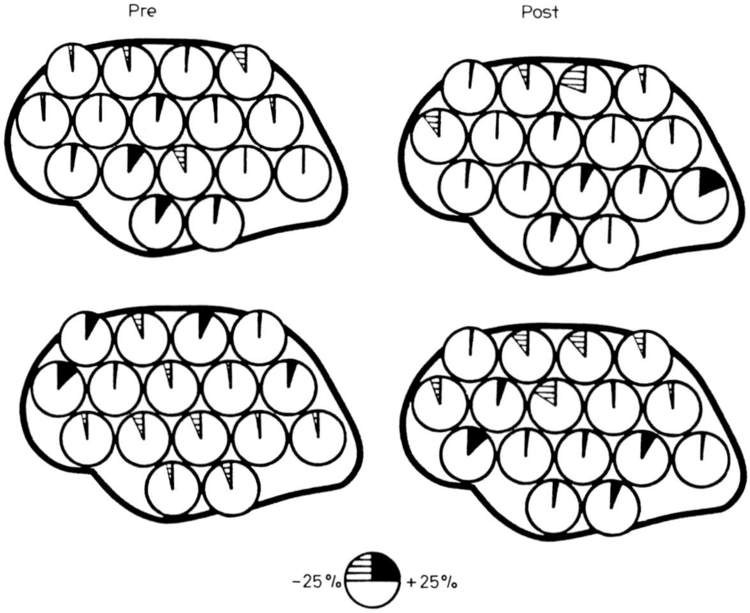

Fig. 1. Interhemispheric differences in rCBF (side of operation minus contralateral side) in 2 patients, before and after operation. Regional flow is expressed as % of hemisphere flow. The preoperative flow differences are of moderate magnitude. After operation there are more marked, negative differences (= lower flow in operated side) in Rolandic and prefrontal regions.

Results

The mean hemisphere flow before and after the operation is shown in table I, comparing the side of operation with the contralateral side. As cerebral blood flow varies in parallel with pCO_2, the corresponding mean pCO_2 values are also given. Comparison of preoperative hemisphere flow with postoperative flow after correction for pCO_2 variations (table II) indicated that a slight flow reduction occurred in the operated hemisphere ($p = 0.05$), whereas the other side did not change significantly. The two hemispheres, measured simultaneously, showed no significant flow difference before the operation. At the postoperative measurement there was, however, a small but significant ($p < 0.001$) interhemispheric difference, the operated side showing a

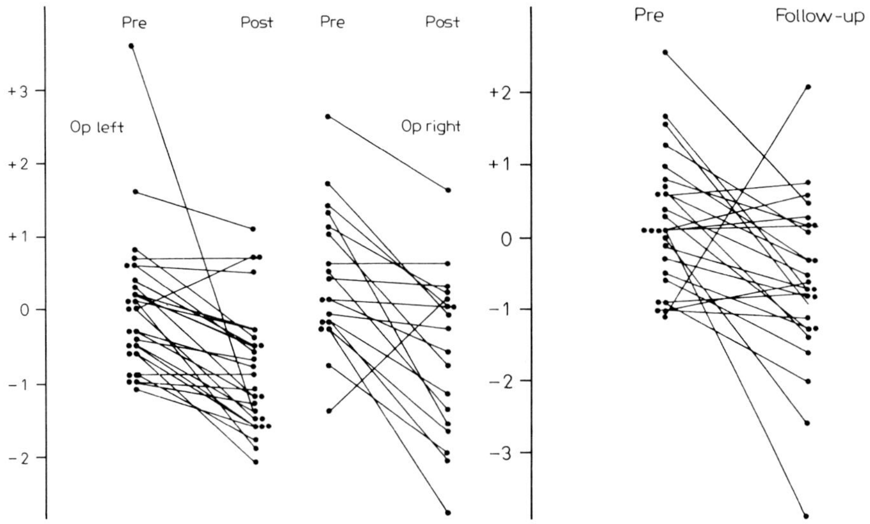

Fig. 2. Individual differences in hemisphere flow (side of operation minus contralateral side): preoperative and postoperative (1–2 weeks), and preoperative and follow-up (½–2 years).

2% lower level compared to the other side. The asymmetry was about the same at follow-up (fig. 1).

The individual interhemispheric differences shown in figure 2 illustrate that, even if the pre- and postoperative values showed considerable overlap, the direction of the change from pre- to postoperative was generally consistent.

The regional flow distribution showed some individual variations, but the average pattern for the group was normal. Thus, no single area emerged as generally responsible for the flow reduction in the operated hemisphere. Some interesting individual changes were noted, however. Some patients showed a postoperative asymmetry in central-parietal and prefrontal regions, with lower flow on the operated side.

Discussion

The results indicate a slight but consistent diminution of the functional activity of the hemisphere operated upon – an operation which involves a lesion in the thalamus as well as penetration of the brain.

One may speculate whether this change is related to the reduction of motor hyperactivity, the desired therapeutic effect of the operation, or whether it reflects some other, probably unwanted, functional alteration related to the operation trauma. No significant correlation between improvement of the motor functions and the rCBF changes, which would have supported the first alternative, was found.

Psychological testing of cognitive functions showed a postoperative decline in performance level in the majority of the patients. However, at follow-up preoperative levels were essentially reestablished. Thus, changes in these mental functions did not parallel the blood flow changes, which persisted at follow-up.

In conclusion, the results indicate a diminished level of activity in the hemisphere subjected to thalamotomy, but the nature and functional importance of the change is unclear.

References

1 Obrist W.D.; Thompson, H.K.; Wang, H.S.; Wilkinson, W.E.: Regional cerebral blood flow estimated by ^{133}Xe inhalation. Stroke *6:* 245–256 (1975).

2 Risberg, J.; Ali, Z.; Wilson, E.M.; Wills, E.L.; Halsey, J.H.: Regional cerebral blood flow by ^{133}Xe inhalation. Preliminary evaluation of an initial slope index in patients with unstable flow compartments. Stroke *6:* 142–148 (1975).

G. Kullberg, MD, Department of Neurosurgery, University Hospital, Lund (Sweden)

Proc. 9th Meeting World Soc. Stereotactic and Functional
Neurosurgery, Toronto 1985
Appl. Neurophysiol. *48:* 367–370 (1985)

Influence of Spinal Cord Stimulation on Peripheral Blood Flow

J. Broseta, G. Garcia-March, M.J. Sanchez, J. Gonçales

Department of Neurosurgery, Hospital Universitario, Salamanca, Spain

Key Words. Spinal cord stimulation · Pain · Blood flow · Peripheral vascular disease

Abstract. In 27 vasculopathic and 9 nonvasculopathic patients who underwent spinal cord stimulation to treat pain in lower extremities, Doppler recordings and thermography were used to study peripheral blood flow changes during stimulation. Generally, poststimulation pain relief coincided with a improvement of Doppler recording, a normalization of morphology and increase of pulse wave amplitude, and a rise of skin temperature in the painful area.

According to previous studies, spinal cord stimulation (SCS) has been highly effective in treating pain of vascular origin resulting from peripheral arterial diseases [1–5]. Nevertheless, there is still disagreement about whether analgesia is related to the peripheral blood flow changes observed. This report concerns findings obtained on peripheral blood flow, measured with Doppler recording and thermography in 27 vasculopathic and 9 nonvasculopathic patients who underwent SCS.

Clinical Materials and Methods

The vasculopathic group consisted of 27 patients with peripheral arterial insufficiency (arteriosclerosis in 18 cases, diabetic angiopathy in 7 and Buerger's disease in 2) presenting day and night pain at rest in distal parts of lower limbs. 8 patients also had cutaneous trophic ulcers. The nonvasculopathic group included 9 patients with pain in lower limbs resulting from arachnoiditis and nerve root avulsion treated with SCS.

Doppler studies were used to measure changes in blood velocity during stimulation to study the hemodynamic conditions of the mean arteries of the lower extremities. They

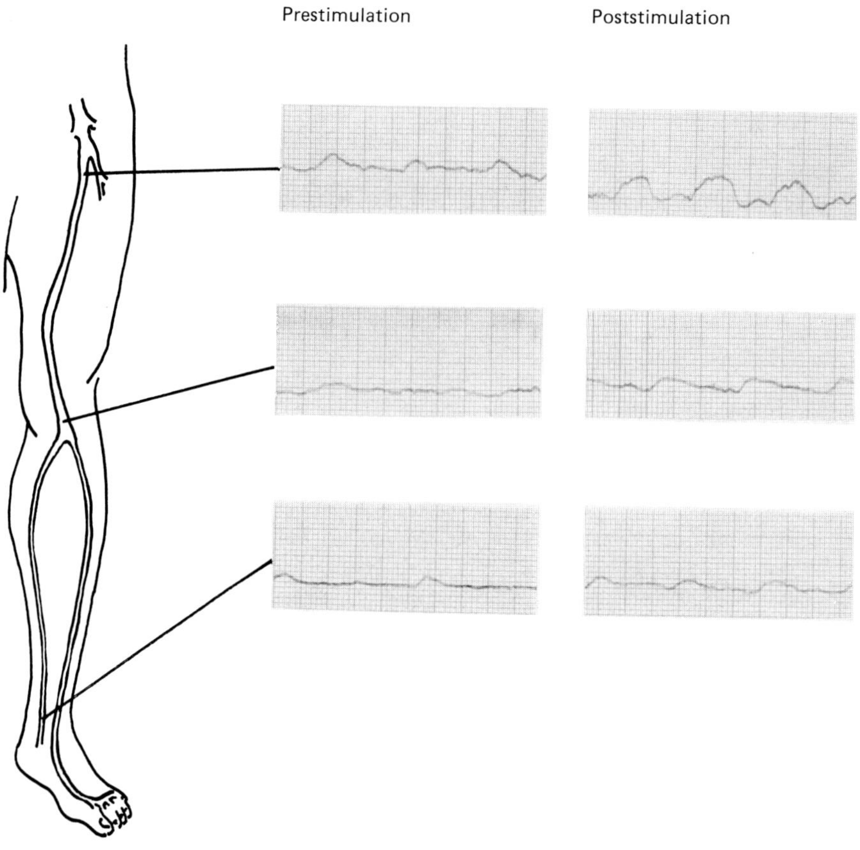

Fig. 1. Pre- and poststimulation Doppler recordings in a vasculopathic case.

were repeated on 2 consecutive days before stimulation, maintaining the incidence angle of the probe in both explorations. In 26 of 27 vasculopathic patients a slow decelerated monophasic pulse wave with absence of the second and third deflection and low maximal systolic velocity was found. In 2 cases Doppler recordings were totally flat. In all nonvasculopathic patients this study was normal.

Telethermography of lower limbs was performed to observe changes in skin temperature during stimulation. Studies were done in an isothermic room after 1 h of rest and keeping the distance between the camera and the explored part constant. In the 16 vasculopathic cases explored, a relative focal decrease in temperature was detected constantly. All nonvasculopathic patients showed normal thermograms.

Considering the previous failure of all conservative and surgical attempts and the impossibility of direct arterial surgery for local or systemic reasons in the vasculopathic patients, SCS was considered as a fair alternative to treat ischemic pain.

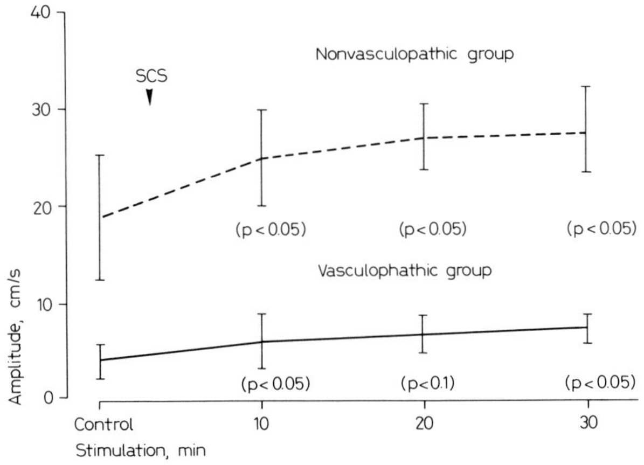

Fig. 2. Mean variations in pulse wave amplitude during 30 min of stimulation in the vasculopathic and nonvasculopathic groups.

SCS was performed by means of one or two percutaneous electrodes inserted in the epidural space following conventional techniques. The final position of the electrodes was usually at the low thoracic spinal cord to the level at which stimulation provoked electric paresthesias in the painful area. A test period of 2 weeks of percutaneous stimulation was standard. The more effective electric parameters were: pulse width of 0,1–0,2 ms, 80–120 Hz according to patient comfort, and amplitude at a low paresthesia threshold. Initially stimulation duration was applied in periods of 1 h on and 1 h off during the day. As all patients benefitted during the test period, the systems were permanently internalized, connecting them to a total implantable device or to a receiver activated by an external transmitter (electrical stimulation equipment was provided by Medtronic Inc., Minneapolis, Minn.).

Results

In general, a 75–100% remission of ischemic pain in 22 out of the 27 vasculopathic patients and significant increase of walking capacity in 18 was obtained. In 16 out of the 26 vasculopathic cases previously explored, Doppler recordings showed a significant improvement of blood flow conditions in lower limb circulation during and after stimulation, expressed by higher blood flow velocity, tendency to normalization of pulse waves and increasing amplitude of same (fig. 1). These changes were recorded after 10 min of SCS and increased throughout 30 min. In nonvasculopathic patients there was a similar to greater tendency to increase pulse wave amplitude, also maintained during the stimulation period. Figure 2 illustrates the mean variations in pulse wave amplitude of the vasculopathic group throughout the stimulation period as compared with the base control as well as in the nonvasculopathic group.

In 11 vasculopathic cases out of the 16 tested, thermography revealed a progressive warming of the painful area during stimulation. These changes, though of lesser degree, were also found in the nonvasculopathic group.

Generally Doppler and thermographic poststimulation improvement coincided in the same cases. Improvement in both studies also occurred in cases with more significant pain relief. Although most peripheral blood flow changes following SCS observed in the vasculopathic patients could be explained via pain relief, the fact that some findings appear in nonvasculopathic cases suggest that spinal cord stimulation has a certain influence on peripheral vascular control, probably mediating on a vasodilation response.

References

1 Augustinsson, L.E.; Carlsson, C.A.; Fall, M.: Autonomic effects of electrostimulation. Appl. Neurophysiol. *45:* 190–194 (1982).

2 Broseta, J.; Barbera, J.; De Vera, J.A.: Spinal cord stimulation in peripheral arterial disease. Cooperative study. J. Neurosurg. (in press, 1985).

3 Fiume, D.: Spinal cord stimulation in peripheral vascular pain. Appl. Neurophysiol. *46:* 290–294 (1983).

4 Meglio, M.; Cioni, B.; Sandric, S.: Spinal cord stimulation and peripheral blood flow; in Indications for spinal cord stimulation, pp. 60–66 (Excerpta Medica, Amsterdam 1981).

5 Tallis, R.C.; Illis, L.S.; Sedwick, E.M.: Spinal cord stimulation in peripheral vascular disease. J. Neurol. Neurosurg. Psychiat. *46:* 478–484 (1983).

Dr. J. Broseta, Department of Neurosurgery, Hospital Clínico Universitario, E-37007 Salamanca (Spain)

Proc. 9th Meeting World Soc. Stereotactic and Functional
Neurosurgery, Toronto 1985
Appl. Neurophysiol. *48:* 371 (1985)

Management of Non-Malignant Chronic Pain Using Stimulators

G. Vijaya, C. Balasubramaniam, T.S. Kanaka

Institute of Neurology, Madras, India

Key Words. Chronic pain · Transcutaneous nerve stimulator

Abstract. A transcutaneous nerve stimulator was used for the management of 220 patients with chronic non-malignant pain and has a definite role in the management.

Patients who were awaiting surgery and patients in whom surgery or analgesics failed to give relief or where there was recurrence of pain after surgery or analgesics were selected for treatment using a transcutaneous stimulator. The chronic painful conditions treated with the Avery transcutaneous nerve stimulator (TNS) include trigeminal neuralgia, post-herpetic neuralgia, hemifacial spasm, etc. Usually the stimulation is given for 1 h once or twice a day depending on the severity of pain. Initially the patients were allowed to take their analgesics and gradually they were then able to reduce them. Trigeminal neuralgia, post-herpetic neuralgia and hemifacial spasm were the conditions best relieved by this method (table I).

Table I. Management of non-malignant chronic pain using stimulators – results of treatment with TNS

Disease	Patients n	Good relief	Partial relief	No improvement
Trigeminal neuralgia	112	84	22	6
Post-herpetic neuralgia	35	25	6	4
Hemifacial spasm	19	14	3	2
Sciatica and low backache	12	–	4	8
Brachial neuralgia	12	2	4	6
Miscellaneous	30	15	5	10

G. Vijaya, MD, Institute of Neurology, Madras 3, 600003 (India)

Proc. 9th Meeting World Soc. Stereotactic and Functional
Neurosurgery, Toronto 1985
Appl. Neurophysiol. *48:* 372–376 (1985)

Electrical Stimulation of the Cervical Spinal Cord Increases Cerebral Blood Flow in Humans

Yoshio Hosobuchi

Section of Functional and Stereotactic Neurosurgery, Department of Neurological Surgery, School of Medicine, University of California, San Francisco, Calif., USA

Key Words. Cerebral blood flow · Cerebrovascular insufficiency · Cervical spinal cord stimulation · Neurostimulation · Thoracic spinal cord stimulation

Abstract. Ten patients were studied to determine the effect of spinal cord stimulation on CBF. In 5 patients using a cervical spinal cord stimulator, the stimulation produced a significant increase in CBF in the hemisphere ipsilateral to the induced paresthesia. Thoracic cord stimulation, used by the other 5 patients, had no effect on CBF. Atropine had no effect on the alteration in CBF produced by cervical cord stimulation. Indomethacin, however, partially blocked the effect. These heuristic observations may have implications for the future treatment of cerebrovascular insufficiency in humans.

Introduction

During the past 8 years there have been reports of patients with peripheral vascular disease whose benefit from spinal cord stimulation was not only pain relief, but also improved peripheral blood flow to a previously ischemic limb, increased skin temperature of the area, and even healing of the ischemic ulcers [1, 2, 4]. No mechanism clearly responsible for this intriguing phenomenon has been proposed. This study was undertaken to determine the effect of spinal cord stimulation on cerebral blood flow in 10 patients.

Materials and Methods

Ten patients, 4 male and 6 female, who underwent implantation of an epidural dorsal cord stimulation system (Medtronic Resume® electrode lead connected to a radiofrequency coupled system) were selected for this study. The mean age of these patients was 43.6 years. All patients had chronic intractable pain involving one limb. The 5 patients who had pain in an upper limb had the electrode implanted at the C3-C4 level. In the other 5 patients who had lower extremity pain the electrode was implanted at the T8-T9 level. The electrode was placed in the epidural space, slightly off midline to the side of the pain, in each case.

Initially the electrode lead was left externalized in order to identify the pair of electrode contacts that produced unilateral paresthesia and satisfactory pain control. After an appropriate pair was identified, the lead was internalized and connected to radiofrequency receiver. The effect of spinal cord stimulation on cerebral blood flow (CBF) was determined 3-4 weeks after the operation to internalize the electrodes.

CBF was measured using the inhaled ^{133}Xe (50 mCi/dose) washout technique [3]. An Anger camera (Nuclear-Chicago) was placed to view the head in the vertex projection in order to record the gamma activity. The washout curves were fitted to a two-exponential model and values for CBF were calculated. Normal values for CBF by this technique range from 35 to 45 ml/min/100 g of brain tissue in adults. The analysis is capable of yielding compartmentalized blood flow estimates in the anterior, middle, and posterior portion of each hemisphere. Three separate CBF measurements were made for each patient over a period of 4 h.

The patients were asked not to use their stimulator for at least 12 h before the initial test. The first CBF measurement was obtained as a baseline control without stimulation. As soon as the first CBF measurement was completed, the patient was instructed to turn the stimulator on to the voltage level used to control their pain; all patients used a frequency of 50 Hz and the pulse duration of the stimulus was 0.3 ms. The patient self-stimulated for 2 h, after which a second CBF determination was obtained while the stimulator was on. As soon as the second CBF measurement was taken, the patients were instructed to turn the stimulation off and leave it off for 2 h. At the end of this period, the third CBF measurement was made.

From 4 patients using cervical cord stimulation, two sets of CBF measurements were obtained during the second CBF determination with the stimulator on. After the first stimulation measurement was taken, 2 of these patients received 0.4 mg atropine and 2 received 25 mg indomethacin, each by intravenous infusion over a period of 30 min while they continued using stimulation. At the end of this 30-min period, CBF measurements were made again.

Results

The initial (baseline control) value for hemispheric CBF in all 10 patients was 34-45 ml/min/100 g of brain tissue. In no patient was there a significant difference in interhemispheric or matched compartmental CBF. The CBF measurements obtained from the other two stimulation conditions were computed in ratio to the control CBF value, which was assigned a value of 1.

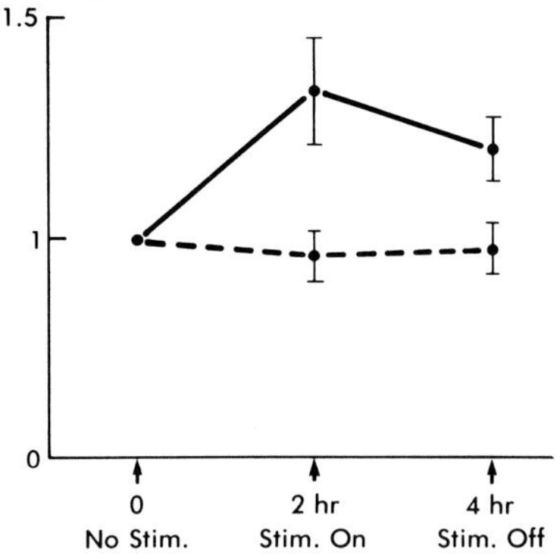

Fig. 1. Hemispheric comparison of findings of a ^{133}Xe CBF study on cervical spinal cord stimulation. The changes are shown in comparison to the control value, which is assigned a value of 1. —— = Ipsilateral hemisphere to the induced paresthesia; --- = contralateral hemisphere to the induced paresthesia ($p < 0.001$).

Among the 5 patients using cervical cord stimulation, there was a significant rise in hemispheric CBF on the side ipsilateral to the induced paresthesia during stimulation; the mean increase over the control value was 34% ($p < 0.001$). There were no changes in CBF values in the contralateral hemisphere (fig. 1). Two hours after the cessation of cervical cord stimulation, this group showed persistently elevated CBF levels in the same hemisphere (fig. 1). When these data were analyzed in a matched compartmental comparison, the significant differences in CBF from control values were found primarily in the middle and posterior compartments (fig. 2). A slight difference in the anterior compartment was insignificant ($p > 0.01$).

Conversely, the patients whose stimulator electrode was implanted in the thoracic cord showed no significant differences between their control and stimulation CBF values in either hemisphere or in a matched compartmental comparison, and showed no significant changes in CBF 2 h after the cessation of the spinal cord stimulation.

In the 2 patients using cervical stimulation who received 0.4 mg of atropine during the second CBF determination (made during stimulation), atropine at this dosage had no effect on the rise in CBF caused by stimulation. Of the 2 other patients using a cervical stimulator who re-

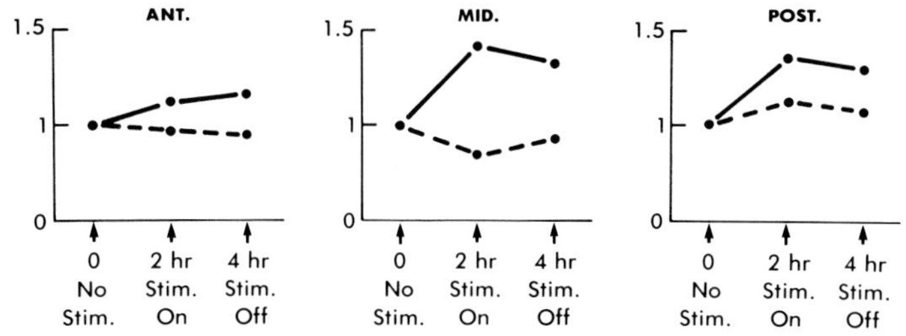

Fig. 2. Compartmental comparison of the anterior, middle, and posterior areas of each hemisphere as determined in the ^{133}Xe CBF study on cervical spinal cord stimulation. The changes are demonstrated in comparison to the control value, which is assigned a value of 1. —— = Ipsilateral to the induced paresthesia; --- = contralateral to the induced paresthesia.

ceived 25 mg indomethacin, both had about a 30% reduction in CBF, as compared to the first CBF measurement taken while the stimulator was on.

Discussion

The reproducibility of CBF measurements determined by the inhaled ^{133}Xe technique has not been established. Nonetheless, it is interesting that cervical spinal cord stimulation produced a significant alteration in CBF values in the patients studied, whereas thoracic cord stimulation had no effect on CBF. The increase in CBF in the patients using cervical cord stimulation was primarily in the hemisphere ipsilateral to the induced paresthesia, suggesting that the alteration in CBF was not related to the increased cerebral metabolic rate resulting from the afferent volley which is produced by artificial stimulation of the spinal cord. The mechanism of this effect is not known.

The third CBF measurement, taken after patients had ceased stimulation for 2 h, was not significantly different from the control value in either hemisphere. This persistent elevation of CBF after cessation of the cervical cord stimulation is very similar to that observed in patients using spinal cord stimulation for peripheral vascular disease [1, 2, 4]. Such a persistent effect on hemodynamics suggests the involvement of humoral factor(s), rather than simply the axonal reflex. The action of indomethacin, which partially blocked the effect of cervical spinal cord stimulation on CBF, may suggest the involvement of prostaglandin or vasoactive intestinal peptide. Further experiments in animals are required to verify the observation and elucidate the mechanism of this fascinating phenomenon. Based on the reported experience regarding the effects of spinal cord stimulation on peripheral vascular diseases, however, cervical spinal cord stimulation may prove useful in treating difficult cases of cerebrovascular insufficiency, particularly those involving the vertebrobasilar system.

Acknowledgement

This work was supported in part by a fund provided by Medtronic, Inc., Neuro Division, Minneapolis, Minn.

References

1 Augustinsson, L.: In Hosobuchi, Corbin, Indications for spinal cord stimulation, pp. 72–75 (Excerpta Medica, Amsterdam 1981).
2 Meglio, M.; Cioni, B.; Lago, A.D.; DeSantis, M.; Pola, P.; Serricchio, M.: Pain control and improvement of peripheral blood flow following epidural spinal cord stimulation. J. Neurosurg. *54:* 821–823 (1981).
3 Obrist, W.D.; Thompson, H.K.; King, H.C.; Wang, H.S.: Determination of regional cerebral blood flow by inhalation of 133-xenon. Circulation Res. *20:* 124–135 (1967).
4 Tallis, R.C.; Illis, I.S.; Sedgwick, E.M.; Hardwidge, C.; Garfield, J.S.: Spinal cord stimulation in peripheral vascular disease. J. Neurol. Neurosurg. Psychiat. *46:* 478–484 (1983).

Yoshio Hosobuchi, MD, Section of Functional and Stereotactic Neurosurgery,
Department of Neurological Surgery, School of Medicine,
University of California, San Francisco, c/o 1360 Ninth Avenue, Suite 210,
San Francisco, CA 94122 (USA)

Proc. 9th Meeting World Soc. Stereotactic and Functional
Neurosurgery, Toronto 1985
Appl. Neurophysiol. *48:* 377–379 (1985)

Complications in Cases of Epidural Stimulation Electrode Implants

K. Sogabe[a], *G. Dieckmann*[b], *G. Veras*[b]

[a] Department of Neurosurgery, Nakamura, Municipal Hospital Kochi, Japan;
[b] Department of Functional Neurosurgery, University of Göttingen, FRG

Key Words. Complication · Spinal cord stimulation

Abstract. Spinal cord stimulation (SCS) is an effective treatment for pain and motor disturbances. We have performed 124 SCS procedures between 1981 and 1984 at the University of Göttingen. Reoperations were required for 69 cases (56%) for various reasons, most frequently changes in electrode position due to the dislodgement (36 cases, 52%.) Analysis of the development of this postoperative repositioning showed that 67% occurred within 1 month after the implantation. Therefore, if patients can be kept at rest during the granulation period of 1 month after operation, we suggest that the frequency of reoperation may be considerably lessend.

Introduction

This report analyzes 124 epidural stimulation cases performed at the University of Göttingen over 3 years since 1981, with particular focus on the cases which required electrode revision.

Materials and Methods

Of 124 patients, 63 suffered from arachnoiditis following intervertebral disc surgery, 16 from spasmodic torticollis, 7 from dystonia, 10 from pain in the upper limb and cervical region, 12 from pain in the lower limb, 11 from motor disturbance in the upper limb and 5 cases from motor disturbance in the lower limb. There were 73 male and 51 female patients. Their ages ranged from 6 to 77 years (mean 48). Implantation was in the cervical region in 44 cases and the lumbar region in 80 cases. Unipolar electrodes were used in 89 cases and bipolar electrodes in 35 cases.

Table I. Types of revisions

Revision	
Repositioning	51
Explantation	43
Wound healing problems	10
Receiver problems	4
Connector problems	4
Total	112

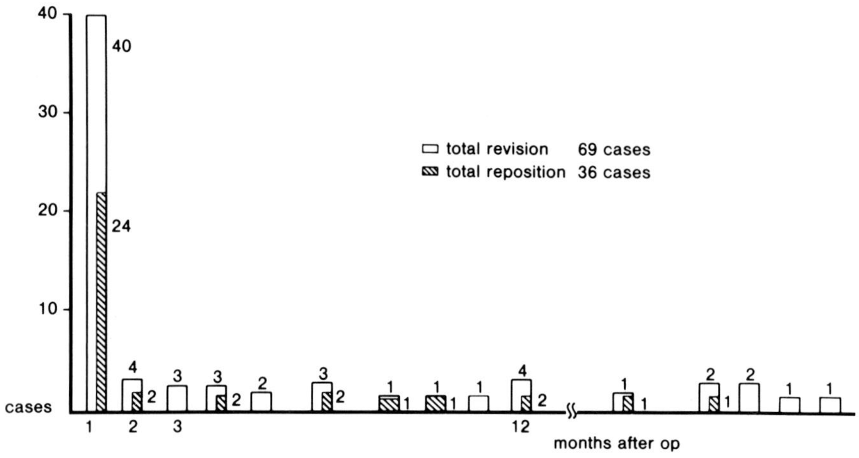

Fig. 1. Postoperative interventions.

For implantation in the cervical region, the electrode was inserted from T_{2-4} and the tip was fixed on the region of C_{2-4}, while the lumbar electrode was inserted from L_{2-3} and the tip was fixed on the region of T_{9-11}.

Results

112 revisions were performed on 69 of the 124 patients implanted with spinal cord stimulators (SCS). 51 revisions were carried out for repositioning, 43 due to ineffective implantation, 10 due to wound infection and 8 due to trouble with receiver or connector (table I). Elec-

trode repositioning was found necessary within 1 month after implantation in a majority of those cases reported in figure 1.

Comparing the frequency of repositions using unipolar and bipolar electrodes, the results indicate reposition developed in 14% of the bipolar electrodes cases as opposed to 21% of the unipolar electrode cases.

Comment

SCS does not cause serious side effects, and has proven to be a very effective and simple method. However, one difficulty is that electrode dislodgement develops easily [1, 2]. Various electrode designs have been studied, but this problem remains. We suggest that the best method is to keep patients at rest for 1 month after operation during the period when granulation occurs. After 2 months postoperatively, it is thought that activity should be allowed because the incidence of dislodgement decreases.

Conclusion

Repositioning was necessary in 36 out of 124 cases of SCS. In 34 cases the repositioning occurred within 1 month after the implantation.

References

1 Ray, C.D.: Percutaneous spinal cord stimulation: Technique; in Hosobuchi, Corbin, Indication for spinal cord stimulation, pp. 17–33 (Excerpta Medica, Amsterdam 1981).

2 Tsuda, T.; Tasker, R.R.: Percutaneous epidural spinal cord electrical stimulation for intractable pain – in regard to the deafferentation pain. Neurol. Surg., Tokyo *13:* 409–415 (1985).

K. Sogabe, MD, Nakamura Municipal Hospital, 1-1 Higashimachi,
Nakamura City, Kochi, 787 (Japan)

Proc. 9th Meeting World Soc. Stereotactic and Functional Neurosurgery, Toronto 1985
Appl. Neurophysiol. *48:* 380–381 (1985)

Indications for Implanted Electrostimulation of the Spinal Cord

D.M. Dooley, J. Karaboyas

Pain Treatment Center, Baptist Hospital of Miami, Fla., USA

Key Words. Blood flow · Electrostimulation · Spasticity

Abstract. Patients with varying complaints of pain and abnormal neurological findings may be suitable candidates for electrical stimulation of the spinal cord. They can be divided into patients with pain and those with arterial disease, movement disorders and neurogenic bladder

Patients suitable for implanted electrical stimulation are those with pain from failed low back and cervical syndrome, peripheral neuropathy, phantom limb pain, postherpetic neuralgia, thalamic syndrome, postcordotomy and postsympathectomy dysesthesias, brachial plexitis, thoracotomy and nephrectomy incisions and demyelinating and degenerative diseases. However, those patients with pain from benign cause should be carefully evaluated by a multidisciplinary Pain Treatment Center team to exclude those persons who are unlikely to respond over the long term due to psychological and/or socioeconomic factors.

Patients who have malignancies producing pain in an upper extremity or in the pelvis and/or lower extremities are excellent candidates. If they do not respond to the temporary stimulation, they can always have a cordotomy or implanted morphine pump. Electrical stimulation of the spinal cord will 'block' only the impulses coming caudal to the electrode and will not affect the descending impulses from more cephalic origins.

The patients who respond most favorably are those with 'denervation' pain. The 'success' rate is 68% of all patients over 5 years.

The temporary testing procedure is not done in patients with spasticity, spasmodic torticollis, dystonia, ataxia and multiple sclerosis if they are ambulatory. The ideal movement disorder patient is one who is disabled by spastic paraparesis and hypotonic neurogenic bladder. Patients with hypotonic neurogenic bladder have a 70% chance of having a significant lessening of symptoms and residual urine. Those with hypertonic bladders have a less likely but still possible chance of help.

In addition, arterial dilatation in an extremity by an electrical impulse applied to the dorsal root or spinal cord segment which innervates that area has been documented by authors dating back to the 19th century. The patients most likely to benefit are those with rest pain and intermittent claudication.

D.M. Dooley, MD, Pain Treatment Center, Baptist Hospital of Miami, Inc.,
Miami, FL 33146 (USA)

Proc. 9th Meeting World Soc. Stereotactic and Functional
Neurosurgery, Toronto 1985
Appl. Neurophysiol. *48:* 382–383 (1985)

Programmed Stimulation in Patients with Chronic Pain and Motor Disturbances

F. Mundinger, H. Neumüller, E. Milios, K. Weigel

Department of Stereotaxy and Neuronuclear Medicine, University Hospital, Freiburg i. Br., FRG

Introduction

Since 1973 we have been performing neurostimulation in cases with chronic pain and motor disturbances. Until February 1980, we used a standard Medtronic device, but then we developed a programmable stimulation device which has been routinely used since 1980.

Methods

The programmed neurostimulators provide a stimulation spectrum of four variable parameters: base frequency, compensatory interval, number of impulses (2–16) per sequence, and pulse width. The parameters are set by the investigator and visualized on an external monitor.

Results

A total of 189 patients were treated with the stimulation technique, 61 patients with the standard device and 128 patients with the programmed neurostimulator. As opposed to the standard stimulation, the programmed neurostimulation clearly shows better results (table I).

Table I

	Number of cases	Results			
		Poor	Fair	Good	Excellent
Results with chronic pain					
Programmed stimulation					
Transcutaneous stimulation	72	0	14	46	12
Subcutaneous stimulation	7	0	2	3	2
Epidural stimulation bipolar	9	0	6	2	1
Deep brain stimulation bipolar	25	0	4	17	4
Standard stimulation					
Epidural stimulation bipolar	17	11	6	0	0
Deep brain stimulation bipolar	20	9	3	8	0
Results with spasticity					
Programmed stimulation					
Transcutaneous stimulation	3	0	0	2	1
Subcutaneous stimulation	1	0	0	0	1
Epidural stimulation unipolar	1	0	0	1	0
Deep brain stimulation bipolar	10	0	5	4	1
Standard stimulation					
Epidural stimulation bipolar	2	1	1	0	0
Deep brain stimulation bipolar	22	10	6	6	0

Prof. Dr. F. Mundinger, Ärztlicher Direktor, Abteilung Stereotaxie und Neuronuklearmedizin, Hugstetter Strasse 55, D-7800 Freiburg i.Br. (FRG)

Session VIII: Epilepsy

Proc. 9th Meeting World Soc. Stereotactic and Functional
Neurosurgery, Toronto 1985
Appl. Neurophysiol. *48:* 384–394 (1985)

Missing Pieces in the Epilepsy Puzzle

Arthur A. Ward, Jr.

Department of Neurological Surgery, University of Washington School of Medicine, Seattle, Wash., USA

Key Words. Epilepsy, surgical therapy · Epileptiogenic focus · Neurotransmitter · Brain grafts · Tissue transplantation · Stereotactic surgery

Abstract. Research regarding the basic mechanisms of the epilepsies has been limited and has generated few clues that have led to dramatic improvements in the surgical therapy of epilepsy. It is now known that the epileptic focus is characterized by a population of pacemaker neurons that fire autonomously in bursts. When this high frequency discharge recruits bursting activity in neighboring neurons, a propagating seizure occurs. Such data as well as other recent data in neurobiology indicate that new forms of surgical therapy may be forthcoming including brain transplantation as well as local application of transmitter compounds which may significantly improve the therapy of epilepsy.

To anyone with an interest in either basic or clinical neuroscience, epilepsy represents an experiment of nature which is unique. It provides opportunities to study properties of the brain which would not otherwise be examined and, for the neurological surgeon, provides an opportunity to undertake sophisticated studies of the awake human brain which can only be justified by the surgical therapy for this condition. On the other hand, progress in our understanding of the mechanisms underlying epilepsy has been slow and progress in therapy has been disappointing. This has been particularly true of the surgical therapy of this condition. Thus it is quite clear that epilepsy continues to be a puzzle and there are many missing pieces.

Research in epilepsy has told us much about neuroscience, but little that leads to new clues regarding therapy. The major concept upon which the surgical therapy of epilepsy is based is the thesis first enunciated by Hughlings Jackson to the effect that an epileptic seizure starts in a localized collection of 'hyperphysiologic neurons'. Thus we have the concept of a 'focus' with the additional extension that a clinical seizure represents a spread of the seizure discharge from the focus to the rest of the brain. This leads to the surgical conclusion that there are two ways to attempt to modify the epileptic process. The first is to remove the source of the seizure discharges – i.e., excise the focus. The second is to block the pathways of spread. The first was developed by Penfield some 50 years ago and, except for some minor technical modifications, has not significantly changed over the past half century. The second surgical approach required the development of surgical techniques to make accurate, localized lesions in the depths of the brain. It was then possible to make stereotactic lesions that hopefully would either block the pathways of spread or modify the input to epileptic circuits to prevent precipitation of seizures. Unfortunately, surgical success based on this principle has been less dramatic.

A significant body of knowledge exists regarding the ways in which signals are propagated throughout the brain. The morphology of the circuits, their physiological properties, the complexities of the transmitters which operate at synapses in these circuits and the chemical properties of the energy sources required to maintain such activity are now modestly well understood. All the evidence indicates that no new properties are operating in the propagation of epileptic discharges although the patterns of discharge in a seizure may be unique.

The same cannot be said about the epileptic focus. It has been apparent that the neurons in a focus must possess properties which represent significant distortions of basic properties of normal neurons. Studies of such properties require a model of human epilepsy in an animal. The chronic monkey model appears to fulfill the desirable criteria [8]. An intracortical scar can be induced in the sensorimotor cortex of these primates which results in the generation of spontaneous clinical seizures at random intervals. Their frequency is relatively constant and the epilepsy appears to last indefinitely. They have many of the clinical properties of human epilepsy of focal cortical origin. These seizures in monkeys may be increased in frequency by behavioral stress, show circadian cycling, and changes in frequency associated with menses. Their profile of response to antiepileptic drugs is the same as in humans. The epileptic focus in both monkey and man contains neurons which autonomously fire in bursts [11]. They are intrinsically hyperexcitable. A single epileptic neuron with such properties obviously cannot generate clinical seizures, but an adequate population of such epileptic neurons in a localized region of cortex appears to constitute the essential feature of an epileptogenic focus.

The neurons in such a focus show a spectrum of intrinsic abnormalities ranging from neurons having normal physiological properties through a sequence to those that are highly epileptic and which appear to serve as pacemakers to the focus. Under such circumstances, it appears that the pacemaker neurons are responsible for the focal cortical epileptogenicity, and they periodically induce clinical seizures by recruiting surrounding neurons into epileptic activity, thereby producing the necessary critical mass in the circuitry to sustain a propagating discharge.

The behavior of such neurons can be studied in the epileptic focus of awake undrugged monkeys for long periods of time, and their behavior can be manipulated by a variety of experimental, physiological, behavioral synaptic inputs as *Wyler* et al. have reported [13]. Extracellular recording from such neurons in man was first undertaken in Seattle some 25 years ago – but even with significant refinements of technique, the observations are necessarily limited because of restricted access to synaptic inputs and because of an already long operation under local anesthesia.

Such extracellular recording of neuronal activity in either monkey or man can be analyzed by a computer which can compute a 'burst index'. The burst index is the percent of interspike intervals less than 5 ms and is computed for consecutive 15-s epochs. Under waking conditions, normal precentral neurons in monkey have mean burst indices of less than 10%, whereas epileptic neurons have burst indices greater than 10%. Epileptic neurons, in turn, can be divided into two groups: Group 1 (strongly epileptic or pacemaker neurons) fire almost exclusively in bursts and their activity is stereotyped and not easily modified by any synaptic inputs. Group 2 (weakly epileptic neurons) exhibit a variable admixture of burst and normal firing patterns and their burst indices are lower and variable. Thus there are quantitative criteria to distinguish epileptic from normal neurons.

The distinction between normal and group I or pacemaker neuronal behavior is shown figure 1. Above we see a sample of normal single cell activity from a pyramidal tract neuron firing at a modestly high tonic rate within normal cortex in the awake monkey. The interspike interval histogram to the right is typical for such cells and shows

A

B

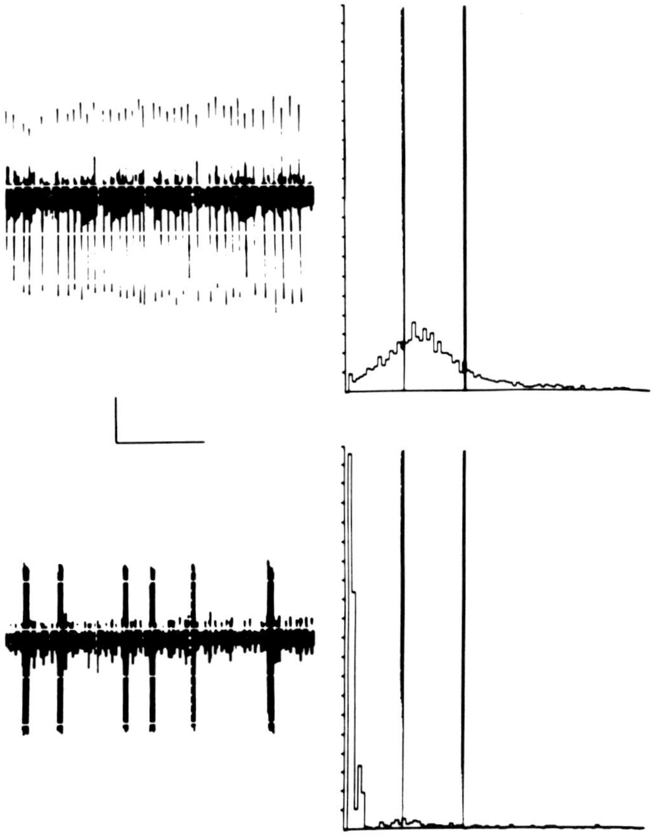

Fig. 1. Activity of single neuron from **(A)** normal and **(B)** epileptic cortical neurons recorded extracellularly. On the right are histograms of 5 min of activity from these units (cursors mark 30 and 60 ms). The individual action potentials which comprise the bursts from the epileptic cell cannot be resolved at this slow sweep speed. Calibration marks, 100 μV, 200 ms [from 14].

only a few interspike intervals less than 5 ms. This cell is illustrated because it is firing at a high rate for a normal cell – but, even so, less than 1% of its interspike intervals are less than 5 ms (cursors at 30 and 60 ms).

In contrast, the lower records show an example of a highly epileptic or pacemaker pyramidal tract neuron in the monkey. The slow sweep speed demonstrates bursts characteristic of such epileptic neu-

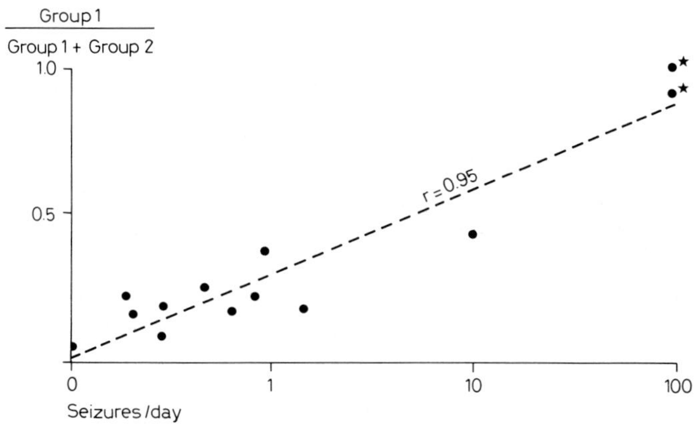

Fig. 2. Plot of 1,617 neurons in 13 monkeys. The proportion of pacemaker neurons is plotted against mean daily seizure frequency for each monkey. The higher the percentage of pacemaker neurons in the focus, the higher the frequency of spontaneous seizures [from 14].

rons. This cell fires only in such bursts. The bursts are composed of interspike intervals less than 5 ms and the interspike interval histogram to the right shows a sharp peak at intervals between 2 and 4 ms. The dramatic difference between the behavior of epileptic and normal neurons is obvious.

Identical patterns of such firing have been repeatedly recorded from human foci. The bursts are autonomous. Their activity is not modified by sleep – which causes profound changes in spontaneous firing of normal cells. It is then not surprising that there is other physiological as well as anatomical evidence that such epileptic neurons are partially deafferented. There is also a reduction of GABA terminals in the focus. In both monkey and man, such cells are embedded in a glial cortical scar.

If, indeed, the epileptogenicity of the focus is maintained by pacemaker neurons, it would be predicted that the density of such neurons within any one focus should correlate with the frequency of clinical seizures [14].

A plot based on the activity of 1,617 neurons recorded from foci in 13 epileptic monkeys is presented in figure 2. Here the ratio of pacemaker neurons in the focus is plotted against the mean daily seizure frequency for each monkey. At the far left is a monkey who was having one seizure about every 10 days - and only 1% of the neurons in his focus were highly epileptic. At the top of the curve are 2 animals showing epilepsia partialis continua - with almost continuous jerking of the fingers of the contralateral hand. Here pacemaker neurons constituted 88 and 99% respectively of cells in the focus. In the animal having slightly less than one seizure per day, 24% of the neurons were pacemaker cells.

This is a log plot - and the correlation between this derived index of epileptogenicity and seizure frequency is highly significant ($p = 0.001$). This logarithmic relationship shows the power such pacemaker neurons have on the recruitment of normal cells into abnormal activity. It is apparent that a modest reduction in the number of such cells would have a major impact on the frequency of clinical seizures. They do not have to be reduced to zero to abolish spontaneous clinical seizures.

The surgical conclusion to be drawn is that the excision of the focus need not ablate all abnormal cells - only reduce their numbers below the critical level necessary to abolish propagating clinical seizures.

Unfortunately, the surgeon is denied information regarding the numbers and exact distribution of such pacemaker neurons in any given patient - and there is no way to determine the number of such pathological cells which can be left in situ without causing clinical seizures. However, these findings would account for the widely recognized fact that, following temporal lobectomy for seizures of temporal lobe origin, residual epileptic spiking can occasionally be recorded in the postresection corticography from the island of Reil. This cortex cannot be safely removed because of the overlying candelabra of the middle cerebral vessels. However, clinical experience has shown that such residual spiking does not influence the long-term favorable outcome in most cases.

How May Future Laboratory Research Point the Way to New Approaches to Surgical Therapy?

Surgical removal of the focus as developed by Penfield has proved to be a very effective surgical therapy which has now been carried out in many centers throughout the world. Many thousands of patients who otherwise would be disabled by this condition now are seizure-free. The surgical approaches and techniques have, however, undergone little modification over the past 50 years. With current knowledge, there is no reason to think that any major changes will occur in the immediate future.

Brain Grafts

It has been pointed out that one of the anatomical abnormalities which characterizes the epileptic focus is a loss of GABAergic synaptic endings in the focus [9]. It is reasonable to presume that the loss of this inhibitory input is related to the hyperactivity that characterizes the focus. This hyperactivity might be reduced or abolished if the population of synaptic terminals in the focus-releasing GABA could be restored.

The new exciting area of research into brain tissue grafts might lead to the development of such a technique. It has been shown that functional input to recipient central nervous system tissue can be provided by brain tissue grafts in experimental animals. Fetal rat dopamine-containing neurons have been implanted adjacent to the caudate nucleus of adult recipients whose endogenous dopaminergic inputs have been destroyed. The grafts show good survival and axonal outgrowth. More importantly, clinical motor abnormalities, which had been induced by the destruction of the endogenous dopaminergic input to the caudate, were significantly reduced after grafting of the fetal brain tissue [2]. It has also been shown that septal grafts implanted into the hippocampus will ameloriate the learning impairments seen in aged rats [4].

Specific brain area transplantation has the significant theoretical advantage that the blood-brain barrier provides protection against rejection of the graft by the host. Thus, it is possible that immune suppressive therapy, with its associated difficulties, may not be necessary in recipients of brain component grafts. A second significant advantage is that spatial localization is conferred by the transplantation site; the transmitter drug is not delivered to all potential receptors in the brain as it would be with parenteral administration of, for instance, a drug that elevates the levels of a given transmitter.

Many fundamental biological problems remain to be solved. Is there a critical period for donor fetal age? Is there selective transplant growth, i.e., do some grafts grow and others do not based on the appropriateness of afferent input to the recipient site? A recent report [7] has suggested that neonatal grafts of cerebral cortex can be preserved for several weeks at low temperature prior to transplantation. This would offer some unique advantages over currently available techniques. Finally, can cultured cells serve as donor material? It is kown that well-characterized cell lines possess characteristics of both cholinergic and catecholaminergic cells [6]. They synthesize, store and release primarily dopamine. Under some circumstances, they can also store, synthesize and release acetylcholine. Thus, cell lines can express transmitter-specific properties and may be useful as donor material. There is no reason to believe that cell lines specific for GABA cannot be developed. It remains to be determined that such cell lines can serve as successful donor material. It is not known what transplantation sites and techniques provide optimal reinnervation of host cells. Three techniques are commonly used in current experimental research: (1) implantation of solid tissue into the ventricular system; (2) implantation of solid tissue, with or without a previously made cavity, into brain tissue, and (3) parenchymal implantation of dispersed cells. Thus, much basic research remains to be done before appropriate surgical strategies can be developed.

Local Drug Perfusion

In the search for new antiepileptic drugs, some drugs of potential interest are currently discarded because they penetrate the blood-brain barrier poorly. Although such a drug may exhibit little antiepileptic effectiveness when administered parenterally, local application to the focus may dramatically reduce seizure frequency [*Lockard*, pers. commun.]. The techniques for accomplishing such local application of drugs exist now. The surgical technology is available and all that remains is the experimental validation of drug action. Thus it is possible that, at some future date, an implanted device can continuously perfuse the focus with potent antiepileptic drugs which will block seizure initiation. This will be accomplished without having to pay the price of secondary side effects (systemic as well as behavioral) that is a necessary property of orally administered drugs.

Utilizing implantable infusion devices would also permit the administration of drugs into the ventricular system or the subarachnoid space. There has been a recent report that, following induced seizures in experimental animals, a peptide is released into the cerebrospinal fluid that has antiepileptic properties [10]. It has been proposed that this opioid compound serves as a natural anticonvulsant. The model is that this compound serves as a mechanism for seizure termination and, in addition, may prevent the recurrence of seizures. The implication is that, were it not for this mechanism, many seizures would progress into status epilepticus. Clearly, surgical techniques can easily be devised that would make such a compound continuously available to the cortex.

Finally, there is an additional potential application of techniques of local perfusion. In the course of development of new antiepileptic drugs, some compounds have been developed that not only reduce seizure frequency when administered systemically but, more importantly, reduction or abolition of seizures is maintained when the drug administration is stopped. The mechanisms by which this apparently irreversible effect is achieved are unknown but it is speculated that conformational changes in neuronal membrane are responsible. There is reason to speculate that such effects could be achieved more dramatically if the drug could be administered in higher concentration to the local site. This requires surgical intervention. Surgeons must obviously be continuously alert to the data developed by such rapidly moving research efforts.

Stereotactic Lesions

Since the development of stereotaxis, the potential to place localized lesions in almost any desired part of the brain has been applied to the therapy of epilepsy. Although some attempts have been made to direct lesions at the presumed source of the seizure discharges, the nature of the underlying pathology in man is such that adequate destruction of a significant number of pacemaker neurons is not easily accomplished. Stereotactic amygdalotomy might be predicted to have the greatest chance of success if cases exist where the focus is confined to the amygdaloid nucleus. Wide experience has confirmed that success is limited. Most of the stereotactic lesions are directed at pathways that presumably are involved in either the spread of the seizure discharge or directed at circuits that somehow play an excitatory role in the precipitation of seizures. Unfortunately the clinical efforts have, for the most part, been based on clinical serendipity rather than on clues developed in the laboratory. This is because the clues developed by research have been few. This is a fertile area for future studies.

Other Surgical Lesions

There has been some recent information obtained in experimental models of epilepsy. Discrete bilateral lesions in the substantia nigra have been reported to significantly attentuate seizures induced either chemically or by kindling [3]. It is not clear why this should be so. Whether this will modify seizures in the human is not known. Unfortunately, even if this should be the case, nonsurgical ways for selective destruction of cells in the nigra are available involving the use of the drug MPTP.

Interestingly enough, the surgical procedure involving section of pathways of spread which appears to be the most effective is also the one that was first described. This is section of the corpus callosum. It was demonstrated some 40 years ago [1] that section of the corpus callosum significantly modified the clinical spread of seizures in a monkey model of epilepsy. Although early clinical experiences with this procedure were only mildly encouraging, recent reports indicate that a more restricted operation as currently performed can provide significant benefit in selected cases [5].

Perhaps the biggest missing piece in the epilepsy puzzle has been the unexplained underutilization of surgical therapy in this condition (Ward). Happily this appears to be in the process of correction. More surgeons now have both the knowledge, interest and skills to provide surgical therapy for epilepsy. This program today is therefore particularly encouraging.

References

1 Erickson, A.E.: Spread of the epileptic discharge. An experimental study of the afterdischarge induced by electrical stimulation of the cerebral cortex. Archs Neurol. Psychiat. *43:* 429–452 (1940).

2 Freed, W.; Perlow, M.; Karoum, F.; Seiger, A.; Olson, L.; Hoffer, B.; Wyatt, R.: Restoration of dopaminergic function in the caudate nucleus by transplantation of fetal rat substantia nigra: long-term behavioral, biochemical and histochemical studies. Ann. Neurol. *8:* 510–519 (1980).

3 Gage, F.H.; Bjorklund, A.; Stenevi, U.; Dunnett, S.B.; Kelly, P.A.T.: Intrahippocampal septal grafts ameloriate learning impairments in aged rats. Science *225:* 533–536 (1984).

4 Gates, J.R.; Leppik, I.E.; Yap, J.; Gumnit, R.J.: Corpus callosotomy. Clinical and electroencephalographic effects. Epilepsia *25:* 308–316 (1984).

5 Greene, L.A.; Tischler, A.S.: PC12 pheochromocytoma cultures in neurobiological research. Adv. cell. Neurobiol. *3:* 373–414 (1982).
6 Houle, J.D.; Das, G.P.: Freezing embryonic neural tissue and its transplantation in the rat brain. Brain Res. *192:* 570–574 (1980).
7 Lockard, J.S.; Ward, A.A., Jr.: Epilepsy: a window to brain mechanisms (Raven Press, New York 1980).
8 MacNamara, J.O.; Rigsbee, L.C.; Galloway, M.T.: Evidence that substantia nigra is crucial to the neural network of kindled seizures. Eur. J. Pharmacol. *86:* 485–486 (1983).
9 Ribak, C.E.; Bradburne, R.M.; Harris, A.B.: A preferential loss of gabaergic symmetric synapses in epileptic foci: a quantitative ultrastructural analysis of monkey neocortex. J. Neurosci. *2:* 1725–1735 (1982).
10 Tortella, F.C.; Long, J.B.: Endogenous anticonvulsant substance in rat cerebrospinal fluid after a generalized seizure. Science *228:* 1106–1107 (1985).
11 Ward, A.A., Jr.: The epileptic neuron: chronic foci in animals and man; in Jasper, Ward, Pope, Basic mechanisms of the epilepsies, pp. 263–288 (Little, Brown, Boston 1969).
12 Ward, A.A., Jr.: Perspectives for surgical therapy of epilepsy; in Ward, Penry, Purpura, Epilepsy, pp. 371–390 (Raven Press, New York 1983).
13 Wyler, A.R.; Ward, A.A., Jr.: Epileptic neurons; in Lockard, Ward, Epilepsy: a window to brain mechanisms, pp. 51–68 (Raven Press, New York 1980).
14 Wyler, A.R.; Burchiel, K.J.; Ward, A.A., Jr.: Chronic epileptic foci in monkeys: correlation between seizure frequency and proportion of pacemaker epileptic neurons. Epilepsia *19:* 475–483 (1978).

A.A. Ward, Jr., Department of Neurological Surgery,
University of Washington School of Medicine, Seattle, Wash. (USA)

Proc. 9th Meeting World Soc. Stereotactic and Functional
Neurosurgery, Toronto 1985
Appl. Neurophysiol. *48:* 395–399 (1985)

The Place of Stereotactic Depth Electrode Recording in Epilepsy

André Olivier, Peter Gloor, Frederick Andermann,
L. Felipe Quesney

Montreal Neurological Institute and Hospital, Montreal, Que., Canada

Key Words. Temporal lobe epilepsy · Stereotactic surgery · Chronic depth electrodes · Epilepsy

Abstract. A series of 70 patients studied with stereotactically implanted depth electrodes is analyzed. Indications and grouping fall into three main categories: (A) the bitemporal series (52 patients), where there is ambiguity as to the lateralization of the focus; (B) the unilateral series (6 patients), where the main problem is one of localization within one hemisphere, and (C) the generalized and/or multifocal series (12 patients), where a primary focus is suspected. The best indication is represented by the group of 'bitemporal cases' which turned out to have a well-lateralized onset with intracerebral recording.

Introduction

Although the role of stereotactic procedures in the surgical treatment of epilepsy remains unresolved, their role in the diagnostic analysis of complex seizure patterns has become clearer. However, there are still many areas of controversy which stem from a combination of factors, namely the invasiveness of the procedure, the selective areas to be covered in relation to the seizure pattern and the availability of other techniques of localization. There is no doubt that, when depth electrodes are inserted stereotactically in low-threshold areas of the brain and used in conjunction with automatic detection of seizures by computer, a large number of attacks can be recorded [4, 6]. We thus have a powerful tool to confirm the suspected focal onset of a seizure. Whatever its value, though, intracerebral recording is an invasive technique which should be used in very specific circumstances and according to specific indications. The role and indications of that procedure are presented by the analysis of the first 70 patients studied at the Montreal Neurological Institute: (A) lateralization of a bilateral focus, mainly bitemporal: 52 patients (74.3%); (B) further localization within one hemisphere: 6 patients (8.6%), and (C) determination of a primary focus in generalized patterns: 12 patients (17.1%).

Material

Categorization of patients: Our total group of 70 patients can be subdivided into three main groups: (A) a bitemporal series of 52 cases (74.3%); (B) a unilateral series of 6 cases (8.6%), and (C) a generalized and/or multifocal series of 12 cases (17.1%).

Out of the 70 patients investigated, 64 later underwent an operation, thus providing a ratio of 91.42% of patients operated against those studied; 6 (8.58%) of these 70 patients were not operated upon. Three were in the bitemporal series and 3 in the generalized-multifocal one. In the bitemporal group, 2 patients showed about an equal amount of epileptic activity in both temporal lobes and one later developed a lymphoma. In the generalized-multifocal group, no epileptic activity was recorded in 1 patient, 1 requested the removal of the electrodes and in another patient the tracings could not be interpreted due to technical failure of the electrodes.

Results

Bitemporal Series

In this series the indication for the procedure was to try to lateralize an epileptic focus which appeared to involve both temporal lobes about equally or with a predominance which was too faint to establish a surgical indication. This bilaterality could take many aspects: bitemporal steady or shifting interictal activity on several EEGs, the onset of a seizure contralateral to the maximum interictal activity, bilateral seizure onset, seizure onset obscured by recording artifacts. In some instances of well-lateralized atrophy of the brain, the seizures appeared to arise from the normal-appearing side of the brain.

Fifty-two patients form the bitemporal series. In 18 of them the electrodes were inserted in both temporal lobes only; in the other 34 patients, the electrodes were inserted in both the temporal and the frontal lobes. In the temporal lobe, multicontact stainless steel electrodes were inserted horizontally through the second temporal gyrus and directed within the amygdala and hippocampus. The multicontact frontal electrodes were inserted through the second and third frontal gyri towards the mesial surface of the first frontal gyrus, the anterior cingulate gyrus and the subcallosal gyrus-orbital area. One striking finding in this group of bitemporal patients was the tendency for the onset of both the electrographic and the clinical seizures to take place in one of the two temporal lobes [3, 5, 6], thus creating a percentage or quotient of lateralization [7]. This quotient of lateralization represents the total number of seizures recorded from the predominant side divided by the total number of seizures recorded. The residual percentage does not necessarily represent seizures arising from the opposite side, but takes into account the seizures where the onset was missed and seizures which were bilateral or impossible to interpret. In our first 10 patients, the percentage of lateralization was in excess of 88% (with ranges of 75–100%) [7]. For the first 35 patients, where this quotient was analyzed, it was 82.3%. This high degree of lateralization was later found in most cases of the bitemporal series. In the analysis of the first 35 patients in the bitemporal series, a retrospective correlation was attempted between the high degree of lateralization to one side of the seizures recorded with depth electrodes and the predominance to one side of both the interictal and ictal activity in the preimplantation tracings. When the interictal activity was considered, a positive correlation (results in agreement) could be found in 65.7% and a negative correlation (results in disagreement) in 34.3%. Correlation with the preimplantation ictal activity was possible and satisfactory in only 15 patients (42.9%); a positive correlation was found in 11 patients (31.5%) and a negative one in 4 patients (11.4%). Out of the 52 patients in the bitemporal series, 49 (94.2%) later underwent a temporal resection.

The results of surgery have been analyzed in the first 27 cases and compared favorably with the so-called 'unilateral' cases. 51.9% were in group I (seizure-free or a maximum of three seizures per year), and 33% were in group II (less than 50% of the original number of seizures). When these two subgroups were added, a success rate of 85.2% was obtained. Four patients (14.8%) remained unchanged and represented the failure group [7].

Unilateral Series

Our unilateral series is made up of 6 patients only. The limited number of patients in this category derives from the insistence in trying to solve the problem of localization within one hemisphere with electrocorticography at surgery. In 2 patients, we tried to determine whether the frontal or the temporal lobe was involved in the onset of the seizures with an ambiguous clinical pattern. In 2 patients, the main ambiguity was between the temporal and the occipital lobes. In 1 case, the posterior extent of the epileptogenic zone was assessed in a patient who had previously undergone two successive temporal resections.

General and/or Multifocal Series

Twelve patients were in this group and presented with difficult seizure problems. We have tried to establish a primary focus (usually thought to be in the frontal lobe in all 12 cases). Three electrodes were inserted in each frontal lobe and two in each temporal lobe. Targets were identical as those of the bitemporal series with frontal implants. Nine patients were operated upon. Five patients (55.5%) are in group A (seizure-free or maximum of 3 seizures per year), 2 patients (22.2%) are in group B (less than 50% of their original number of attacks) and 2 patients (22.2%) are in group C (not helped by surgery).

Discussion and Conclusion

Intracerebral recording of seizures with chronically implanted depth electrodes and computer detection programs is a powerful tool in determining the side and site of onset in cases where such a focus is suspected but not proven. However, the working hypothesis of lateralization and localization should be clearly established after all the conventional investigative procedures (including radiology and psychology) and the modalities of standard recording have been worked out.

In our experience, the best indication for stereotactic depth electrode monitoring is the group of patients with a so-called 'bitemporal focus' where one temporal lobe can usually be shown as clearly dominant in the seizure process. These patients who had been rejected for surgery in the past [1, 2] will show, following a temporal lobectomy, a decrease in their seizure tendency comparable with the so-called 'unilateral' cases [2, 5]. Another indication for this procedure is the persistence of ambiguity in the localization within one hemisphere where there is a clear hemispheric lateralization. This is an approach we have probably underutilized.

Finally, a selected group of patients presenting with either a generalized or a multifocal pattern can benefit from this technique. They have actually displayed a primary focus in one of the frontal lobes. When this focus was resected, a beneficial result has been obtained in over three quarters of the cases.

References

1 Bloom, D.; Jasper, H.; Rasmussen, T.: Surgical therapy in patients with temporal lobe seizures and bilateral EEG abnormality. Epilepsia *1:* 351-365 (1959/1960).

2 Crandall, P.H.; Walter, R.D.: Clinical applications of studies in stereotactically-implanted electrodes in temporal lobe epilepsy. J. Neurosurg. *20:* 822–840 (1963).

3 Gloor, P.; Olivier, A.; Ives, J.: Prolonged seizure monitoring with stereotaxically-implanted depth electrodes in patients with bilateral interictal temporal foci: How bilateral is bitemporal epilepsy? in Wada, Penry, Advances in epileptology. 10th Int. Symp. on Epilepsy (Raven Press, New York 1980).

4 Ives, J.R.; Thompson, C.J.; Gloor, P.: Seizure monitoring: a new tool in electroencephalography. Electroenceph. clin. Neurophysiol. *41:* 422–427 (1976).

5 Olivier, A.; Gloor, P.; Ives, J.: Investigation et traitement chirurgical de l'épilepsie bitemporale. Un. méd. Can. *109:* 247–250 (1980).

6 Olivier, A.; Gloor, P.; Ives, J.; Thompson, C.J.; Andermann, F.: Chronic multiple depth electrodes in 'bitemporal epilepsy': a clinical appraisal in ten patients (Abstract). Can. J. neurol. Sci. *2:* 339 (1975).

7 Olivier, A.; Gloor, P.; Quesney, L.F.; Andermann, F.: The indications for and the role of depth electrode recording in epilepsy. Appl. Neurophysiol. *46:* 33-36 (1983).

A. Olivier, MD, Montreal Neurological Institute and Hospital,
3801 University Street, Montreal, Que. H3A 2B4 (Canada)

Proc. 9th Meeting World Soc. Stereotactic and Functional
Neurosurgery, Toronto 1985
Appl. Neurophysiol. *48:* 400–403 (1985)

Radiosurgical Treatment of Epilepsy

J.L. Barcia Salorio, P. Roldan, G. Hernandez, L. Lopez Gomez

Department of Neurosurgery, University Hospital, Valencia, Spain

Key Words. Epilepsy · Radiosurgery

Abstract. Focal irradiation of epileptic foci has been performed in a group of 6 epileptic patients, of whom 2 presented with epilepsy and 4 with epileptic psychoses. The epileptic focus was localized by means of conventional scalp EEG, electrocorticography and stereoelectroencephalography. Radiosurgery was performed by coupling a stereoguide to a ^{60}Co unit using a 10-mm diameter collimator. An estimated dose of 10 Gy was administered. Results are presented and the mechanism of action of radiation discussed.

The reasons which have led to the treatment of focal epilepsy by radiosurgery are the following: (1) There is clinical evidence that focal irradiation may be beneficial in the clinical evolution of such attacks, as in irradiation of arteriovenous malformations and low-grade tumors [7]. (2) *Elomaa* [4] proposed the radiosurgical treatment of epilepsy based on nonsynaptic mechanisms of epileptogenesis. We have seen the disappearance of convulsive crises after focal irradiation in an experimental cobalt epileptic model in the cat [3]. (3) Low-dose radiation does not produce the sequelae sometimes seen after extirpation of some foci. Consequently, we have carried out radiosurgery since 1982 in 6 patients, all of whom had received lengthy medical treatment previously, but were resistant to anticonvulsants and presented a single and well-defined focus.

Materials and Methods

Our series consisted of 6 epileptic patients, 4 male and 2 female, from 17 to 30 years old, with an average age of 24 years. Two were epileptic and 4 had epileptic psychoses.

Table I. Clinical data and results of radiosurgery for epilepsy

Case	Sex	Age	Diagnosis	EEG	ECoG	SEEG	Radiosurgery		Follow-up	Results
1/FSP	M	30	E. psy.	lTF	lTF	lTF	lTF	10/82	3 y	exc.
2/MDN	F	21	E+Beh. dis.	BD	lTF, rTF	lTF, rTF	lTF	1/83	2 y	exc.
3/RRL	M	26	E. psy.	BD	lTF	–	lTF	7/83	2 y	exc.
4/CSA	F	21	E.	BD	lTF	–	lTF	2/85	4 m	exc.
5/FGA	M	17	E. psy.	BD	rTF	rTF	rTF	2/85	4 m	–
6/ASO	M	30	E. psy.	BD	rTF	rTF	rTF	12/84	6 m	poor

ECoG = electrocorticography; SEEG = stereoelectroencephalography; E = epilepsy; E. psy. = epileptic psychosis; Beh. dis. = behavioral disturbances; lTF/rTF = left/right temporal focus; BD = bilateral discharges.

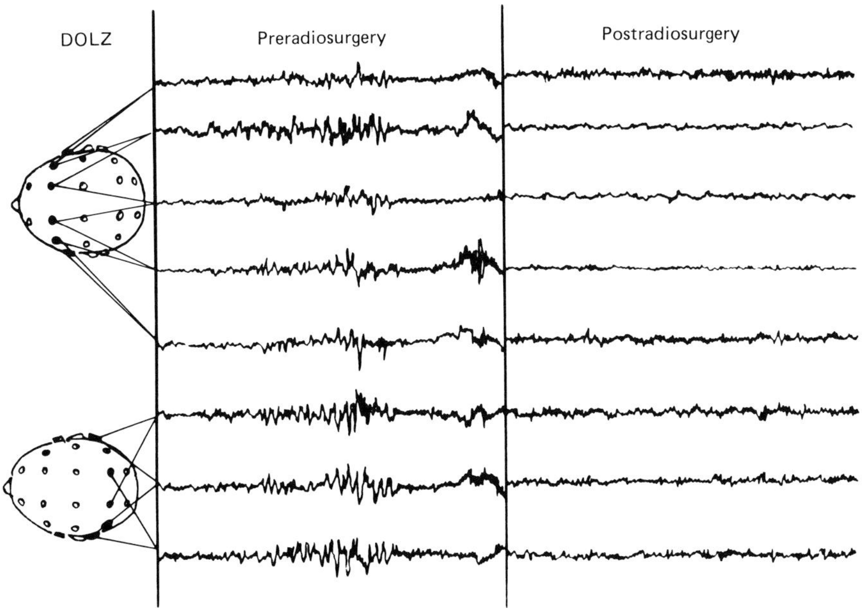

Fig. 1. Case No. 2: preoperative EEG and postradiosurgery control EEG. Left temporal focus. Postoperative disappearance of epileptiform activity.

The localization of the focus was done by means of stereoelectroencephalography (SEEG). In the first stage, a CT and EEG were done in order to isolate the area concerned and justify more detailed study. Secondly, burr-hole electrocorticography (ECoG) was performed introducing cortical electrodes into the subarachnoid space [2], which allowed the exact delimitation and localization of the focus. This was carried out by multiterminal electrodes, each with 7 contacts separated by 7 mm, allowing for the exploration of an area 4.5 cm long.

Radiosurgery was performed by coupling a stereoguide to a conventional ^{60}Co unit (Theratron) using a 10-mm diameter collimeter which produces 90% isodose of 1 cm diameter [1], and by the cross-fire method an estimated dose of 10 Gy was administered.

Results

The results (table I) were excellent except in case 6 who continues to have mild attacks. Patient No. 1 is a 30-year-old male with grave psychic disturbances who required hospital admission every 6 months over several years. After radiosurgical treatment and during a 3-year follow-up period he remains treatment-free, has married and works in a normal job. Case No. 4, a 20-year-old women, had several daily crises and reactive depression; at 5 months' postradiation she is symptom- and medication-free. Patient No. 2, a 21-year-old female with a low IQ, epileptic crises and behavioral disturbances, who, postirradiation, is symptom- and medication-free after a follow-up of 2 years (fig. 1).

Discussion

We must emphasize that a very minimal dose was used, only 10 Gy, which would suppose a very specific action of ionizing radiations on epileptic neurons. *Elomaa* [4] proposed an action upon somatostatin and the loss of its effects on the cell membrane. However, our results with focal cobalt radiation in experimental epilepsy in the cat, also a synaptic model, led us to think of another mechanism of ionizing radiation. Most authors believe in deafferentation as the basic mechanism involved in epileptogenesis, the most striking feature being the loss of dendritic spines. On the other hand, *Malis* et al. [5] observed a great dendritic proliferation a few days after producing a deuteron laminar lesion in the IV cortical layer of the rabbit.

Multiple hypotheses may therefore be presented. The epileptic neurons are hypersensitive to irradiation, or irradiation would induce synaptic neoformation, or rather, as *Monnier and Krupp* [6] pointed out, 10 Gy irradiation diminishes cortical activity.

References

1 Barcia Salorio, J.L.; Cerdá, M.; Hernandez, G.; Bordes, V.; Beraha, J.; Calabuig, C.; Broseta, J.: Pathological findings in acoustic neurinoma after stereotactic irradiation. Acta neurochir. *33:* suppl., pp. 317–321 (1984).

2 Barcia Salorio, J.L.; Roldan, P.; Ramos, S.; Lopez Gomez, L; Broseta, J.: Chronic burr-hole ECoG and SEEG in the assessment of surgical treatment for epilepsy. Acta neurochir. *33:* suppl., pp. 79–83 (1984).

3 Barcia Salorio, J.L.; Vanaclocha, V.; Cerdá, M.; Roldan, P.: Focal irradiation in epilepsy. Experimental study in the cat. Appl. Neurophysiol. (in press, 1985).

4 Elomaa, E.: Focal irradiation of the brain: an alternative to temporal lobe resection in intractable focal epilepsy. Med. Hypoth. *6:* 501–503 (1980).

5 Malis, L.I.; Rose, J.E.; Kruger, L.; Baker, C.P.: Production of laminar lesions in the cerebral cortex by deuteron irradiation; in Haley, Snider, Response of the nervous system to ionizing radiation, pp. 359–368 (Academic Press, New York 1962).

6 Monnier, M.; Krupp, P.: Action of gamma radiation on electrical brain activity; in Haley, Snider, Response of the nervous system to ionizing radiation, pp. 607–620 (Academic Press, New York 1962).

7 Rossi, G.F.: Epileptogenic cerebral low-grade tumours: effect of interstitial stereotactic irradiation on seizures. Appl. Neurophysiol. (in press, 1985).

J.L. Barcia Salorio, MD, Department of Neurosurgery,
University Hospital, E-46010 Valencia (Spain)

Proc. 9th Meeting World Soc. Stereotactic and Functional Neurosurgery, Toronto 1985
Appl. Neurophysiol. *48:* 404–407 (1985)

Surgery for Epilepsy
Selective Partial Microsurgical Callosotomy for Intractable Multiform Seizures: Criteria for Clinical Selection and Results

Raul Marino, Jr.

Division of Functional Neurosurgery, University of Sao Paulo, Medical School, Brazil

Key Words. Callosotomy · Generalized epilepsy · Multiform seizures

Abstract. A series of 35 patients have been submitted to microsurgical callosotomy since February 1978, their age ranging from 6 to 42 years. The surgical procedure consisted either of a frontal parasagittal trephination or a larger frontoparietal rectangular craniotomy to allow the investigation of the surgical areas of the hemispheres with electrocorticography under local anesthesia. This allowed us to better follow the electrographic abnormalities and plan the extent of the callosal section suited to each case, in particular rostral and genual section, section of the trunk only or subtotal section sparing the splenium. In 2 cases, cortical resection was associated with the split. The callosal fibers which were divided by careful section under the resected portion provided a critical postoperative control of the extent of the lesion. Results and selection criteria will also be analyzed.

Until recent years, functional neurosurgery had very little to offer to patients with intractable generalized seizures. In 1940, *Van Wagenen and Herren* [4] first proposed central commissurotomy for control of spread of epileptic discharge from one hemisphere to the other. This previously empirical procedure was later reviewed by *Bogen and Vogel* [1] in 1962, and their patients became the subjects of *Sperry and Gazzaniga's* [6] studies on disconnection of the hemispheres in 1962. In 1977, *Wilson* et al. [6], based on their own experience, concluded that anterior and/or complete section of the corpus callosum without breaching the ventricles could be the procedure with least morbidity and greatest benefit from the epilepsy point of view.

The present study will review some of our data obtained from this procedure, findings that have helped us improve our selection criteria, and our results, using a more selective and functional procedure. This procedure has also served us as a research tool to study brain and mind mechanisms since it will also produce important changes in psychiatric, neurophysiological, neuropsychological and cognitive functions of the human brain, findings that we have reported elsewhere [4].

Material and Methods

Thirty-five patients have been submitted to partial microsurgical callosotomy since February 1978, their age ranging from 6 to 42 years. In 6 cases an extension of the section involved also the trunk of the callosum, sparing the splenium, and in 3 cases a selective split of the trunk only was performed. In 2 patients, unilateral mesial cortical resection was also accomplished. All remaining patients were submitted to anterior callosotomy, its extension being determined by the EEG findings.

The *selection criteria* for surgery were based on patients presenting uncontrollable *multiform seizures* (a combination of minor generalized fits with focal seizures and tonic-clonic generalized attacks) with duration of the epilepsy of at least 4 years, and EEG demonstrating generalized bisynchronous spike and slow-wave discharges with or without focal or multifocal accentuation and with normal or abnormal background activity. Based on our EEG findings, we tentatively divided our patients into four groups: *Group I:* generalized epilepsies with fast spike-and-wave discharges and normal background activity. *Group II:* secondary generalized epilepsy with slow spike-and-wave discharges and slow background activity. *Group III* (or 'hemispherectomy' group): patients with large hemispheric lesions, who would have an indication for subtotal hemispherectomy. *Group IV* (or 'miscellaneous' group): they composed a nonhomogeneous group which did not meet the strict selection criteria listed above, including an 18-year-old patient with petit mal, one mesial focus with focal seizures alone, and 1 patient with continuous focal motor seizures and startle-induced myoclonus.

After exposure of the mesial surface of both hemispheres, flat 8-lead platinum electrodes were inserted into the mesial aspect of the hemispheres for recording, and callosal section was carried up to the point where disruption of the bisynchrony was obtained.

Results

In group I, an important decrease of the frequency of seizures occurred in all patients. The rare remaining seizures are now of shorter duration and less disruptive of the patient's contact. This was parallel by dramatic disruption of the bisynchrony, leading to asynchronous discharges, occurring in one or the other hemisphere. Prolonged slow-wave discharges may still be seen restricted to one hemisphere or during several records, accompanied by concomitant discharges of different morphology in the contralateral hemisphere, usually not followed by overt seizure behavior. There was great improvement in neuropsychological performance, particularly in attention.

All group II patients showed important improvement in their clinical status despite the fact that some of them still present generalized epilepsies with multiform accentuation. The best improvements in this group, however, do not parallel similar cases in group I; yet, they are also associated with a marked disruption of bisynchrony.

Group III patients also showed a remarkable improvement with almost total disappearance of startle-induced myoclonic phenomena. This was followed by partial isolation of focal discharges with few remaining bisynchronous episodes.

Group IV represents poor therapeutic results, except for the patient presenting with startle myoclonus, who improved markedly.

Discussion

Experimental demonstration by *Marcus and Watson* [3], *Naquet* et al. [5] and *Gloor* [2] that section of the callosum, even when incomplete, will partially prevent the bilateral synchronization of discharges in cat and monkey has also been demonstrated in our clinical cases, where marked disruption of bisynchrony was found after partial section of the callosum. This was accompanied clinically by marked reduction in the frequency of absences, atonic fits, tonic axial seizures and myoclonic seizures, startle-induced or not. This may be related to a decreased capacity of the newly separated hemispheres to organize bisynchronous discharges, leading to a marked decrease in the frequency of generalized seizures.

This improvement related to seizure frequency and duration was also accompanied by a global improvement in attention and neuropsychological performance and adaptation. Some patients resumed their formal education after surgery, became more active, organized their thoughts better, showing marked improvement over their previous epileptic cognitive dysfunctions. These findings allow us to propose microsurgical functional callosotomy as a valuable alternative procedure to treat multiform epilepsy which does not respond to medical treatment.

References

1 Bogen, J.E.; Vogel, P.J.: Neurologic status in the long term following complete cerebral commissurotomy; in Michel, Scott, Les syndromes de disconnection calleuse chez l'homme (1975).
2 Gloor, P.: Generalized corticoreticular epilepsies - some considerations on the pathophysiology of generalized bilaterally synchronous spike-and-wave discharges. Epilepsia *9:* 249–263 (1968).
3 Marcus, E.M.; Watson, C.W.: Bilateral synchronous spike-wave electrographic patterns in the cat: interaction of bilateral cortical foci in the intact, the bilateral cortical callosal and adiencephalic preparation. Archs Neurol. *14:* 601–610 (1966).
4 Marino, R., Jr.; Regazzo, P.C.: Selection criteria and results of partial callosotomy; in Reeves, Epilepsy and the corpus callosum, pp. 281–301 (Plenum Press, New York 1985).
5 Naquet, R.; Menini, C.; Cartier, J.: Photically induced epilepsy in *Papio papio:* the initiation of discharges and role of frontal cortex and corpus callosum; in Petsche, Brazier, Synchronization of EEG activity in epilepsies, pp. 347–365 (Springer, New York 1972).
6 Wilson, D.H.; Reeves, A.; Gazzaniga, E.: 'Central' commissurotomy for intractable generalized epilepsy 2. Neurology *32:* 687–697 (1982).

R. Marino, MD, Rua Maestro Cardim, 808, Sao Paulo, SP 01323 (Brazil)

Proc. 9th Meeting World Soc. Stereotactic and Functional Neurosurgery, Toronto 1985
Appl. Neurophysiol. *48:* 408–417 (1985)

Foramen Ovale Electrodes: A New Technique Enabling Presurgical Evaluation of Patients with Mesiobasal Temporal Lobe Seizures

J. Siegfried[a], *H.G. Wieser*[b], *S.R.G. Stodieck*[b]

Departments of [a] Neurosurgery and [b] Neurology, University Hospital, Zürich, Switzerland

Key Words. Preoperative recording · Foramen ovale electrode · Temporal lobe epilepsy

Abstract. A recently developed technique to record from the mesiobasal aspect of the temporal lobes by subdural electrodes inserted through the foramen ovale is described. Experience with this technique in 13 candidates for surgical epilepsy therapy is presented. Our results indicate that interictal epileptiform potentials as well as ictal discharges are reliably picked up by the foramen ovale electrode whenever nucleus amygdalae, hippocampus and parahippocampal gyrus show synchronous epileptic activity. The advantages of this technique are discussed.

The limbic structures, particularly the amygdala-hippocampus complex, play a key role both in the origin and spread of complex partial seizure. The exact localization and delineation of the epileptogenic focus is an indispensable prerequisite for successful neurosurgical treatment. To date, in many instances, the most reliable method to answer the question as to the possible mesiobasal limbic origin of such seizures is to record directly from these structures by means of stereotactically implanted depth electrodes (SEEG). Because of the invasive nature of this approach, however, rigid selection criteria must be used. Noninvasive or less invasive recording with nasopharyngeal or sphenoidal electrodes may help but usually cannot provide the precise information on which to base a sound surgical judgement, e.g., should an anterior temporal lobectomy be performed or will a selective restricted medial temporal lobe (TL) resection suffice to cure a given patient.

Therefore, a technique of epicortical recordings from the mesiobasal aspect of the TLs by electrodes placed through the foramen ovale

(FO) was developed. Our aim was to improve the preoperative evaluation of candidates for a selective amygdalohippocampectomy because of drug-resistant complex partial seizures of suggested mesiobasal TL origin. Because this procedure of placing an electrode through the FO is relatively simple and does not injure the brain itself, it was furthermore hoped that in certain cases FO recording might substitute for the more invasive SEEG evaluation which requires an exact neuroradiological examination under stereotactic conditions and the implantation of several electrodes into the brain itself [6].

Animal Experiments

Evaluation of the FO electrode technique was started with experiments in 2 dogs. Interictal and ictal focal epileptic activity in one hippocampus was induced by local penicillin application. The EEG was recorded by hippocampal depth, subdural strip, scalp, and the FO electrodes. Comparison of the differently recorded EEG signals showed that the FO electrode recorded the hippocampal epileptiform activity with a high degree of accuracy and reliability, whereas many spikes and seizure discharges could be recorded neither by the subdural strip electrodes (placed over the lateral temporal cortex), nor by the scalp electrodes. Using Ag-AgCl ball electrodes (insulated by teflon except for the tip), as an appropriate reference and conventional DC mode amplification, the DC shift accompanying the seizure discharges was clearly reflected in both hippocampal and FO recordings [9].

Human Recording

Because of these favorable animal experiments, it seemed justified to apply this technique to human epileptics. The first application, however, was in a nonepileptic patient suffering from drug-resistant trigeminal neuralgia, who, following a short recording period, underwent a therapeutic electrocoagulation of the third trigeminal branch of the Gasserian ganglion [3]. Since then, 13 candidates for surgical therapy because of drug-resistant complex partial seizures have been evaluated using the FO recording method. Nine patients had FO electrodes in addition to SEEG.

Table I shows that the first 9 patients had only unilateral implantation. To date, 4 patients underwent bilateral implantation. For obvious reasons, bilateral insertion of FO electrodes was performed only after it was ascertained that no complications had occurred with unilateral FO electrodes.

With the exception of 2 patients who had very short lasting painful or tingling sensations during withdrawal of the FO electrodes and minor trouble during eating, no side effects and no effect on the trigeminal nerve was observed during or after the recording period. Withdrawal of electrodes did not require any anesthesia.

Table I. Data of patients who underwent foramen ovale electrode recording

Pat. No.	Sex	Age	Diagnosis	SEEG Evaluation, placement and number ( ) of electrodes	FO electrode, side and recording period		Therapeutical operation[1]	Outcome	Follow-up (months) since	
									FO	operation
1	f	60	trigeminal neuralgia	–	R	1 h	percutaneous trigeminal rhizotomy	–	14	(14)
2	m	35	drug-resist. TLE	R:T(4)F(1)P(1)O(1) L:T(2)	R	6 days	causal R AHE	seizure-free	14	14
3	m	25	drug-resist. TLE	R:T(3)F(2)P(1) L:T(2)	R	5 days	palliative R AHE	improved	13	10
4	f	43	calcified AVM R P, drug-resist. cps	–	R	4 days	palliative R AHE	improved	13	13
5	m	9	drug-resist. multifocal epilepsy	R:T(1)F(1) L:T(2)F(1)P(1)	L	4 days	–	–	12	–
6	m	33	drug-resist. TLE	R:T(2)F(1)P(1) L:T(3)F(2)P(1)	R	9 days	palliative R AHE	improved	12	10
7	f	10	drug-resist.	–	L	3 days	causal L AHE and removal of insular oligodendroglioma	seizure-free	10	6
8	f	22	drug-resist. multifocal epilepsy with progressive atrophy of R hemisphere and left hemiparesis	R:T(3)F(2)C(3)P(2) L: –	L	4 days	palliative R AHE	improved (no further cps with strong vegetative signs)	10	6

Table I (continued)

Pat. No.	Sex	Age	Diagnosis	SEEG Evaluation, placement and numbers ( ) of electrodes	FO electrode, side and recording period		Therapeutical operation[1]	Outcome	Follow-up (months) since: FO	Follow-up (months) since: operation
9	m	14	drug-resist. cps and focal motor seizures with sec. generalization	– later: R:T(2)F(3)C(1) L:T(1)	R	1 day	removal of R F-opercular cavernoma	seizure-free	10	3
10	f	34	drug-resist.	R:T(1)F(1)P(1) L:T(3)F(1)P(1)	L	11 days	causal L AHE	seizure-free	8	6
11	m	22	drug-resist. TLE	–	R&-L	4 days	removal of R insular cavernoma	seizure-free	7	6
12	f	21	drug-resist. TLE	R:T(3)P(1) L:T(1)	R&-L	5 days	waiting for (causal R AHE)	–	3	–
13	m	17	multiple cavernoma with cps	–	R&-L	3 days	removal of L T cavernoma	(seizure-free)	½	½
14	m	35	drug-resist. TLE	R:T(2)F(1)P(1) L:T(1)F(1)	R&-L	6 days	waiting for (causal R AHE)	–	¼	–

R = right; L = left; T = temporal; F = frontal; C = central; P = parietal; O = occipital; AHE = selective amygdalohippocampectomy; cps = complex partial seizures.

[1] With exception of trigeminal rhizotomy all resective surgery was done by Prof. *G. Yasargil*.

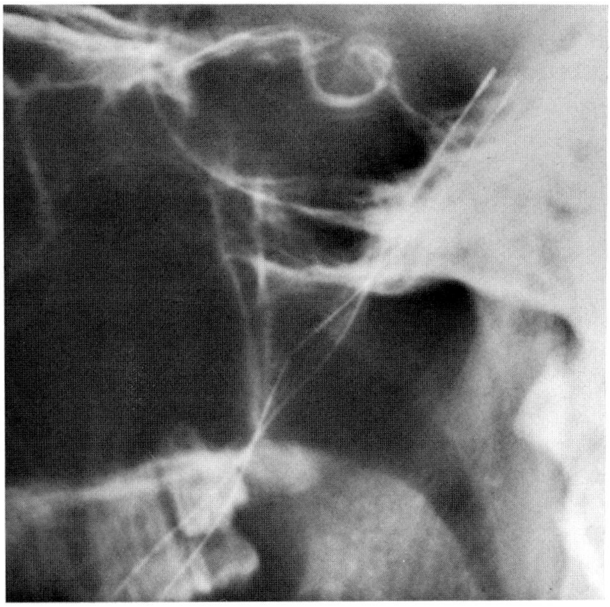

Fig. 1. X-ray showing the bilateral foramen ovale electrodes.

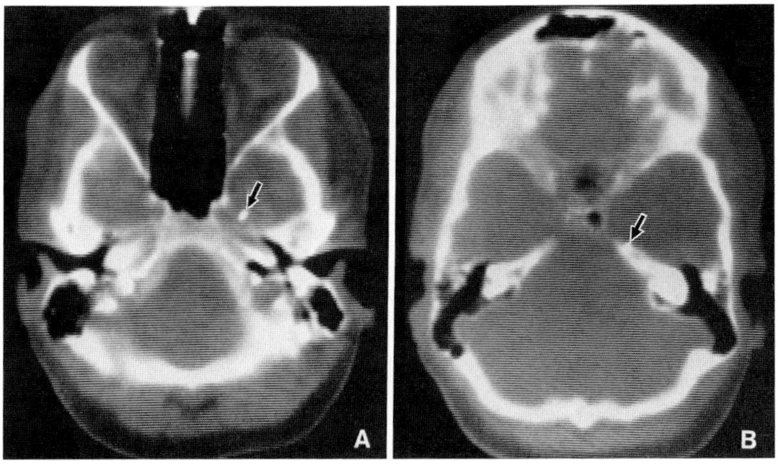

Fig. 2. CT of a patient with right foramen ovale electrode (arrow).

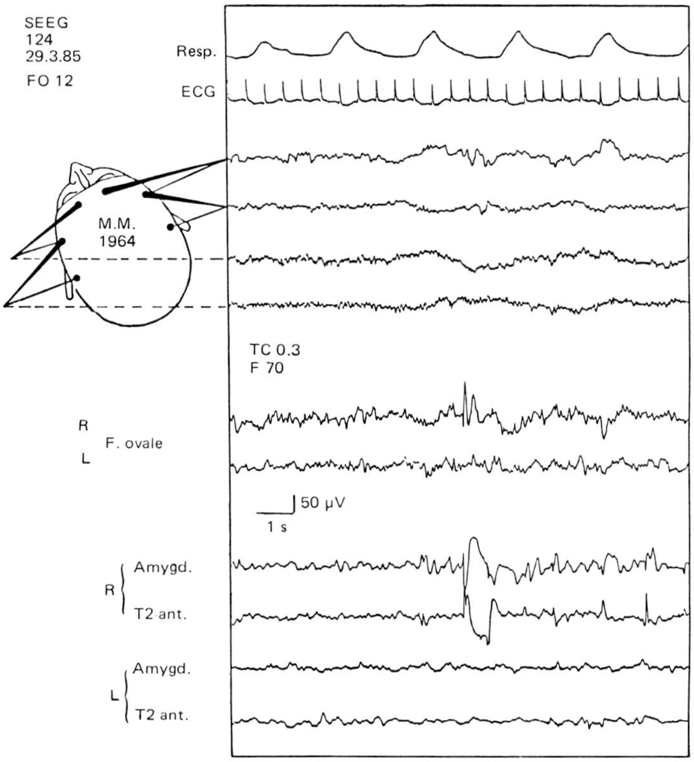

Fig. 3. Selected channels out of a simultaneously recorded 32-channel, surface and depth EEG showing a spontaneous interictal epileptiform event originating at the right basolateral amygdala. Note that the epileptiform spike is well reflected by the right FO electrode (T2 ant. = second temporal convolution, anterior part).

Technique of FO Electrode Positioning and Recording

Positioning of the FO electrode follows the technique of the so-called 'percutaneous trigeminal rhizotomy', as originally described by *Kirschner* [2]. After the patient has been anesthetized with 30–50 mg methohexital, i.v., a 19-gauge spinal needle is inserted 3 cm lateral to the oral commissure and directed by freehand manipulation to the FO. Cutaneous landmarks are used, according to the technique of *Härtel* [1]. After perforating the dura, the recording electrode is introduced through the cannula. Depending on the electrode type (single or multicontact stainless steel or sintered Ag-AgCl), the tip of the electrode may be advanced as far as to the ambient cistern (fig. 1, 2).

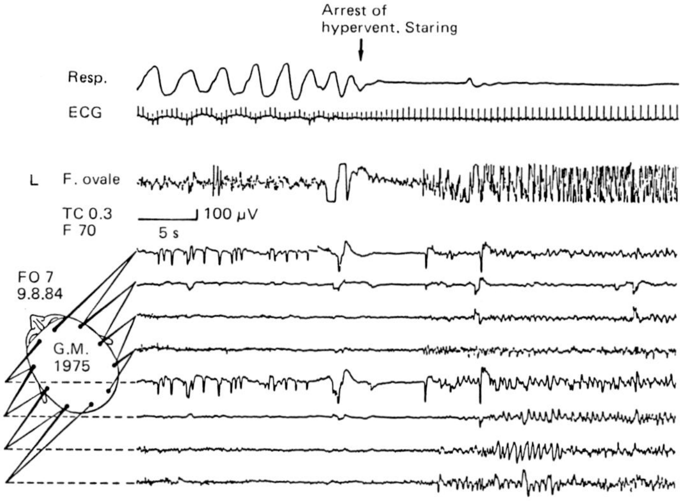

Fig. 4. Surface and left FO electrode recording at the onset of a complex partial seizure, clinically characterized by an arrest (↓) and vegetative signs. Note that the 'initial complex' in the left FO electrode (AC mode) recorded EEG corresponds well with the clinical seizure onset, whereas the scalp EEG does not indicate the exact time and site of the seizure onset (pat. No. 7 in table I).

For DC recording we used electrodes which consisted of a cylindrical Ag-AgCl pellet (0.4 mm diameter, 4 mm length) sintered around the tip of a silver wire of 0.25 mm diameter. As reference, a disk-shaped sintered Ag-AgCl electrode (of 2.5 mm diameter) was implanted subgaleally at the vertex (fig. 5).

Results

Evaluation of FO electrode recorded activity was possible in 8 patients by comparing it with simultaneously recorded direct intracerebral EEG obtained by depth electrodes implanted in mesiobasal limbic (amygdala, hippocampus, parahippocampal gyrus) and other structures (table I). Interictal epileptiform activity (fig. 3) as well as seizure discharges (fig. 4, 5) were reliably reflected when a larger mesiobasal limbic brain volume displayed spike activity. However, seizure discharges narrowly confined to either amygdala or hippocampus only, in some cases, escaped detection by the FO electrodes. The negative

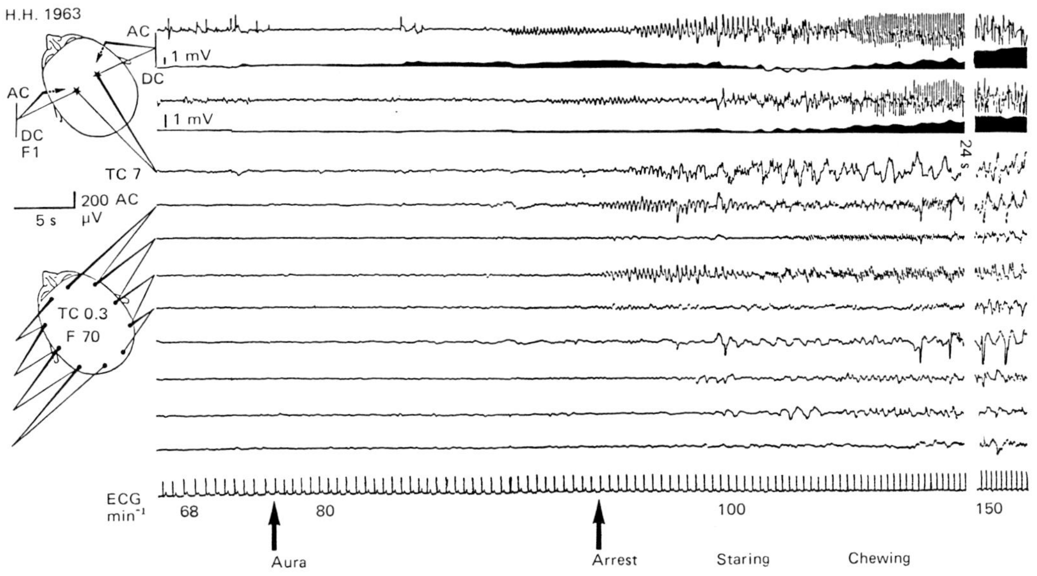

Fig. 5. Two sections of a complex partial seizure originating at the right TL and recorded by scalp EEG and bilateral FO electrodes in AC and DC mode. Note that the negative DC shift of the right FO electrode activity (black) corresponds well with the warning of the patient (↑ Aura) and precedes the rhythmic seizure activity picked up first by the right FO electrode (AC mode recording). Later, the seizure discharges propagate to the contralateral mesiobasal TL. We concluded that seizure origin was in the right TL, but not in mesiobasal limbic structures which obviously were affected only secondarily. Therefore at operation only the right insular cavernoma was removed (pat. No. 11 in table I).

epicortical DC shift, that is well known to accompany seizures in experimental animals [5], was clearly picked up by the special FO electrode that enables DC recording. These findings proved to be especially helpful in lateralizing the seizure origin in cases with bilateral TL foci (fig. 5).

Discussion

The main advantages of the FO electrode are (1) FO electrode recording is atraumatic to the brain itself. (2) Insertion of the FO electrode is a free-hand manipulation performed within minutes; no stereotactic frame and no endotracheal anesthesia are needed. (3) FO electrodes allow for almost artifact-free, extremely stable recordings which are superior to that obtained by sphenoidal electrodes. (4) When sintered Ag-AgCl FO electrodes are used, reliable recordings in DC mode can be obtained. (5) The FO electrodes are well tolerated and no major side effects or complications have occurred so far.

We conclude that FO electrode recordings are very useful to confirm the laterality of mesiobasal temporal epileptogenic foci and exactly localize the site where the seizure originated. In certain epilepsy candidates for surgery, FO electrode recording may provide sufficient information to give the indication for surgical resection either by anterior temporal lobectomy or by selective amygdalohippocampectomy [7, 8]. In those cases where an insular, a neocortical lateral-posterior TL, or an extratemporal seizure origin has to be ruled out or ascertained, FO electrodes help to reduce the number of depth electrodes necessary for SEEG exploration of the TLs. In patients with morphological TL lesions (tumors, AVMs, etc.), FO electrode recording might suffice to document the epileptogenicity of the lesions. Furthermore, it may provide clues as to whether in addition to the lesion itself the seizure-prone mesiobasal TL structures should also be resected in order to guarantee postoperative seizure control.

References

1 Härtel, F.: Über die intracranielle Injektionsbehandlung der Trigeminusneuralgie. Med. Klin. *10:* 582–584 (1914).

2 Kirschner, M.: Electrocoagulation des Ganglion Gasseri. Zentbl. Chir. *47:* 2841–2843 (1932).

3 Siegfried, J.: Percutaneous controlled thermocoagulation of Gasserian ganglion in trigeminal neuralgia. Experiences with 1,000 cases; in Samii, Jannetta, The cranial nerves (Springer, Berlin 1981).

4 Siegfried, J.; Vosmansky, M.: Technique of the controlled thermocoagulation of trigeminal ganglion and spinal roots; in Krayenbühl, Advances and technical standards in neurosurgery, vol. 2 (Springer, Wien 1975).

5 Speckmann, E.J.; Caspers, H.; Janzen, R.W.: Relations between cortical DC shifts and membrane potential changes of cortical neurons associated with seizure activity; in Petsche, Brazier, Synchronization of EEG activity in epilepsies, pp. 93–111 (Springer, New York 1972).

6 Wieser, H.G.: Electroclinical features of psychomotor seizure (Fischer-Butterworths, Stuttgart 1983).
7 Wieser, H.G.; Yasargil, G.: Selective amygdalohippocampectomy and a surgical treatment of mesiobasal limbic epilepsy. Surg. Neurol. *17:* 445–457 (1982).
8 Wieser, H.G.; Yasargil, G.: Selective amygdalohippocampectomy: indications, investigative technique and results; in Symon et al., Advances and technical standards in neurosurgery, vol. 13 (Springer, Vienna 1985).
9 Wieser, H.G.; Elger, C.E.; Stodieck, S.R.G.: The 'foramen ovale electrode': a new recording method for the preoperative evaluation of patients suffering from mesiobasal temporal lobe epilepsy. Electroenceph. clin. Neurophysiol. (in press, 1985).

Prof. Dr. J. Siegfried, Neurochirurgische Klinik, Universitätsspital,
CH-8091 Zürich (Switzerland)

Proc. 9th Meeting World Soc. Stereotactic and Functional Neurosurgery, Toronto 1985
Appl. Neurophysiol. *48:* 418–422 (1985)

Dynamic EEG Topography and Analysis of Epileptic Spikes and Evoked Potentials following Thalamic Stimulation

Hiroshi Takahashi, Masaharu Yasue, Buichi Ishijima

Department of Neurosurgery, Toky Metropolitan Neurological Hospital, Tokyo, Japan

Key Words. Dynamic EEG topography · Epileptic spikes · Evoked potentials · Thalamic stimulation · Electroencephalograms · Epilepsy · Stereotactic surgery

Abstract. Dynamic EEG topography is used to study evoked potentials following thalamic stimulation as well as epileptic spikes and spike-wave complexes during stereotactic operations. Dynamic EEG topography is an effective method for displaying the distribution pattern of evoked potentials following thalamic stimulation. This technique makes it possible to observe successive increases in augmenting responses and to define the localization of epileptic foci.

Introduction

A system for displaying EEG and evoked potentials topographically has been developed by *Duffy* et al. [1, 2] and *Matsuoka* et al. [4]. The term dynamic EEG topography implies a topographical display of the EEG images or evoked potentials which changes with respect to time. In the present study, dynamic EEG topography is used to analyze evoked potentials following thalamic stimulation and to define the localization of epileptic foci.

Materials and Methods

Evoked potentials were recorded following stimulation of the thalamus on 18 trajectories in 13 patients who underwent stereotactic surgery to alleviate tremor, spasmodic torticollis, rigidity or thalamic pain. The targets of the stereotactic operations

a

b

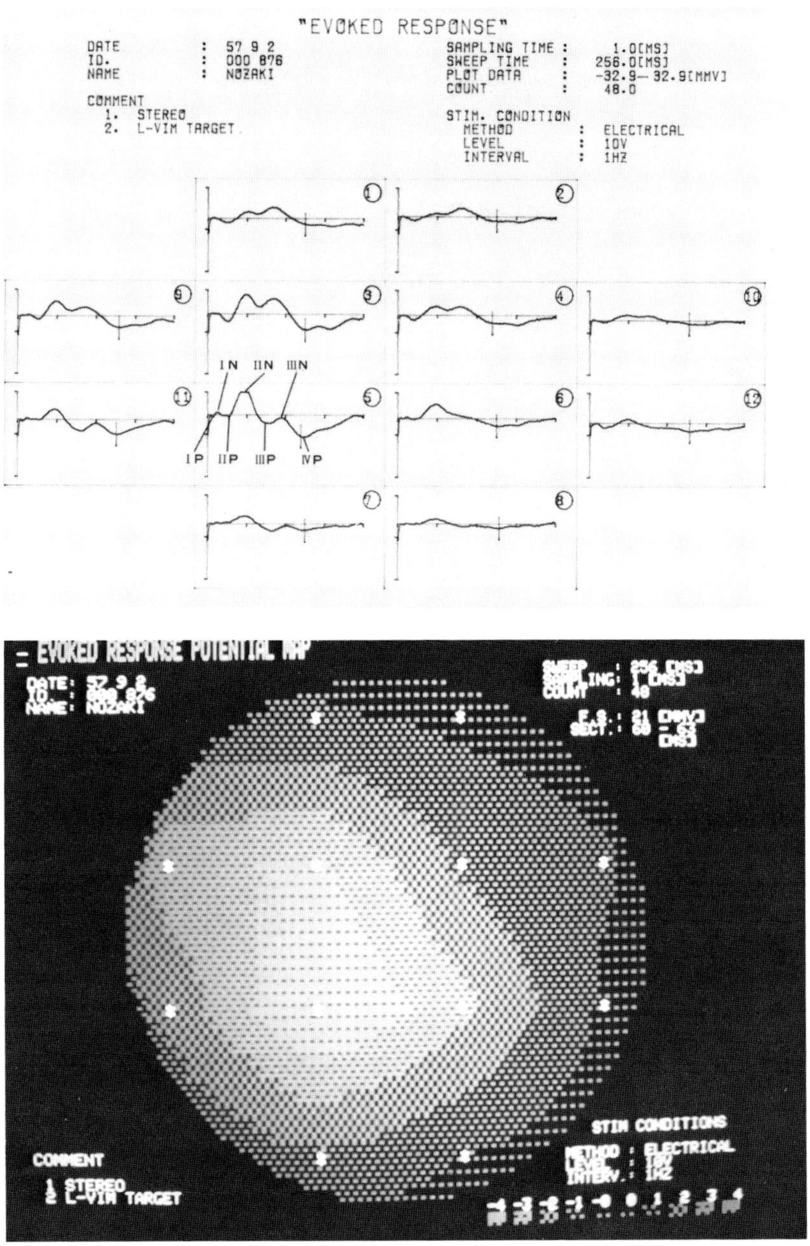

Fig. 1. a 12-channel evoked potentials following stimulation of the left Vim. Each component of the evoked potential is shown using the nomenclature of *Matsumoto* [3]. P means positive wave and N negative wave. Analysis time: 256 ms; full scale: 32.9mm V. **b** Topographical image of IIn peak on the scalp.

were the Vim for tremor, Voi for spasmodic torticollis, Voa-Vop for rigidity and Vc for thalamic pain. Epileptic spikes or spike-wave complexes were recorded in 18 patients with epilepsy and 25 with symptomatic seizures.

12-channel evoked potentials and 12-channel EEGs were recorded and fed to a data recorder. The data were transferred off-line to an ATAC 450 medical computer (Nihonkoden Co. Ltd.), and the topographical amplitude image of each address point was displayed on a color monitor. These serial images were then photographed using a 16-mm movie camera, which made it possible to visualize dynamic changes. The course of each secondary generalized seizure was divided into 15 EEG segments, each with a duration of 2,048 ms. When the 15 segments were processed serially, the entire course of the secondary generalized seizure could be displayed with an analysis time of 30,720 ms using dynamic EEG topography.

Results

Evoked Potentials following Thalamic Stimulation

Evoked potentials resulting from stimulation of specific thalamic nuclei usually consist of Ip, In, IIp, IIn, IIIp, IIIn and IVp [3] within 256 ms (fig. 1). IIn usually exhibited maximum amplitude and was distributed ipsilaterally over the centroparietal area when Vim was stimulated (fig. 1), but when either Voa-Vop or Vc was stimulated, there was a tendency for the distribution pattern of IIn to shift to the central or parietal area, respectively. With the moving images, topographical increases in augmenting responses could be demonstrated dynamically. For example, when a point on the trajectory 4 mm rostral to the target of Voi was stimulated at 6 Hz, successive increases in the amplitude and distribution of IIn were dynamically displayed over the central part of the scalp.

Epileptic Spikes and Spike-Wave Complexes

Focal spikes always originated from the epileptic foci and spread to the surrounding region but the highest potentials were consistently seen at the foci throughout the course. Figure 2 shows the serial topographical distribution of a spike in a patient with a subcortical gangliocytoma in the right parietal lobe. In this case, the theta focus was found to coincide with the origin of the spikes, where CT revealed a calcified solid mass lesion.

3 Hz spike-wave complex originated from the frontal pole bilaterally and spread posteriorly and laterally, rapidly covering the entire scalp. However, in a case with secondary generalized seizures, focal

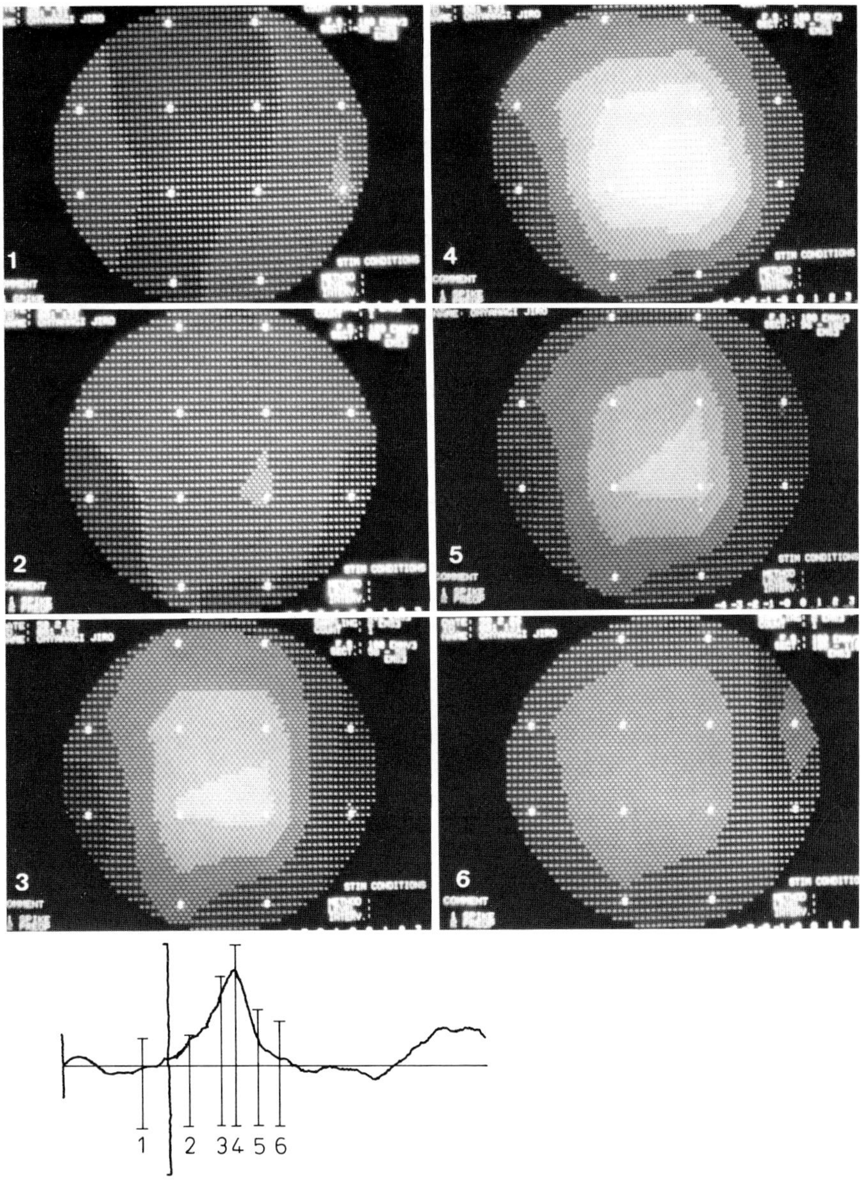

Fig. 2. Amplitude scalp topography for a spike in a case with gangliocytoma. The topographical images correspond to the wave form shown below: 1 shows the state just before the appearance of the spike. In 2, 3 and 4 the spike appears in the right parietal region, its amplitude increases, and the spike spreads to the neighboring area. 5 and 6 show the decay phase of the spike.

spikes appeared first, with multifocal spikes gradually predominating, finally culminating in an ictal state. At the same time, dynamic EEG topography showed rapidly alternating changes in polarity between the two hemispheres.

Conclusion

Dynamic EEG topography provides useful information by displaying the distribution patterns of evoked potentials elicited by thalamic stimulation, so that augmenting responses can be visualized. It is especially useful in defining the locus of epileptic foci where spikes or spike-wave complexes originate and where maximum amplitude peaks appear.

References

1 Duffy, F.H.; Burchfiel, J.L.; Lombroso, C.T.: Brain electrical activity mapping (BEAM): a new method for expanding the clinical ability of EEG and evoked potential data. Ann. Neurol. *5:* 307–321 (1978).
2 Lombroso, C.T.; Duffy, F.H.: Brain electrical activities in the epilepsies; in Akimoto, Kazamatsuri, Seino, Ward, Advances in epileptology. 13th International Symposium on Epilepsy, pp. 173–179 (Raven Press, New York 1982).
3 Matsumoto, K.: Thalamo-cortical relation in man; analysis of evoked cortical responses following stimulation of the thalamic VL nucleus and the centro-median area (in Japanese); in Matsumoto, Proceeding of the Japanese Conference of Topographic Electroencephalography, Tokyo 1984, pp. 11–22.
4 Matsuoka, S.; Arakaki, Y.; Numaguchi, K.; Ueno, S.: The effect of dexamethasone on electroencephalograms in patients with brain tumors. With special reference to topographic computer display of delta activity. J. Neurosurg. *48:* 601–608 (1978).

H. Takahashi, MD, Department of Neurosurgery,
Tokyo Metropolitan Neurological Hospital,
2-6-1 Musashidai Fuchi-shi, Tokyo 183 (Japan)

Proc. 9th Meeting World Soc. Stereotactic and Functional
Neurosurgery, Toronto 1985
Appl. Neurophysiol. *48:* 423–426 (1985)

Absence Attacks Controlled by Thalamic Stimulation

O.J. Andy, M. Jurko

Department of Neurosurgery, Medical Center, University of Mississippi,
Jackson, Miss., USA

Key Words. Absence attacks · Epilepsy · Pain · Seizures · Thalamic stimulation

Abstract. Thalamic electrical stimulation in 3 patients alleviated chronic pain, absence attacks and spontaneously occurring delta and theta EEG discharges. It is suggested that diencephalic discharges may activate and/or lower the threshold for pain at the level of the diencephalon.

Introduction

Three adult patients with major complaints of chronic intractable pain also had absence attacks. They had spontaneously occurring bilateral delta and theta discharges. Daily thalamic electrical stimulation suppressed both the pain and the absence attacks. These findings support the thesis that diencephalic electrical discharges may activate pain [1–3].

Results

Patient 1 is a 20-year-old girl with seizures since 3 years of age. The attacks consisted of loss of consciousness for 30 min or longer, followed by a return to normal. There were transient attacks of looking into space, and she 'would not pay any attention' to her mother. At puberty she developed recurring brief periods of pain radiating in the

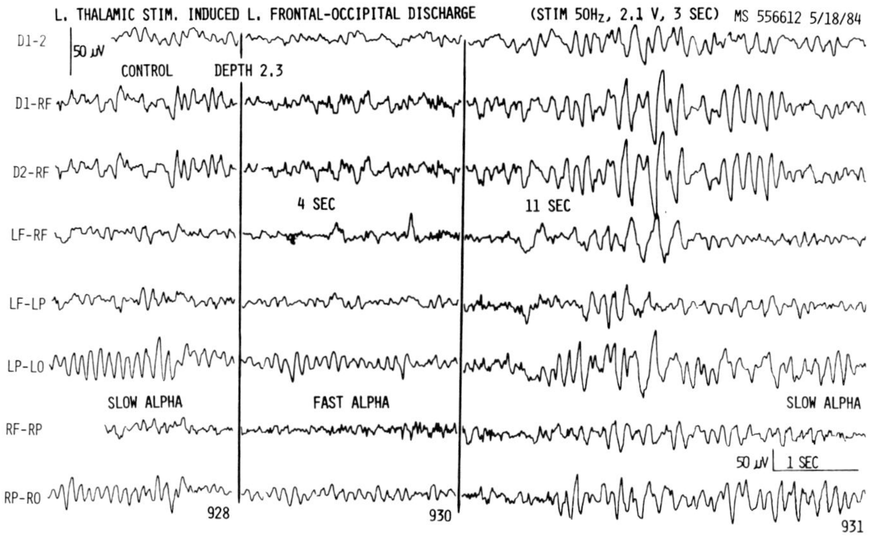

Fig. 1. Thalamic stimulation-induced discharge. Note mixture of sharp wave and theta discharges in thalamus and ipsilateral frontal and occipital areas 11 s after stimulation. D 1–2 = bipolar thalamic recording.

arms, head, chest, abdomen, legs, vagina and feet, which began on the left and later spread to the right.

EEG revealed delta and theta discharges predominantly in the frontal and parietal areas. Touching the face, hyperventilation and photic stimulation precipitated the discharges. Thalamic stimulation at Fp 5.5; H 0; L 7.2 of 5s elicited discharges, whereas 10 s stimulation suppressed them. Thalamic electric stimulation at 50 Hz, 200 ms, 1–2 V, 3–4 times/day and Dilantin 100 mg t.i.d. for the past 3 years have markedly reduced the spontaneous discharges and prevented the recurrence of both the pain and the absence attacks.

Patient 2 is a 53-year-old woman who had several lumbar laminectomies for chronic pain which became progressively worse with each procedure. She also had severe migraine headaches since childhood. EEG revealed bilateral paroxysmal delta and theta wave discharges, predominantly frontal, although temporal and parietal areas were also involved. Thalamic stimulation at Fp 6; H –1.5, L 5.5 of short duration

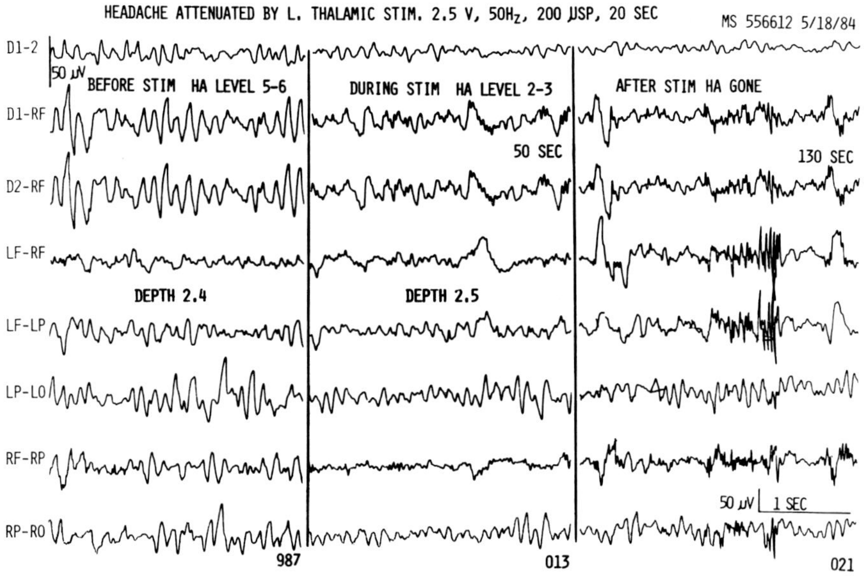

Fig. 2. Thalamic stimulation attenuates pain and coexisting thalamic and scalp discharge activity. HA = headache is evaluated by patient according to a range of no pain to the most severe, being 0–10.

activated the discharges (fig. 1). Long-duration thalamic stimulation suppressed the discharges and the pain (fig. 2). Electrical stimulation for 10–20 min once or twice per day prevents recurrence of pain and the absence attacks.

Patient 3 is a 36-year-old woman diagnosed as having migraine headaches since childhood. The headaches have become more intense and persistent. She also had attacks of falling out, especially at night when she was tired, and periods of memory lapses. Since childhood she had chronic ear infections with recurrent episodes of drainage. EEG revealed bilateral paroxysmal high and low voltage bursts of theta and delta activity. Thalamic recordings revealed irregular low voltage delta and theta patterns with occasional sharp waves. Thalamic electrode implant at Fp 4.5; H 0; L 7.5 with unipolar stimulation of 100 Hz, 200 ms, 2 V, 3 times/day for 10–20 min suppressed the discharges and has abolished the absence attacks and the severe headaches for the past 9 months.

Discussion

Whether the genesis of pain associated with seizures is cortical and/or subcortical remains unknown [3]. If subcortical, is it limbic and/or diencephalic [2]? The present observations further support the hypothesis that diencephalic generated discharges can both activate pain and/or decrease the threshold for pain [1]. Note that these patients had a concomitant reduction of the absence attacks, pain and electrographic discharges in response to thalamic stimulation.

References

1 Andy, O.J.: Thalamic stimulation for chronic pain. Appl. Neurophysiol. *46:* 116–123 (1983).
2 Gates, P.; Nayernouri, T.: Epileptic pain: a temporal lobe focus. J. Neurol. Neurosurg. Psychiat. *47:* 319–320 (1984).
3 Young, G.B.; Blume, W.F.: Painful epileptic seizures. Brain *106:* 537–554 (1983).

Dr. O.J. Andy, Department of Neurosurgery, Medical Center,
University of Mississippi, 2500 N. State St., Jackson, MS 39216 (USA)

Proc. 9th Meeting World Soc. Stereotactic and Functional Neurosurgery, Toronto 1985
Appl. Neurophysiol. *48:* 427–430 (1985)

CT-Guided Stereotactic Aspiration of Intracerebral Hematoma – Result of a Hematoma-Lysis Method Using Urokinase

Hiroshi Niizuma, Taisuke Otsuki, Hidefumi Johkura, Nobukazu Nakazato, Jiro Suzuki

Division of Neurosurgery, Institute of Brain Diseases, Tohoku University School of Medicine, Sendai, Japan

Key Words. Intracerebral hematoma · Computed tomography · Stereotactic aspiration · Urokinase · CT stereotaxis · Stereotactic surgery

Abstract. CT-guided stereotactic aspiration was performed in the CT room on 97 patients with hypertensive intracerebral hematomas, using a standard ventricular cannula. Residual hematomas were liquefied by urokinase and aspirated through the drainage tube. Major and minor rebleeding were seen in 7 cases. Two out of the 4 major rebleeding cases were followed by craniotomy, while the other cases were treated conservatively. More than 80% of the hematomas were aspirated in 68 cases, 50–70% in 19 cases and 30–40% in 6 cases. Operation in the CT room and hematoma lysis with urokinase is very useful for the aspiration of intracerebral hematomas.

Introduction

There are two methods for aspirating intracerebral hematomas stereotactically: one method uses a special aspiration instrument with a rotating helical mandrel inside a cannula [1, 4, 5], while the other employs a standard needle and urokinase for lysis of the hematoma [3, 7]. We adopted the latter method in treating 97 cases of hypertensive intracerebral hematomas using the CT-guided stereotactic system. This paper reports upon the effectiveness of this CT-guided stereotactic operation in the CT room and hematoma lysis with urokinase in cases of intracerebral hematoma.

Table I. Sites of the hematoma and preoperative consciousness levels

Site of hematoma	Preoperative consciousness level					Total
	alert	confused	somnolent	stuporous	semicomat.	
Putamen	14	26	6	9	5	60
Thalamus	2	8	5	6	2	23
Subcortex	2	4				6
Cerebellum	1	3		2	1	7
Pons					1	1
Total	19	41	11	17	9	97

Clinical Materials and Method

The patients ranged in age from 28 to 76 years. The sites of the hematoma and preoperative consciousness levels are shown in table I. The estimated hematoma volume was 6–20 ml in 36 cases, 21–40 ml in 33 cases and 41–100 ml in 28 cases. Among the operated cases with estimated volumes of less than 20 ml, there were 18 thalamic and 15 putaminal hemorrhage cases, all of whom were incapable of raising and lowering the limbs of the affected side, and 3 cases of posterior fossa hematoma. Thirty-three cases were operated upon within 24 h of onset, 22 between 25 and 48 h, 28 between 3 and 7 days, 11 between 8 and 14 days and 3 after 15 days.

Operations were performed under local anesthesia in the CT room. The three-dimensional coordinates of the target point (center of the hematoma) were directly measured from the CT using Leksell's CT-guided stereotactic system [6]. The long axis of the hematoma was considered in making the burr hole but naturally a burr hole on the motor cortex was avoided. In 8 cases of posterior fossa hematoma, the head was tilted 30–40° towards the healthy side and a burr hole was made in the retromastoid area. Aspiration of the hematoma was done manually using a syringe and a lengthened Dandy ventricular cannula (3 mm in diameter). After initial aspiration, a silastic drainage tube was inserted into the hematoma cavity and 6,000 units of urokinase dissolved in 2–3 ml of saline solution was injected. Twenty-four hours later, the dissolved hematoma was aspirated through the drainage tube. If required, injection of urokinase can be repeated several times until the bulk of the hematoma has been removed. CT-guided stereotactic ventricular drainage was also done in 8 cases with ventricular enlargement or hematoma.

Results

By initial aspiration, it was possible to remove more than 50% of the estimated hematoma in 56 cases (58%), between 30 and 49% in 29 cases (30%) and less than 29% in 12 cases. In the first 10 cases, there were 5 cases in which aspiration of less than 29% was possible. In the remaining 87 cases, those in which less than 29% was removed numbered only 7. Five out of these 7 cases were operated upon 28 h to 14 days after the onset, and the blood clot was very hard to aspirate. However, at least 2 or 3 ml of the hematoma could be removed and urokinase was administered. Aspiration of the hematoma was relatively easy in the cases in which the operation was performed within 24 h of onset.

Rebleeding occurred in 7 cases (7%). Reaccumulated hematomas were larger than preoperative hematomas in 4 cases (major bleeding), and smaller in 3 cases (minor bleeding). Two of the cases underwent conventional craniotomy, while the others received continued aspiration or were treated conservatively. Rebleeding just after the operation was seen in only 1 case. In the other 6 cases, rebleeding occurred while urokinase was being used postoperatively. Rebleeding seems to have been due to excessive aspiration and changes in the position of the drainage tube while urokinase was being used postoperatively.

More than 80% of the hematoma was removed in 68 cases (70%) by the hematoma lysis method with urokinase. Between 50 and 70% was removed in 19 cases (20%) and between 30 and 40% was removed in 6 cases (6%).

In comparison with conservative treatment or conventional craniotomy, the postoperative recovery following stereotactic aspiration is rapid in many cases and more than two-thirds of our patients showed improvement in symptoms on the day following surgery. The drainage tube was left in place for 1–6 days, but no cases of meningitis were experienced. There were 3 deaths (3%). Deaths were caused by rebleeding, pneumonia and cerebral infarction of the contralateral side.

Among the 58 patients who have been followed for more than 6 months postoperatively, 41 have returned to normal social lives or are in good condition and capable of unassisted domestic life. Thirteen patients are partially disabled and living at home, and 4 are totally disabled or bedridden.

Discussion

Various instruments with rotating helical mandrels for aspiration of hematomas have been reported [1, 4, 5]. However, the rate of rebleeding has been relatively high (13–16%) [2, 5]. When the CT-guided stereotactic system is used, however, special aspiration instruments seem not to be necessary. Since the operation is carried out entirely in the CT room, it is possible to check the position of the cannula by CT and aspirate the hematoma with confidence. More than 30% of the hematoma could be aspirated initially in 88% of our cases. If a hematoma can be approached along its long axis, some 50–80% of the hematoma can be aspirated during surgery using a lengthened ventricular cannula, even in cases in the acute stage. By injection of urokinase to dissolve the residual hematoma, the majority of hematomas can be finally removed in most cases.

The hematoma lysis method was introduced by *Doi* et al. [3]. We confirmed its effectiveness. However, its hematoma-dissolving effect also seems to have a little relation to rebleeding. We delayed the administration of urokinase 3–12 h in cases in which surgery was performed within 24 h of onset. Excessive aspiration or frequent changes in the position of the drainage tube should be avoided while using urokinase. Administration of urokinase should be minimized and subtotal evacuation (80–90% of the hematoma) is safe and sufficient.

References

1 Backlund, E.O.; Holst, H.: Controlled subtotal evacuation of intracerebral hematomas by stereotaxic technique. Surg. Neurol. *9:* 99–101 (1978).

2 Broseta, J.; Gonzalez-Darder, J.; Barcia-Salorio, J.L.: Stereotactic evacuation of intracerebral hematomas. Appl. Neurophysiol. *45:* 443–448 (1982).

3 Doi, E.; Moriwaki, H.; Komai, N.; Iwamoto, M.: Stereotactic evacuation of intracerebral hematomas. Neurol. Med. Chir. *22:* 461–467 (1982).

4 Higgins, A.C.; Nashold, B.S., Jr.: Stereotactic evacuation of large intracerebral hematoma. Appl. Neurophysiol. *43:* 96–103 (1980).

5 Kandel, E.I.; Peresedov, V.V.: Stereotaxic evacuation of spontaneous intracerebral hematomas. J. Neurosurg. *62:* 206–213 (1985).

6 Leksell, L.; Jernberg, B.: Stereotaxis and tomography. A technical note. Acta neurochir. *52:* 1–7 (1980).

7 Matsumoto, K.; Hondo, H.: CT-guided stereotaxic evacuation of hypertensive intracerebral hematomas. J. Neurosurg. *61:* 440–448 (1984).

H. Niizuma, MD, Division of Neurosurgery, Institute of Brain Diseases,
Tohoku University School of Medicine, Seiryo-cho 1-1, Sendai 980 (Japan)

Proc. 9th Meeting World Soc. Stereotactic and Functional
Neurosurgery, Toronto 1985
Appl. Neurophysiol. *48:* 431–439 (1985)

CT-Guided Stereotactic Surgery for Evacuation of Hypertensive Intracerebral Hematoma

T. Tanikawa, K. Amano, H. Kawamura, H. Kawabatake, M. Notani, H. Iseki, T. Shiwaku, T. Nagao, Y. Iwata, T. Taira, Y. Umezawa, T. Shimizu, K. Kitamura

Department of Neurosurgery, Neurological Institute, Tokyo Women's Medical College, Tokyo, Japan

Key Words. Hypertensive intracerebral hematoma · CT stereotaxis · Archimedes' screw · Stereotactic surgery

Abstract. During the last 3 years, 46 cases of hypertensive intracerebral hemorrhage were treated by CT-guided stereotactic surgery. Our present report is concerned with the evaluation of this procedure in the treatment of hypertensive intracerebral hematoma, in terms of the rate of aspirated hematoma and follow-up study of patients. It is difficult to draw any definite conclusion about the operative indications. CT-guided stereotactic aspiration, however, can be evaluated as a less invasive and more definitive treatment of intracerebral hematoma in the basal ganglia and thalamus.

Introduction

In recent years, many papers have been published on CT-guided stereotactic brain surgery. During the last 3 years, 46 cases of hypertensive intracerebral hematoma were treated by this technique. Our present report is concerned with the evaluation of this procedure in a treatment of hypertensive intracerebral hematoma, in terms of the rate of aspirated hematoma and follow-up study of patients.

Materials and Methods

The subjects in this study were 46 patients, with 28 putaminal hemorrhage and 18 thalamic hemorrhage (fig. 1). They ranged in age from 45 to 79 years, averaging 56 years. Most of the intracerebral hematomas considered for this procedure were medium in size.

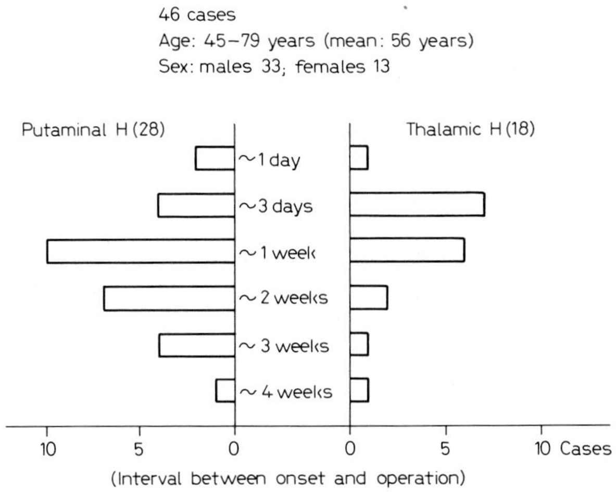

Fig. 1. Cases of hypertensive intracerebral hematoma.

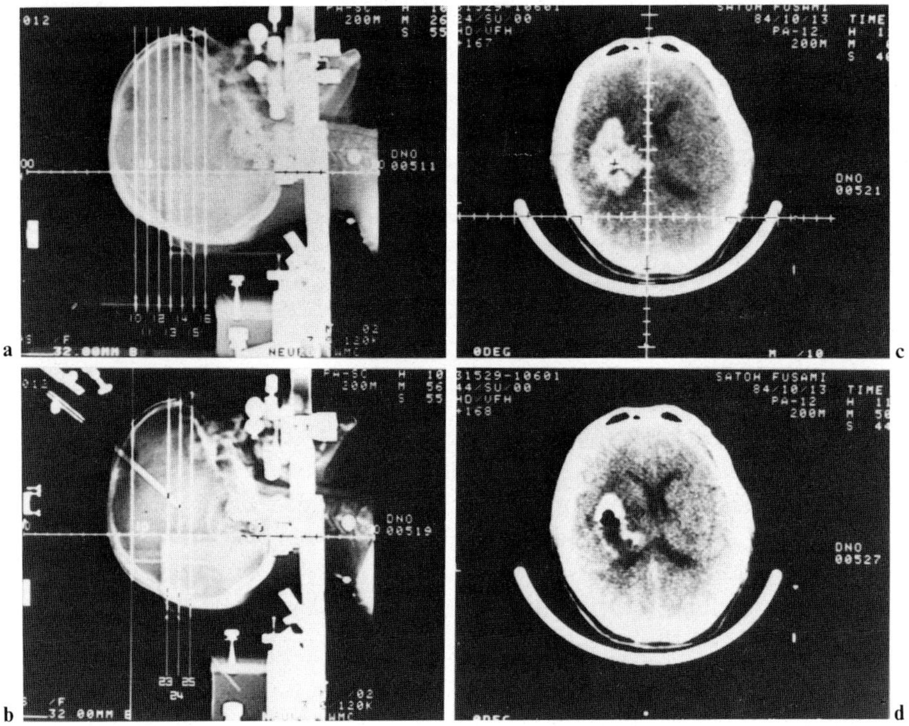

Fig. 2. Lateral scanogram and CT during operation: **a** scanogram for the measurement of Z axis; **b** scanogram confirming the position of the tube; **c** CT at the target point; **d** CT after aspiration.

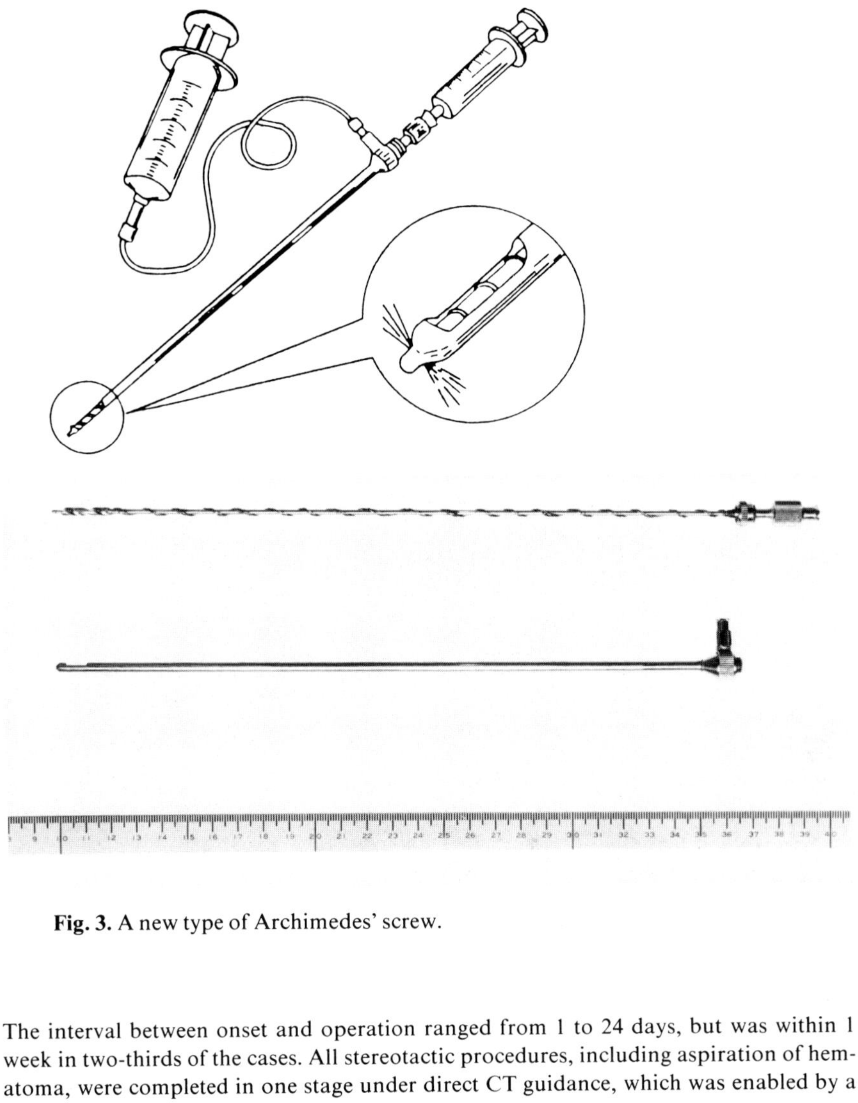

Fig. 3. A new type of Archimedes' screw.

The interval between onset and operation ranged from 1 to 24 days, but was within 1 week in two-thirds of the cases. All stereotactic procedures, including aspiration of hematoma, were completed in one stage under direct CT guidance, which was enabled by a new apparatus developed by *Iseki* [4].

With the head correctly positioned in the apparatus, the X, Y and Z axis coordinates were measured by lateral scanogram and CT images (fig. 2). In most cases, the center of hematoma was chosen as the target point. Aspiration of the hematoma was carried out gradually with a suction tube of 4 mm diameter with a rotating Archimedes' screw mandrel (fig. 3) first introduced by *Backlund and von Holst* [1].

The outcome of the cases in terms of the change of consciousness and the recovery of motor and sensory function was investigated in the follow-up periods ranging from 1

Table I. Classification of hypertensive intracerebral hematoma according to CT findings

Class	Criteria
Putaminal hemorrhage	
I	localized in the outside of internal capsule
II	extended to the anterior limb of internal capsule
IIIa	extended to the posterior limb of internal capsule
IIIb	IIIa with V
IVa	extended to the anterior and posterior limb of internal capsule
IVb	IVa with V
V	extended to the thalamus or subthalamus
Thalamic hemorrhage	
Ia	localized in the thalamus without V
Ib	localized in the thalamus with V
IIa	extended to the internal capsule without V
IIb	extended to the internal capsule with V
IIIa	extended to the hypothalamus or midbrain without V
IIIb	extended to the hypothalamus or midbrain with V

V = massive ventricular hemorrhage.

year to 3 years and 4 months. In these studies, overall motor function of extremities was assessed by voluntary movement or walking and graded, from a score of 0 for no movement to a score of 5 for normal movement in the upper extremity, and from a score of 0 for inability to walk to a score of 4 for normal walking. Fine movements were assessed by the ability of taking a meal with a spoon or chopsticks, tying a string and buttoning. Sensory functions were assessed by the impairment of touch and temperature sensation, as well as the appearance of dysesthesia and paresthesia. These results were evaluated separately in each type of hematoma, being classified according to the criteria proposed by the Japanese Association for the Study of Surgical Treatment of Stroke in 1978 (table I).

Results

The volume of hematoma in 30 cases measured on CT ranged from 6 to 37 ml, the average being 23.1 ml. Aspirated hematoma volume in these cases ranged from 5 to 34 ml, the average being 19.6 ml. The percentage of aspirated volume ranged from 54 to 100%, the average being 81%.

Table II. Neurological grading (NG) and CT classification **(A)** and criteria of NG **(B)**

A

NG grade	CT classification														
	putaminal type								thalamic type						
	I	II	IIIa	IIIb	IVa	IVb	V	total	Ia	Ib	IIa	IIb	IIIa	IIIb	total
1	10	1	6		2			19			1	2	1	2	6
2			3				1	4			2	2		2	6
3	2	1	1		1			5				2		1	3
4a													1	1	2
4b														1	1
5															
Total	12	2	10		3		1	28			3	6	2	7	18

B

Grade	Criteria	Grade	Criteria
1	alertness or confusion	4a	semicoma without herniation signs
2	somnolence	4b	semicoma with herniation signs
3	stupor	5	deep coma

As for the neurological functions, preoperative consciousness was not dramatically changed in most of the cases (table II). In patients with putaminal hemorrhage, 19 were alert or confused, 4 somnolent, 5 stuporous, while in thalamic hemorrhage, 6 were alert or confused, 6 somnolent, 3 stuporous and the remaining 3 were semicomatose. During the follow-up periods, all but 2 remained in an appallic state, 1 (graded I) had recurrent bleeding immediately after the procedure, and the other (grade II) had been appallic preoperatively. In the 18 thalamic hemorrhage cases, 3 died, 2 (grades II and IVb) from gastrointestinal bleeding or DIC, and 1 (grade III) from rehemorrhage 2 months after the operation. Another semicomatose patient (grade IVa) remained appallic. The remaining 14 cases recovered to an alert or confused state within a short term.

Preoperative motor and sensory functions were moderately or severely disturbed in all cases. In putaminal hemorrhage, most of the pa-

Table III. CT classification **(A)** and outcome of neurological function **(B)** in putaminal hemorrhage

A

CT class	Motor function of upper extremity												Motor function of lower extremity									
	preoperation						follow-up						preoperation					follow-up				
	5[1]	4	3	2	1	0	5	4	3	2	1	0	4	3	2	1	0	4	3	2	1	0
I		2	2	3	3	2	4	5	1		1	1		2	2	2	6	5	2	2	2	1
II					1	1		1	1								2		1	1		
IIIa		1			6	3	1	2	1	1	3	2				2	8	1	1	1	3	4
IIIb																						
IVa				1		2		1				2			1		2		1			2
IVb																						
V						1						1					1					1

B

CT class	Fine movement			Sensory function			
	good[1]	fair	poor	good	fair	poor	D/P
I	4	5		8	2		2
II	1		1	2			
IIIa	2	1	3	1	4	2	2
IIIb							
IVa		1					
IVb							
V							

[1] Evaluation (D/P = dysesthesia or paresthesia).

tients in class I or II with an intact posterior limb of internal capsule showed fairly good recovery of motor function of both extremities (table III). On the other hand, two-thirds of the patients with severe motor weakness remained hemiplegic. The outcomes of fine movement were evaluated as 'good' or 'fair' in 14 cases out of 18 investigated. The recovery of sensory function was excellent in most cases, although it remained poor in 2 cases of class IIIa where the posterior limb of internal capsule was severely damaged.

Table IV. CT classification **(A)** and outcome of neurological function **(B)** in thalamic hemorrhage

A

CT class	Motor function of upper extremity												Motor function of lower extremity									
	preoperation						follow-up						preoperation					follow-up				
	5[1]	4	3	2	1	0	5	4	3	2	1	0	4	3	2	1	0	4	3	2	1	0
Ia																						
Ib																						
IIa		1		1		1	1	2								1	2			3		
IIb		2		1		2	3		1	1					2		3	2	1		2	
IIIa				1		1		1			1					1	1			1		1
IIIb					2	3	1	2		1	1						5		1	1	2	1

B

CT class	Fine movement			Sensory function			
	good[1]	fair	poor	good	fair	poor	D/P
Ia							
Ib							
IIa	1	2		2	1		2
IIb	3	1	1	2	3		3
IIIa		1			2		
IIIb	2	1			2	1	2

[1] Evaluation (D/P = dysesthesia or paresthesia).

In thalamic hemorrhage, regardless of preoperative poor motor function, two-thirds of cases showed excellent recovery as high as score 4 of 5 in the upper extremity and being able to walk without a cane and support (better than score 1) (table IV). The outcome of fine movement was also excellent as well as overall motor function. The recovery of sensory function, however, was insufficient in many cases, and over 50% of patients have been suffering not only from sensory loss but also from development of dysesthesia and paresthesia.

Discussion

Attempts to aspirate intracerebral hematoma stereotactically have been made for a long time. Successful aspiration of hematoma in the acute stage, however, was first described by *Backlund and von Holst* [1] in 1978, who designed the Archimdes' screw for this procedure. Since, CT-guided stereotactic surgery has been established and is being applied to intracerebral hematoma as well as brain tumor.

As far as hypertensive intracerebral hematomas are concerned, this procedure has been almost exclusively applied to the large hematoma in the acute stage. On the contrary, most intracerebral hematomas considered for this procedure in the present report were medium in size with considerable local mass effect on CT. The operation was carried out for the purpose of improved recovery in neurological function in patients with moderate or severe neurological deficits.

The Archimedes' screw has been indicated as an effective instrument in aspirating hematomas composed of primarily solid clot. For more gentle evacuation, authors have developed a new type of Archimedes' screw, with which both aspiration and irrigation of the hematoma at the same time are possible (fig. 3). The high percentage of hematoma aspirated in the present study confirmed the safety and effectiveness of this new Archimedes' screw.

No complications immediately related to the operation were observed, except in 1 case operated 10 days after onset where recurrent bleeding in the same site occurred immediately after this procedure.

Improvement of consciousness was obtained within a short postoperative period in most cases. Perifocal edema in these cases diminished much earlier than in those patients treated conservatively. In addition, some cases operated in the chronic stage showed alteration of consciousness, in terms of increased spontaneous activity and diminished hypersomnia. Based on these results, it can be said for certain that CT-guided stereotactic aspiration affords faster recuperation, which allows motor exercise to begin sooner.

The outcome of motor and sensory function in cases of putaminal hemorrhage indicates the usefulness of this operation, particularly in patients with partial or no involvement of the internal capsule. In thalamic hemorrhage, it is noteworthy that all of the cases had extension of the hematomas into the internal capsule. In this respect, we can say that CT-guided stereotactic aspiration of hematoma can increase the likelihood of recovery of motor function, even in patients with involvement of the internal capsule after thalamic hemorrhage.

Finally it is difficult to draw any definite conclusion about operative indication of this procedure from this limited number of patients. CT-guided stereotactic aspiration, however, can be evaluated as a less invasive and more definitive treatment for intracerebral hematoma in the basal ganglia and thalamus.

References

1 Backlund, E.O.; Holst, H. von: Controlled subtotal evacuation of intracerebral hematomas by stereotactic technique. Surg. Neurol. *9:* 99–101 (1978).
2 Broseta, J.; Gonzales-Darder, J.; Barcia-Salorio, J.L.: Stereotactic evaluation of intracerebral hematomas. Appl. Neurophysiol. *45:* 443–448 (1982).
3 Higgins, A.C.; Nashold, B.S., Jr.: Stereotactic evacuation of large intracerebral hematoma. Appl. Neurophysiol. *43:* 96–103 (1980).
4 Iseki, H.: CT-guided stereotactic brain surgery: an application to evacuation of intracerebral hematoma. Neurol. Surg. *12:* 663–671 (1984).
5 Kandel, E.; Peresedov, V.V.: Stereotaxic evacuation of spontaneous intracerebral hematomas. J. Neurosurg. *62:* 206–213 (1985).

Dr. T. Tanikawa, Department of Neurosurgery, Neurological Institute, Tokyo Women's Medical College, 10-Kawachacho, Tokyo (Japan)

Proc. 9th Meeting World Soc. Stereotactic and Functional
Neurosurgery, Toronto 1985
Appl. Neurophysiol. *48:* 440–443 (1985)

Cryptic Vascular Malformations Diagnosed by Stereotactic Biopsies – A Preliminary Study

C. Daumas-Duport[a], *M. Mann*[a], *C. Munari*[b], *S. Blond*[b], *A. Musolino*[b], *V. Monsaingeon*[a], *J.P. Chodkiewicz*[b]

Departments of [a] Neuropathology and [b] Neurosurgery, Centre Hospitalier Sainte-Anne, Paris, France

Key Words. Vascular malformations · Stereotactic surgery · CT stereotaxis

Abstract. A series of 14 cryptic vascular malformations (CVM) deeply situated or localized in functional cortical areas were diagnosed by serial stereotactic biopsies. No history was suggestive of hemorrhage, despite a substantial hematoma being evacuated during biopsy procedures in 4 patients. Retrospectively, CVM without hematoma were found to have certain characteristics that should raise the suspicion as to the correct diagnosis. At the time of discharge from the hospital, only 1 patient had mild aggravation of a preexisting motor deficit, which further improved. Serial stereotactic biopsies provided the required histological diagnosis with relatively low risk.

Introduction

Cryptic vascular malformations (CVM) are small angiographically occult vascular malformations. Diagnosis of these lesions requires histologic examination. In the past, CVM were considered rare clinically and usually discovered in autopsy material.

With the availability of CT scanning, which demonstrates these lesions, patients with CVM are more frequently explored surgically [1, 8]. Since they are frequently misinterpreted to be low grade gliomas [2, 4, 5, 11], we are reporting 14 cases of CVM diagnosed by serial stereotactic biopsies in patients with deeply situated or important functional area lesions, who are part of a series of patients who underwent serial stereotactic biopsies in Sainte-Anne Hospital in Paris.

In this series, CVM accounted for 255 of the nontumoral lesions. The Talairach and Szikla stereotactic methodology was used, and includes systematic intraoperative stereotactic stereoscopic lateral and anteroposterior teleangiographies [9, 10].

Case Reports

CVM were localized in functional cortical areas in 5 patients, diencephalon and basal ganglia in 7, mesencephalon and metencephalon in 2. One patient had a double location. Only one lesion was situated in a nonfunctional cortical area in a patient evaluated for epilepsy surgery. Presenting symptoms were: neurologic deficit in 8 patients, progressive in 6 of them, seizures in 5 patients, headache in 1. No patient had arterial hypertension. None presented with a typical hemorrhage, but substantial hematomas were evacuated in 4 patients at the time of the biopsy procedures.

Ages ranged from 15 to 62 years; 8 patients were male, 6 female. The duration of symptoms ranged from 1 month to 11 years. The preoperative CT scan was misinterpreted as glioma in all cases.

Results

As other authors, we found retrospectively that CVM without hematoma shows certain characteristics on CT scanning which should raise the suspicion as to the correct diagnosis: in 8 of our cases noncontrast CT revealed a hyperdense lesion, with no or mild mass effect and no surrounding edema. After contrast infusion, 7 of the 8 cases showed a moderate or mild contrast enhancement that may be demonstrated only after measuring the absorption coefficient [3, 7, 8]. The volume of the lesion was not increased after contrast infusion.

Following biopsy procedures, 5 patients had a mild and transitory aggravation of a preexisting motor deficit. One patient with a pontine telangiectasia experienced a transient extrapyramidal syndrome. However, at the time of discharge from the hospital, mild aggravation of a preexisting motor deficit persisted in only 1 patient which further improved. Follow-up ranged from 1 to 62 months, with an average of 19 months. Six patients are unchanged, 8 are improved. No evidence of significant bleeding or rebleeding has been observed in any patient at follow-up.

Serial stereotactic biopsies of CVM have a relatively low risk and provide the correct diagnosis in lesions thought to be gliomas on CT scanning. However, CVM have characteristic features on CT that may raise suspicion for the diagnosis. An appearance identical in 5 patients which correlated with the presence of a substantial hematoma was hyperdensity before contrast infusion, ring contrast enhancement, and mass effect with or without edema. In only 1 case was the lesion hypodense, circumscribed, and nonenhancing. Angiographies disclosed no evidence of a vascular malformation in any of our patients. In 5 cases, angiography showed nonspecific abnormalities related to mass effect. In 1 patient only discrete abnormalities occurred during the venous phase. Lastly, in 1 case, abnormalities were related to angiographic spasm.

CVM in this series have been classified according to the commonly accepted classification of *Russel and Rubinstein* [6]. Cavernous angioma was found in 5 patients, capillary telangiectasia in 2, venous angioma in 3. Arteriovenous malformation, as proven by the presence of elastic fibers, was only found in 1 patient. A calcified vascular malformation likely to be part of an AVM was found in 2 patients. One case failed to enter any classification. This vascular hamartoma was composed of a network of capillaries. This atypical case corresponded to the only hypodense lesion on CT. Surgical removal of the CVM was not performed in any case. Hematomas were evacuated in 4 patients: 2 underwent ventriculocysternostomy for obstructive hydrocephalus and radiotherapy was administered in the other 2 patients.

References

1 Becker, D.H.; Townsend, J.J.; Kramed, R.A.: Occult cerebrovascular malformations: a series of 18 histologically verified cases with negative angiography. Brain *102:* 249–287 (1979).

2 Bell, B.A.; Kendall, B.E.; Symon, L.: Angiographically occult arteriovenous malformations of the brain. J. Neurol. Neurosurg. Psychiat. *41:* 1057–1064 (1978).

3 Cohen, H.C.M.; Tucker, W.S.; Humphreys, R.P.: Angiographically cryptic histologically verified cerebrovascular malformations. Neurosurgery *10:* 704–714 (1982).

4 Golden, J.B.; Dramer, R.A.: The angiographically occult cerebrovascular malformation: report of three cases. J. Neurosurg. *48:* 292–296 (1978).

5 Leblanc, R.; Ethier, R.: The computerized tomographic appearance of angiographically occult arteriovenous malformations of the brain. Can. J. neurol. Sci. *8:* 7–13 (1981).

6 Russel, D.S.; Rubinstein, L.J.: Pathology of tumors of the nervous system; 4th ed. (Arnold, London 1977).

7 Shuey, H.M.; Day, A.L.; Quising, R.G.: Angiographically cryptic cerebrovascular malformations. Neurosurgery *5:* 476–479 (1979).

8 Steiger, H.J.; Tew, J.M.: Hemorrhage and epilepsy in cryptic cerebrovascular malformations. Archs Neurol. *41:* 722–724 (1984).
9 Szikla, G.; Blond, S.: Bilan stéréotaxique des tumeurs cérébrales. Encycl. Méd.-Chir. 31660 E (1981).
10 Szikla, G.; Blond, S.; Daumas-Duport, C.; Missir, O.; Miyahara, S.; Munari, C.; Musolino, A.; Schlienger, N.: Stereotaxis in the management of brain tumors. Three-dimensional angiography, sampling biopsies and focal irradiation using the Talairach stereotactic system. Ital. J. neurol. Sci. *2:* suppl., pp. 83–96 (1983).
11 Wharen, R.E.; Scheithauer, B.W.; Laus, E.R.: Thrombosed arteriovenous malformations of the brain: an important entity in the differential diagnosis of intractable focal seizure disorders. J. Neurosurg. *57:* 520–526 (1982).

C. Daumas-Duport, MD, Department of Neuropathology,
Centre Hospitalier Sainte-Anne, 1, rue Cabanis, F-75674 Paris Cedex 14 (France)

Proc. 9th Meeting World Soc. Stereotactic and Functional
Neurosurgery, Toronto 1985
Appl. Neurophysiol. *48:* 444–447 (1985)

Physiological Monitoring of Stereotactic Biopsy

R.R. Tasker

Toronto General Hospital, Toronto, Ont., Canada

Key Words. CT stereotactic biopsy · Impedance

Abstract. It is helpful to have direct confirmation during a CT-guided stereotactic procedure that the intended target has been reached without operating under imaging. This can be simply accomplished with readily available equipment by serial monitoring of electrical impedance as a probe is directed to the target because the impedance of hematomas, cysts, and most neoplasms is conspicuously below that of normal brain.

The stereotactic technique, particularly guided by modern imaging, is increasingly useful for definitive treatment of lesions such as colloid cysts, biopsy or aspiration of lesions in deep or inaccessible locations or in patients unsuited for more major procedures, for multiple and/or differential biopsy, and for interstitial therapy. It is helpful to have confirmation that the stereotactically guided probe has reached target during such procedures, confirmation that can be provided by working under imaging, using a 'phantom', employing a computer graphics display or with an ultrasound probe. Such confirmation can also be provided more cheaply and simply by following electrical impedance along the probe tract.

It has been established that [3,4] electrical resistance between a roving electrode in brain and a remote fixed point on the body can be manipulated so that the impedance recorded reflects mainly neural features, a fact exploited by us [1, 2] to produce an 'impedance profile' of the brain traversed by a stereotactically directed probe. Whereas such a profile proved insufficient to identify individual brain structures, the impedance of gray matter averaging $1{,}180 \pm 160\,\Omega$, of white,

1,440 ± 155 Ω, the impedance of cerebrospinal fluid averaged a sharply disparate 650 ± 120 Ω which low level was approached in most types of pathological brain lesions. For example, the impedance of 7 malignant gliomas and 1 metastasis averaged 0.5 times that of normal brain. Tissue, including capsule, which was physically tough, however, exhibited higher levels of impedance, that of 1 metastasis and 3 meningiomas measuring 1.0, 1.3, 1.3 and 1.6 times that of normal brain respectively (fig. 1). However, most neoplasms, cysts, infarcts, hematomas and infectious lesions are strikingly revealed by impedance monitoring.

Technique

Impedance monitoring during stereotactic operations can be simply and cheaply accomplished by manually advancing a stereotactic macrostimulating (1.1 mm diameter, 0.5 mm bare tip) or lesioning (1.1 mm diameter, 3.0 mm bare tip) electrode (Diros Technology Inc., Toronto, Ont., Canada) along the intended trajectory before the introduction of any other instrument, recording electrical impedance monopolar against a surface electrode using the electronics backup for percutaneous cordotomy such as the 'Owl' instrument (Diros Technology Inc.).

Results

Figure 1a and b presents our experience monitoring electrical impedance 18 times during 9 conventional and 18 CT-guided consecutive stereotactic interventions with appropriate models of the Leksell frame. The target was missed in 1 conventional procedure, attained in the remaining 26. One colloid cyst could not be aspirated; biopsy was not diagnostic for one astrocytoma; all other 24 procedures achieved their purpose. One patient with a pinealoblastoma died from postoperative hemorrhage and infection delayed recovery in the 2 patients with arachnoid cysts of the quadrigeminal plate after stereotactic shunting for the cyst-induced hydrocephalus and brainstem compression. The cardiac status of 1 patient with cyanotic heart disease and pyogenic abscess worsened temporarily following general anesthesia used in the procedure. There were no neurological sequelae.

Equipment failure occurred once. Conspicuous drops in impedance occurred as the probe entered 13 of the 17 targets, in 5 out of 6 astrocytomas of varying degrees of malignancy, 1 lymphoma, 1 crani-

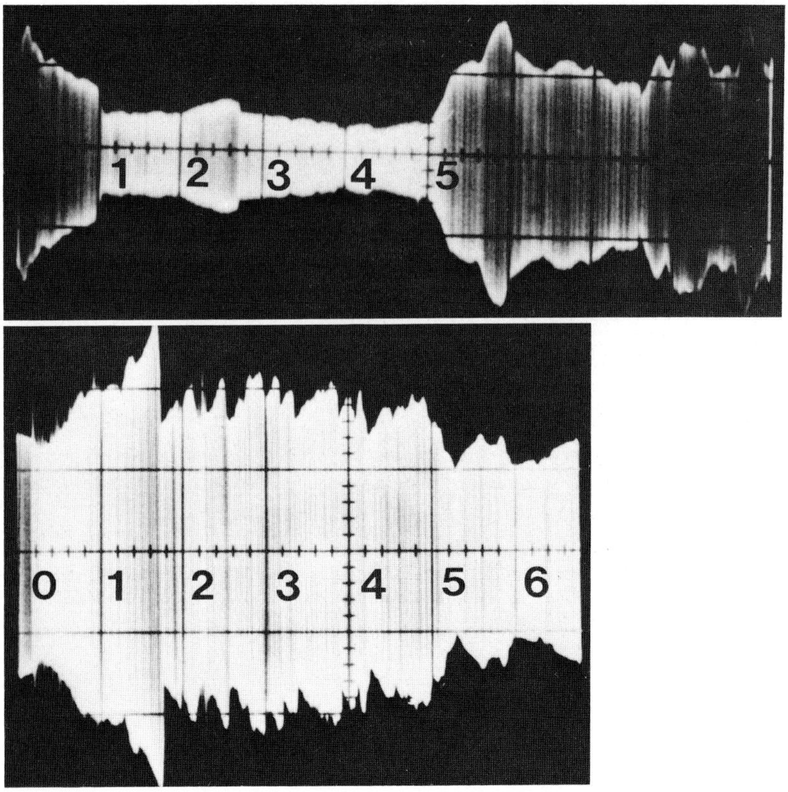

Fig. 1. Impedance profiles of a patient with **(a)** a right frontal glioblastoma multiforme and **(b)** a syncytial meningioma of the outer third of the left sphenoid wing measured at craniotomy by advancing a stereotactic macrostimulating electrode (see text) perpendicularly into the tumor with an electric motor (1). Numbered squares record depth in centimeters from the surface. A striking impedance fall to half that of brain occurred in the glioblastoma between 1.0 and 5.0 cm below the surface indicating precisely the gross extent of the tumor. A less well-defined rise occurred in the physically tough meningioma between 0.4 and 5.3 cm below the surface.

opharyngioma cyst, 1 colloid cyst, 2 arachnoid cysts, 1 granuloma, 1 hematoma, and the ventricle. One astrocytoma also contained a calcified area of high impedance. In 1 malignant astrocytoma, 1 malignant ependymoma, and 2 pyogenic abscesses, less striking elevation of impedance occurred.

Conclusion

Electrical impedance drops in a striking fashion between surrounding brain and a wide variety of but not all brain lesions. Though more data must be collected to fully define the relationship, impedance monitoring using readily available equipment can be simply used to confirm that a stereotactically guided probe has reached its target in a majority of cases.

References

1 Organ, L.W.; Tasker, R.R.; Moody, N.F.: The impedance profile of the human brain as a localization technique in stereoencephalotomy. Confinia neurol. *29:* 192–196 (1967).
2 Organ, L.W.; Tasker, R.R.; Moody, N.F.: Brain tumor localization using an electrical impedance technique. J. Neurosurg. *27:* 35–44 (1968).
3 Robinson, B.W.: Localization of intracerebral electrodes. Expl Neurol. *6:* 201–223 (1962).
4 Robinson, B.W.; Bryan, J.S.; Rosvold, H.E.: Locating brain structures. Extensions to the impedance method. Archs. Neurol., Chicago *13:* 477–486 (1965).

Dr. R.R. Tasker, Room 14–215 EN, Toronto General Hospital,
200 Elizabeth Street, Toronto, Ont. M5G1L7 (Canada)

Proc. 9th Meeting World Soc. Stereotactic and Functional
Neurosurgery, Toronto 1985
Appl. Neurophysiol. *48:* 448–453 (1985)

Correlation between Stereo-EEG, CT-Scan and Stereotactic Biopsy Data in Epileptic Patients with Low-Grade Gliomas

C. Munari[a, d], *A. Musolino*[a], *C. Daumas-Duport*[b], *O. Missir*[c], *P. Brunet*[d], *A.T. Giallonardo*[d], *J.P. Chodkiewicz*[a], *J. Bancaud*[a, d]

Hôpital Sainte-Anne, Service de [a] Neurochirurgie, [b] d'Anatomo-pathologie et [c] Radiologie, Paris, et [d] Inserm U 97, Paris, France

Key Words. Stereo-EEG · Depth electrodes · CT scan · Stereotactic surgery · Partial epilepsy · Cerebral gliomas · Stereotactic biopsies

Abstract. Stereo-EEG activity, which was recorded precisely from the same location as stereotactic biopsies, was studied on 11 patients with low-grade glioma and severe partial epilepsy. The volume of the lesions varied from 6 to 72 cm^3 (mean 23 cm^3). A very depressed activity was recorded in all the 25 specimens of solid tumor and in more than half of infiltrated white matter. The background activity was still conserved in all 'normal' fragments, while it is never found in solid tumor; sometimes it could be found in the infiltrating tumors of white or gray matter. High voltage theta and delta activity was recorded in neither 'normal' nor solid tumors. We emphasize the importance of considering the stage of evolution when we evaluate the significance of the stereo-EEG activity.

Introduction

The current use of CT scanning in patients with severe drug-resistant partial epilepsies enables one to discover a relatively high number of lesions. A correct diagnostic approach should permit one to (a) clarify the type of the lesion, (b) define its limits, and (c) plot the topographic relationships between the lesion and the epileptogenic area(s) [6]. Stereotactic methodology allows two techniques to attain the above mentioned three goals: serial biopsies and stereo-EEG [1, 2, 5].

The aim of this paper is to study if and how a comparative study of the data obtained from both biopsies and stereo-EEG may improve the anatomical-functional definition of the lesions and of the neigh-

Table I. Diagnosis, spatial configuration and volume (cm^3)

		Spatial configuration (4)		
		I	II	III
Oligodendrogliomas	G.A.		9	
	L.J.			24
	C.G.		8	
	B.C.			8
Astrocytomas	B.M.		72	
	P.C.			40
	T.J.		54	
Oligoastrocytoma	T.E.		10	
Pilocytic astrocytoma	D.F.	6		
Cerebellar astrocytoma	J.S.	15		
Dysembryoneuroepithelioma (dysplasia)	M.J.	11		
Total number		3	5	3

boring areas. We selected 11 patients with severe drug-resistant epilepsy, in whom the CT scan demonstrated a hypodensity, who were submitted to a stereo-EEG as well as to a stereotactic biopsy investigation.

Patients and Methods

Clinical Findings

This study concerns 11 patients (10 m, 1 f) aged 12–50 years (mean 29). The epilepsy history started 2–11 years before the admission to the Neurosurgical Department of the S. Anne Hospital. All presented with so-called complex partial seizures with a daily frequency in 9, and weekly in 2. The interictal neurological examination showed a slight motor deficit in 1 patient, speech disturbances in 1, unilateral hyperreflexia in 2, and an initial papilledema in 2. 6 were neurologically normal.

Neuroradiological Data

The CT scan (with and without enhancement) showed a hypodensity in all 11, with partial enhancement in 2. The lesions were in the dominant hemisphere in 8 (4 frontal, 2 temporal, 1 parietal and 1 frontoparietal), and in the nondominant hemisphere in 3 (1 frontal, 1 temporal, 1 central). In all patients, after the clinical, EEG and CT scan examination, we performed a neuroradiological study under the stereotactic protocol, according to the Talairach methodology [8]. The data obtained by the CT scan were always manually reconstructed on stereotactic coordinates. The volume of the lesions varied from 6 to 72 cm^3 (mean 23 cm^3) (table I).

Stereo-EEG Investigations

All patients underwent a 3- to 6-hour stereo-EEG exploration with 4–8 multilead (10–20) intracerebral electrodes to define the extent of the lesion and the epileptogenic areas.

We used 66 electrodes with 448 useable leads. The diameter of the electrodes was 1.8–2.4 mm; the length of the leads was 2 mm and the interlead distance 1.5 mm. Stereo-EEG findings were considered valid only when (1) it was possible to identify the following types of patterns: (a) persisting background activity; (b) high voltage permanent theta-delta activity; (c) very depressed activity ($<10\ \mu V$), and (2) the leads exactly correspond to the biopsy samples (274).

Stereotactic Biopsies

Stereotactic biopsies were performed (a) to define the type of lesion, (b) to determine (when necessary) the volume of the lesions, (c) to obtain specimens of the different areas identified by the CT scan, avoiding of course, as much as possible, hazardous approaches.

Thus, we realized a total of 35 tracks: 27 of them corresponded to the trajectory of an electrode. We obtained a total of 165 samples (length 3–8 mm, diameter 1–1.8 mm). The diagnosis was oligodendroglioma in 4, astrocytoma in 3, and, in the other 4, oligoastrocytoma, pilocytic astrocytoma, cerebellar astrocytoma and dysembryoneuroepithelioma. According to the spatial configuration of *Daumas-Duport* et al. [4], there were 3 of type I, 5 of type II and 3 of type III (table I). For this retrospective study, we considered only (a) the specimen corresponding to 1 or more leads of the deep electrodes, and (b) those of the following types: (1) solid tumor; (2) dense tumoral infiltration; (3) identifiable cerebral cortex infiltrated by tumor cells with more or less edema; (4) white matter infiltrated by tumor cells with more or less edema; (5) cerebral cortex and white matter with edema, but without tumor infiltration; (6) 'normal' tissue – meaning a specimen characterized by the absence on any histopathological abnormality, even though close to the lesion and to the epileptogenic areas.

Results

Stereo-EEG Findings and Histopathological Data

(1) Very depressed activity (10 μV) was recorded in 87 specimens, 25 corresponding to a solid tumor. In 55, this activity was observed in the white matter, either infiltrated by tumor cells (44) or only with

edema (11). In 7 specimens we found an infiltrated cerebral cortex with various degrees of edema.

(2) Permanent high voltage theta-delta activity (with or without spikes) was recorded in 75 specimens. It never corresponded to normal tissue or to solid tumor, but may be found in dense tumor infiltration (15), in the white matter, infiltrated (33) or edematose (9), as well as in cerebral cortex, infiltrated (11), or edematous (3) or in peritumoral tissue with gliosis (4).

(3) In 51 specimens, the background activity was well conserved, 13 were considered 'normal'. 24 corresponded to an infiltrated white matter. The other specimens corresponded to the other histopathological groups, except solid tumor.

Histopathological Data and Stereo-EEG Findings

(1) In all the 25 specimens of a solid tumor we recorded only very depressed activity (10 μV).

(2) In the 21 specimens with dense tumor infiltration the electrical activity was characterized 15 times by permanent slow theta-delta activity (with or without spikes). Background activity persisted in 3. In the 28 specimens of infiltrated cortex, the activity was very depressed in 7 and characterized by permanent slow waves in 11. A well-conserved background activity persisted in only 2. In about one-half (44) of the infiltrated white matter specimens (89), we recorded very depressed activity. In 17 there were permanent slow waves. The edema of the cerebral cortex (10 specimens) often corresponds to well conserved background activity with interictal spikes [7]. In the 17 specimens of 'normal' tissue, the background activity was always well conserved, with or without interictal spikes.

CT Scan Data and Histopathological Findings

In all patients, 3 or more specimens were obtained in hypodense areas: all these specimens were more or less infiltrated by tumor cells. In two-thirds of them more or less significant edema also exists.

CT Scan Data and Stereo-EEG Findings

In two-thirds of the leads exploring a hypodense area the electrical activity was very depressed (< 10 μV). Well conserved background activity was recorded in only 3% of the leads exploring such hypodense areas.

Discussion

In order to define the spatial volume of small intracerebral slow growing tumors we use stereotactic biopsies (as many people in the world). The utilization of intracerebral electrodes to study the epilepsy of such patients allowed us to compare these different data.

The first limitation of this study is the small number of patients. The second, less important in our mind, is that the reconstruction of the CT scan data in stereotactic coordinates is 'manual'. The third is that the evaluation of the stereo-EEG data was not done with the help of modern information technology.

Despite these limitations our data seem to show that in a solid tumor the electrical activity is always very depressed (like so-called 'electrical silence'), but this type of activity may also be recorded in different histopathological conditions, more particularly in the infiltrated white matter. In 'normal' tissues the background activity is always well preserved, but it may also persist in different histopathological situations, except solid tumors. A high-voltage permanent theta-delta activity may be recorded in very different histopathological patterns, except solid tumors and normal tissue. Interictal spikes may be recorded in very different histopathological situations, varying from normal tissue to infiltrated gray or white matter. An inversion of polarity may, however, help in the definition of the limits of the lesion. The hypodensity shown by the CT scan in such tumor cases seems to correspond to the real extent of the tumor, with or without edema. Very depressed activity is found in two-thirds of the CT scan hypodensities. The fact that a background activity may persist in a small percent of such specimens may be linked to the rate of expansion of the lesion. Thus, we did not find any 'typical' electrical pattern permitting a correct diagnosis only on the basis of the stereo-EEG findings. This conclusion is in agreement with the results of *Bancaud* et al. [3] and *Musolino* [7]. However, a more sophisticated study on a greater number of patients could permit better identification of other factors potentially modulating the intracerebral electrical activity.

References

1 Bancaud, J.: Apport de l'exploration fonctionnelle par voie stéréotaxique à la chirurgie de l'épilepsie. Neurochirurgie *5:* 55–112 (1959).

2 Bancaud, J.; Talairach, J.: Macro-stereo-electro-encephalography in epilepsy; in Bancaud, Handbook of electroencephalography and clinical neurophysiology, vol. 10, part B, pp. 3–33 (Elsevier, Amsterdam 1975).
3 Bancaud, J.; Talairach, J.; Szikla, G.: Stereo-EEG exploration in interstitial irradiation of gliomas; in Szikla, Stereotactic cerebral irradiation. Inserm Symp. No. 12, pp. 57–62 (Elsevier/North-Holland, Amsterdam 1979).
4 Daumas-Duport, C.; Monsaingeon, V.; Szenthe, L.; Szikla, G.: Serial stereotactic biopsies: a double histological code of gliomas according to malignancy and 3-D configuration as an aid to therapeutic decision and assessment of results. Appl. Neurophysiol. *45:* 431–437 (1982).
5 Munari, C.; Bancaud, J.: The role of the stereo-EEG in the evaluation of partial epileptic seizures; in Morselli, Porter, The epilepsies, pp. 267–306 (Butterworths, London 1985).
6 Munari, C.; Talairach, J.; Musolino, A.; Szikla, G.; Bancaud, J.; Chodkiewicz, J.P.: Stereotactic methodology of 'functional' neurosurgery in tumoral epileptic patients; in Broggi, Gottlieb, Slow-growing cerebral tumors (Masson, Milan 1983); Ital. J. neurol. Sci. *2:* suppl., pp. 69–82 (1983).
7 Musolino, A.: Definizione spaziale di alcuni tumori gliali cerebrali: approccio stereotassico ed esplorazione stereo-elettroencefalografia. Tesi di specializzazione in neurofisiopatologia, 135 pp. (Sept. 1984).
8 Talairach, J.; Szikla, G.; Tournoux, P., et al.: Atlas d'anatomie stéréotaxique du télencéphale (Masson, Paris 1967).

C. Munari, MD, Hôpital Sainte-Anne, Service de Neurochirurgie,
1, rue Cabanis, F-75014 Paris (France)

Proc. 9th Meeting World Soc. Stereotactic and Functional Neurosurgery, Toronto 1985
Appl. Neurophysiol. *48:* 454–459 (1985)

Use of Intraoperative Stimulation in the Selection of Target Sites for CT-Guided Stereotactic Biopsies

Dennis E. Bullard, Thad T. Makachinas, Blaine S. Nashold, Jr.
Duke Medical Center, Durham, N.C., USA

Key Words. CT-stereotaxis · CT-guided biopsy · Brain tumors · Intraoperative stimulation · Stereotactic surgery

Abstract. We have utilized intraoperative stimulation to establish the functional nature of tissue to be biopsied in 20 patients undergoing CT-guided stereotactic biopsies. We have performed from 1–4 stimulations at 2–100 Hz using a monopolar and/or bipolar electrode at the intended target sites. Thresholds for motor and sensory response have been obtained. Stimulation results have ranged from sensory changes to tonic/clonic motor activity of the contralateral body and face.

Introduction

The marriage of computed tomography (CT) to conventional stereotactic technology has allowed CT-guided stereotactic biopsies of deep-seated intracranial lesions [1–4]. While the morbidity and mortality associated with this type of procedure is significantly better than that previously reported with free-hand biopsies, a certain percentage of cases are associated with postoperative morbidity, often in association with small intracranial hemorrhages [2]. We have utilized intraoperative stimulation prior to performing biopsies to determine if this can be of benefit in predicting and thereby preventing these postoperative functional defects with the rationale that the results of stimulation should predict the functional potential of tissue within a 2–5 mm radius.

Table I. Patient population

Patient	Diagnosis	Location
1	anaplastic astrocytoma	parietal
2	glioblastoma multiforme	parietal
3	malignant glioma	frontal
4	glioblastoma multiforme	frontal
5	tumor	parietal
6	astrocytoma	parietal
7	glioblastoma multiforme	frontal
8	astrocytoma	parietal
9	anaplastic astrocytoma	thalamus
10	inflammation	thalamus
11	anaplastic astrocytoma	thalamus
12	infarction	thalamus
13	glioblastoma multiforme	thalamus
14	glioblastoma multiforme	basal ganglia
15	lymphoma	basal ganglia
16	astrocytoma	basal ganglia
17	lymphoma	basal ganglia
18	glioblastoma multiforme	basal ganglia
19	encephalitis	basal ganglia
20	glioblastoma multiforme	corpus callosum

Materials and Methods

Stereotactic biopsies were performed on 20 patients with deep, surgically inaccessible lesions, or lesions in exquisite subcortical areas (table I). All surgical procedures were performed utilizing either the Gildenberg technique [4] and a Todd-Wells stereotactic frame or a Brown-Roberts-Wells frame (Trent-Wells Co., Southgate, Calif.) [1, 3]. CT-stereotactic coordinates were selected prior to the actual operation utilizing a GE-8800 scanner. Target points were selected to avoid potentially functional areas, such as the internal capsule. With the initial target point centered in the frame, a stimulating electrode was inserted. Tissue impedance was monitored at various depths from the cortex to the target. Stimulation was performed at 2–100 Hz and 1 ms pulse duration using a Radionics Lesion Generator (Radionics, Inc., 76 Cambridge, Burlington, Mass.). Biopsies were performed with a blunt-tipped, metal biopsy needle with a 1 cm side port [3]. Routinely, four quadrant biopsies are performed at each target point with one of the samples being sent for frozen section and the others saved for permanent analysis.

Table II. Results of monopolar stimulation

Patient	Location	Target	Frequency, Hz	Threshold, V	Response	Postoperation exam
1	P	A	5, 20,50, 100	10	NR	–
2	P	A	5	9	↑ tone CL body	–
			100	7		
3	F	A	5	6	clonic hand movement	no biopsy taken
		B	5, 100	10	NR	–
4	F	A	2	8	masseter contraction	–
			100	4	↑ tone CL arm	
		B	2	6	masseter contraction	
			100	4	masseter contraction	
5	P	A	2	8	BL blepharospasm	–
			100	4	'funny feeling' head	
6	P	A	2	8	clonic CL body movement	no biopsy taken
			100	4	↑ tone CL body	
		B	2	5	BL blepharospasm	
			100	4	BL frontalis contraction	
7	F	A	2	7	'twitching' head	
			100	6	nystagmus	
8	P	A	2	10	pain, head	hemiparesis
			100	3	pain, head	
9	T	A	5	5	↑ CL tone	–
			100	5	↑ CL tone	
10	T	A	5	6	CL eye deviation	–
			100	6	CL tonic contraction	
11	T	A	2	6	frontalis contraction	–
			100	10	↑ CL tone leg	
12	T		2	10	NR	–
			100	10	↑ CL tone	
13	T	A	5	7	frontalis contraction	
			100	5	frontalis contraction	
14	BG	A	2	10	NR	–
			100	10	NR	
15	BG	A	2	5	CL arm movement	transient ↑
			100	5	↑ CL tone	hemiparesis
16	BG	A	2	8	↑ CL tone	–
			100	6	masseter	
17	BG	A	2	7	facial paresthesias	–
			100	6	facial paresthesias	
18	BG	A	2	3	CL body movement	transient ↑
			100	0.5	↑ CL tone	hemiparesis

Table II (continued)

Patient	Location	Target	Frequency, Hz	Threshold, V	Response	Postoperation exam
19	BG	A	2	1	CL facial movement	
			100	1	CL facial movement	no biopsy taken
		B	2	5	CL facial movement	
			100	5	CL facial movement	–
20	CC	A	2	8	'funny feeling' head	–
			100	4	L body paresthesias	

* P = Parietal; F = frontal; T = temporal; BG = basal ganglia; CC = corpus callosum; NR = no response; CL = contralateral; BL = bilateral; L = left.

Results

In 8 patients with subcortical lesions in the frontal or parietal lobes, monopolar stimulation was performed (table II). At 2–5 Hz, thresholds for response ranged from 5 to 10 V. In 5 of 8 patients, a nonspecific response was seen at high voltage. In 1 patient, increased contralateral body tone was seen at 9 V. In 2 patients, clonic contralateral movements were seen at 6 and 8 V, respectively. In both of these patients, the target site was changed to a point where a nonspecific response was seen. At 100 Hz, thresholds ranged from 3 to 10 V. Nonspecific responses were seen in 4 patients, nystagmus in 1, and increased contralateral tone in 3. In 7 of 8 patients, no postoperative deficit was noted. In the 8th patient, a large hematoma developed with a secondary hemiparesis.

Five patients with thalamic lesions were stimulated. At 2–5 Hz, thresholds ranged from 5 to 10 V. In 1 of 5 patients, increased contralateral tone was noted at 5 V and in another patient contralateral eye deviation was seen at 6 V. In the remainder, nonspecific responses occurred. At 100 Hz, thresholds ranged from 5 to 10 V. Increased tone was seen contralaterally in 4 patients and a nonspecific response in 1. In none of these 5 patients was a postoperative deficit noted.

In 6 patients, basal ganglia lesions were stimulated and biopsied. At 2 Hz, thresholds ranged from 1 to 10 V. In 1 patient, a nonspecific response was seen, in 1 patient increased tone, in 3 patients contralateral tonic movement, and in 1 patient paresthesias were noted. At 100 Hz, nonspecific responses were seen in 2 patients, increased contralateral tone in 2, paresthesias in 1, and clonic facial movement in 1. In the 2 patients who noted contralateral movement at 2 Hz and increased tone contralaterally at 100 Hz at 0.5 and 5 V, respectively, transient postoperative hemiparesis was noted. In both, this resolved within 5 days. In 1 patient, the biopsy site was altered because of contralateral facial movement at low voltage. No neurologic deficit was noted postoperatively in this patient.

In 1 patient with a corpus callosum lesion, stimulation at 2 Hz resulted in a nonspecific response a 8 V. Stimulation at 100 Hz resulted in paresthesias in the left body at 4 V and the right body at 5 V. No postoperative deficit was noted.

Discussion

The development of CT-guided stereotactic procedures has allowed exquisite areas of the brain to be biopsied with relatively low morbidity and mortality [2]. Small hemorrhages, however, can be associated with major deficits. The ability to predict the functional potential of the tissue to be biopsied would help to avoid such misfortunes. In functional neurosurgery, intraoperative stimulation prior to lesioning has long been employed for this pourpose and low-voltage monopolar stimulation has been valuable in identifying motor and sensory structures around the target area within a 3-mm range [5]. The goal of this study was to see if such stimulation would be of benefit in CT-guided stereotactic biopsies. We used monopolar stimulation at the site of planned biopsy in 20 patients. The patients all had lesions in functional areas of the brain with relative preservation of functioning. Stimulation at 2–5 Hz resulted in tonic contralateral movements in 5 patients with subcortical or basal ganglia lesions. In 2 of these patients, biopsies were taken with resulting mild but definite transient neurologic deficits. In the remaining 3 patients, the target site was altered to a point where no localizing response was found. In these patients, no postbiopsy deficit was noted. In the remaining patients, a nonspecific response to stimulation was seen. In only 1 of these 15 patients was a postoperative deficit noted. This was in association with a large hematoma which extended well beyond the area stimulated. While the small number of patients evaluated precludes detailed analysis, we believe that this data suggests a predicitive value for intraoperative stimulation which warrants further evaluation.

Acknowledgements

The authors would like to thank Mrs. *Rose Hagan* for her editorial assistance and her help in preparation of the manuscript. This work was supported by Research Grant CA-11898 and CA-32672 from the National Cancer Institutes and PO2-NS0023 from the National Institute of Neurologic and Communication Disorders and Stroke, National Institutes of Health. *D.E.B.* holds Teacher-Investigator Development Award 1 KO7NS00800 from the NINCDS.

References

1 Brown, R.A.: A stereotactic head frame for use with CT body scanners. Invest. Radiol. *14:* 300–304 (1979).
2 Bullard, D.E.: The role of stereotaxic biopsy in the management of patients with intracranial lesions. Semin. Neurol. (in press, 1985).
3 Bullard, D.E.; Nashold, B.S.; Osborne, D.; Burger, P.C.; Dubois, P.: CT-guided stereotactic biopsies using a modified frame and Gildenberg techniques. J. Neurol. Neurosurg. Psychol. *47:* 590–595 (1984).
4 Gildenberg, P.L.; Kaufman, H.H.; Murthy, K.S.K.: Calculation of stereotactic coordinates from the computed tomographic scan. Neurosurgery *10:* 580–586 (1982).
5 Molina-Negro, P.: Functional surgery of abnormal movements; in Rasmussen, Marino, Functional neurosurgery, pp. 89–121 (Raven Press. New York 1979).
6 Schaltenbrand, G.; Wahren, W.: Electroanatomical observations; in Schaltenbrand, Walker, Stereotactic surgery of the human brain, pp. 390–409 (Thieme-Stratton, New York 1982).

Dennis E. Bullard, MD, Duke Medical Center, Box 3128,
Durham, NC 27710 (USA)

Proc. 9th Meeting World Soc. Stereotactic and Functional
Neurosurgery, Toronto 1985
Appl. Neurophysiol. *48:* 460–462 (1985)

Correlation of CT-Directed Target Site with Histology and Cell Culture in Cerebral Glioma

D.G.T. Thomas, M.P. Powell, R. Bradford, J.L. Darling, J. Olney, R.O. Barnard

National Hospitals, London, UK

Key Words. Glioma · Intralesion variation · Local treatment · Stereotactic biopsy · Tissue culture · Stereotactic surgery · CT-stereotaxis

Abstract. The Brown-Roberts-Wells stereotactic system has been used to remove multiple samples from both the tumour centre and the CT-enhanced edge of intracranial tumours in 44 patients. Histological studies indicate that there is considerable variation between biopsies taken from select spatial sites within a single tumour. The tissue culture studies, using the coverslip overlay explant technique, will ultimately provide fundamental information on the biological variability of human gliomas. Although there was histological variation between multiple samples taken from a single tumour, in many cases the enhancing edge of the tumour was found to be free of infiltrating tumour cells, suggesting that radical local treatment may be warranted for tumour control.

Introduction

By using computer tomographic (CT)-directed stereotactic procedures, targets defined on the CT scan can be biopsied with an accuracy of better than 2 mm [1]. With this method, areas within a cerebral tumour with varying appearances on the CT scan can be biopsied and studied histologically, with good spatial correlation. In addition, material taken from various biopsy sites can be assessed for its ability to be grown in tissue culture.

We present the results of 44 cases of cerebral glioma in which multiple biopsies were taken from within the enhancing edge of the tumour and from the enhancing edge itself.

Patients, Materials and Methods

Between 1980 and 1985, 118 patients referred to the National Hospitals with a suspected cerebral tumour underwent CT-directed stereotactic biopsy using the BRW (Brown-Roberts-Wells) system (Radionics Ltd., Burlington, Mass.). CT scan images were used to select targets from within the body of the tumour and from the enhancing edge. The operative procedures involved in the collection of tumour biopsies have been reported in detail elsewhere [2]. Material obtained from the various biopsy sites was subjected to routine histological examination and, in addition, samples were sent to the tissue culture laboratory where cultures were initiated using the coverslip overlay explant technique. This technique has also been described in detail elsewhere [3].

Results

Of the 118 patients who underwent CT-directed biopsy, 44 (37%) had multiple biopsies taken from a tumour which was subsequently proven to be a cerebral glioma. The results of the histological examination of biopsies taken from the tumour edge are as follows: 20/44 (46%) tumour-free edge; 4/44 (9%) tumour edge biopsy diagnostic. Where biopsies taken from the enhancing edge of the tumour were histologically tumour free the diagnosis was made on samples taken from the body of the tumour. 29 biopsies were sent for tissue culture. The overall success rate of the coverslip overlay technique for these 29 biopsies was as follows: 29/44 (66%) biopsies submitted for tissue culture; 24/29 (83%) grown in tissue cultures; 5/29 (17%) failed to grow.

Discussion

CT-directed stereotactic biopsy enables targets which have been located on the CT scan to be sampled with precision. Cerebral tumours often have zones of varying appearance on the CT scan and these can be studied histologically by employing this technique. The series of 44 cases reported here confirms our previous finding of intratumour histological variability [2]. In a substantial percentage of patient samples obtained from the enhancing edge of the tumour were histologically tumour free. It follows that in selected cases the brain beyond the apparent enhancing boundary on CT scan may be free of tumour and that in these cases radical local treatment of cerebral glioma may be potentially curative.

This study also confirms that cell cultures can be obtained from small biopsy samples of cerebral glioma using the explant coverslip overlay technique. This opens up the possibility of using cultured biopsy samples for detailed in vitro studies of intratumoral variability.

References

1 Brown, R.A.: A computerized tomography-computer graphics approach to stereotaxic localization. J. Neurosurg. *50:* 715–720 (1979).

2 Thomas, D.G.T.; Anderson, R.E.; Boulay, G.H. du: CT-guided stereotactic neurosurgery: experience in 24 cases with a new stereotactic system. J. Neurol. Neurosurg. Psychiat. *47:* 9–16 (1983).

3 Thomas, D.G.T.; Darling, J.L.; Watkins, B.A.; Hine Maria, C.: A simple method for the growth of cell cultures from small biopsies of brain tumours taken during CT-directed stererotactic procedures. Acta neurochir. *33:* suppl., pp. 243–245 (1984).

D.G.T. Thomas, MD, Gough Cooper Department of Neurological Surgery,
Institute of Neurology, National Hospital for Nervous Diseases,
Queen Square, London WC1 (UK)

Proc. 9th Meeting World Soc. Stereotactic and Functional
Neurosurgery, Toronto 1985
Appl. Neurophysiol. *48:* 463–466 (1985)

Accuracy of CT Scans in Identifying Tumor Tissue

P.W. Hitchon[a], *R.L. Schelper*[b], *T. Barloon*[c]

[a] Division of Neurosurgery, [b] Division of Neuropathology, and
[c] Department of Radiology, University of Iowa Hospitals, Iowa City, Iowa, USA

Key Words. Stereotactic surgery · Computerized tomography · Brain tumor · Brain biopsy · CT-stereotaxis

Abstract. The authors present their experience with stereotactic biopsy of brain tumors. Biopsies were obtained sequentially at different depths from the center of the tumor according to coordinates derived from computerized tomography (CT). Biopsies were obtained from 23 brain tumors: 17 gliomas, 5 metastases, and 1 lymphoma. In all a total of 137 biopsies were studied from both enhancing and nonenhancing areas. The tumor yield from these biopsies was 68 and 73%, respectively. It appears that tumor tissue may be obtained from both the enhancing periphery as well as the nonenhancing center of tumors.

The indications for stereotactic biopsies of brain tumors are now well established. Utilizing information derived from computerized axial tomography (CT), it is now possible to obtain biopsies with an accuracy not heretofore possible. CT adapted stereotactic biopsies are ideal in small lesions, particularly when deep seated or close to vital brain structures, e.g., Broca's area, precentral gyrus. Since these biopsies are generally performed under local analgesia, they have proven appropriate in patients carrying a relatively high surgical risk. The question presenting to us was that of the ideal location from which to obtain a biopsy. Should the biopsies be obtained from the enhancing periphery, the nonenhancing center of tumors as they appear on CT scans, or both? Studies to date comparing whole brain sections with antemortem CT scans have shown that the central areas of tumors generally consist of necrotic tumor [2, 3, 5]. The ring enhancing periphery comprises vascular and viable tumor. The peritumoral zone, on the other hand, consists of edematous brain where tumor cells may yet be encountered. With this autopsy material available to us, we elected to compare the tumor yield in our serial biopsies.

Materials and Methods

For the past 2 years the authors have employed CT stereotaxy utilizing the Brown-Roberts-Wells system. In all, 43 procedures were performed upon 39 patients. The diagnosis in these was gloima (18), metastasis (8), abscess (7), lymphoma (2), cyst (2), radiation necrosis (1), and normal caudate (1). Eight of the recurrent gliomas have also undergone stereotactic implantation with ^{125}I seeds.

Twenty-three of the above tumors were selected in this study in whom sequential biopsies at 2–5 mm intervals, both superficial and deep to the center of the tumor, were obtained. The tissue diagnoses of these were glioma (17), metastasis (5), and lymphoma (1). Most tumors comprised both enhancing and nonenhancing components on their scans. The total number of biopsies obtained was 137 of which 104 were from enhancing and 33 from nonenhancing areas, including the cystic fluid when encountered.

There was only 1 operative mortality among the 39 patients who underwent stereotactic biopsy, a 75-year-old male with metastatic lung cancer to the pineal region. The cause of death was cardiac arrest following a tension pneumothorax on the side of the large bronchogenic carcinoma.

Results

Our technique failed to establish the true tissue diagnosis in 3 cases of lymphoma, malignant ependymoma, and metastasis. The incorrect diagnosis made from our specimens was toxoplasmosis, reactive gliosis, and necrosis. Of the 23 tumors subjected to serial biopsies at various depths, the tumor yield was 68% from the enhancing and 73% from the nonenhancing areas.

Discussion

Our mortality of 1 patient is comparable to that of *Mundinger* [6] (1.4%) and *Ostertag* et al. [7] (2.3%). Our failure to establish the true diagnosis in 3 cases, though seemingly high, is not dissimilar from that encountered by others [7].

A similar analysis regarding biopsy sites was undertaken by *Boethius* et al. [1]. In 9 patients with gliomas, tumor was identified in biopsies from the enhancing, nonenhancing, as well as the peripheral zones of low attenuation. The best yield, however, was found in biopsies from the enhancing rim. *Lewander* et al. [4] subjected 13 patients with gliomas to the same analysis. Tumor tissue was encountered in areas that were identified on CT scan as compatible with edema, necrosis, and cystic formation. Furthermore, areas on CT scan that were suggestive of tumor were on occasion free of abnormality or consisting of necrosis only. Thus, of 45 biopsies, 36 were predicted correctly from the CT scan, a yield of 80%.

Obtaining serial biopsies at various depths with respect to the tumor as apparent on CT is mandatory if we are to confirm the diagnosis of a neoplastic process. The yield of tumor tissue from enhancing and nonenhancing areas was about 70% in each. One would have expected the positive results to be far greater in specimens obtained from the enhancing rim. This rim, however, consisting of viable tumor, may be quite narrow, so that obtaining a specimen from it may not always be successful. Furthermore, cystic fluid, when encountered, should be analyzed for malignant cells, as was found in 3 of our 4 cysts. Our only negative result was the fluid associated with a cystic glioma. Whether or not new diagnostic techniques such as magnetic resonance imaging will improve the yield of stereotactic biopsies remains to be seen.

References

1 Boethius, J.; Collins, V.P.; Edner, G.; Lewander, R.; Zajicek, J.: Stereotactic biopsies and computer tomography in gliomas. Acta neurochir. *40:* 223–232 (1978).

2 Burger, P.C.; Dubois, P.J.; Schold, S.C.; Smith, K.R.; Odom, G.L.; Crafts, D.C.; Giangaspero, F.: Computerized tomographic and pathologic studies of the untreated, quiescent, and recurrent glioblastoma multiforme. J. Neurosurg. *58:* 159–169 (1983).

3 Jacobs, L.; Kinkel, W.R.; Heffner, R.R.: Autopsy correlations of computerized tomography: experience with 6,000 CT scans. Neurology *26:* 1111–1118 (1976).

4 Lewander, R.; Bergstrom, J.; Boethius, J.; Collins, V.P.; Edner, G.; Greitz, T.; Willems, J.: Stereotactic computer tomography for biopsy of gliomas. Acta radiol. Diag. *19:* 867–888 (1978).

5 Lilja, A.; Bergstrom, K.; Spannare, B.; Olsson, Y.: Reliability of computed tomography in assessing histopathological features of malignant supratentorial gliomas. J. comput. assist. Tomogr. *5:* 625–636 (1981).

6 Mundinger, F.: Implantation of radioisotopes (curietherapy); in Schaltenbrand, Walker, Stereotaxy of the human brain: anatomical, physiological and clinical applications; 2nd ed., pp. 410–435 (Thieme-Stratton, New York 1982).
7 Ostertag, C.B.; Mennel, H.D.; Kiessling, M.: Stereotactic biopsy of brain tumors. Surg. Neurol. *14:* 275–283 (1980).

P.W. Hitchon, MD, Division of Neurosurgery, University of Iowa Hospitals, Iowa City, IA 52242 (USA)

Proc. 9th Meeting World Soc. Stereotactic and Functional
Neurosurgery, Toronto 1985
Appl. Neurophysiol. *48:* 467–471 (1985)

Diagnosis and Treatment of Brainstem Mass Lesions by CT-Guided Stereotactic Surgery

R.J. Coffey, L.D. Lunsford

Department of Neurological Surgery, JHM Health Center, Gainesville, Fla., and
Department of Neurological Surgery, Presbyterian University Hospital,
Pittsburgh, Pa., USA

Key Words. Brain biopsy · Brainstem surgery · Computed tomography · Mesencephalon · Pons · Stereotactic surgery · CT stereotaxis

Abstract. Current neuroradiographic techniques including computed tomographic scanning (CT) and magnetic resonance imaging (MRI) when added to the clinical neurologic examination can localize precisely even small lesions within the brainstem. While the clinical-radiographic diagnosis is accurate with respect to locale, it is often in error with respect to the pathologic nature of the solitary brainstem lesion. Therefore, empiric treatment without the benefit of a tissue diagnosis will often be inappropriate. CT-guided stereotactic surgery can safely and reliably provide a tissue diagnosis in such cases. Furthermore, in selected cases, therapeutic interventions can be of substantial and lasting benefit to the patient.

Materials and Methods

The Leksell Model CT Stereotactic Frame (AB Elekta Instruments, Decatur, Ga.) was used in combination with the GE 8800 CT/T Scanner (General Electric Medical Systems, Milwaukee, Wisc.) in 13 operations on 12 patients with mass lesions involving the midbrain and/or pons (table I). The 9 most recent cases were operated upon in a dedicated CT operative suite. Table I summarizes the clinical and radiographic finding in these patients. A transfrontal trajectory via a coronal burr hole (or twist drill hole) was used in 9 patients with biopsy targets in the midbrain or rostral pons. Local anesthesia with the patient awake on the CT table was employed in these cases. An additional 3 patients with biopsy targets in the lateral or ventrolateral pons at the level of the middle cerebellar peduncle underwent surgery in the prone position via a laterally placed suboccipital burr hole. General anesthesia was employed in these 3 cases. The prone rather than the sitting position was employed to allow the actual operation to be performed on the CT table.

Table I

Patients, n	Clinical presentation	Location of mass
Transfrontal approach		
5	Weber's or Benedikt's syndrome	cerebral penducle (± thalmus; ± pons)
2	Parinaud's syndrome	pineal/periaqueductal region
1	ataxia and hemiparesis	pontomesencephalic junction
1	mixed midbrain/pontine syndrome	brainstem and thalmus extensively involved
Transcerebellar approach		
3	pontine cranial nerve deficits with cerebellar and pyramidal signs	lateral-ventral pons at the level of middle cerebellar peduncle

a b c

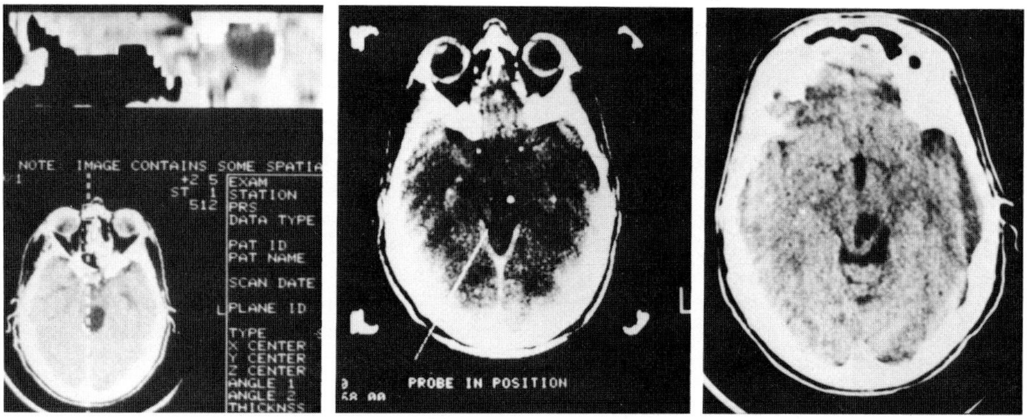

Fig. 1. Percutaneous twist-drill aspiration of midbrain cyst. **a** Preoperative contrast CT ventriculogram and parasagittal reformation; the patient's status is postventriculoperitoneal shunt. An intraparenchymal cyst of the midbrain displaces the aqueduct and does not communicate with the ventricular system or basal cisterns. **b** Intraoperative CT scan showing the aspiration cannula within the partially collapsed cyst; 1 ml of additional fluid was then removed. **c** CT scan performed 6 months postoperatively. The cyst has remained collapsed, and the aqueduct has resumed its normal position.

CT image reformation in multiple planes was used to select the safest and most productive biopsy probe trajectory through the lesion in all cases. A spiral biopsy needle and a fine aspiration needle were employed to sample or aspirate the lesions along a single probe trajectory. In 2 patients intraoperative CT scanning was performed with the probe held in position within the lesion (fig. 1), and, in another 2 patients, contrast CT ventri-

Table II

Preoperative clinical diagnosis	Number correct	Number in error
Primary glial neoplasm	2	4
Metastatic carcinoma	2	0
Infection, abscess	0	1
Hematoma (primary)	1	1
Nonneoplastic cyst	1	0
Total	6	6

Table III

Postoperative histologic diagnosis	Number of cases
Astrocytoma	2
Anaplastic	1
Malignant	1
Metastatic carcinoma	4
Lymphoma	1
Hepatoma	2
Non-neoplastic cyst	2
Inflammation/vasculitis	1
Total	12

culography was performed after biopsy and aspiration of tissue. In all cases immediate postoperative scanning confirmed accurate location of the biopsy site and excluded hemorrhagic complications.

Results

CT-guided stereotactic biopsy yielded adequate tissue for pathologic diagnosis in all cases. No new neurologic deficit appeared as a result of surgery. The 6 patients who underwent aspirations of intra-axial cysts, hematomas, or necrotic tumors all improved in the early postoperative period. While this effect was only temporary in the cases of cystic malignancies, it was of lasting benefit in those patients with benign tissue diagnoses.

Tables II and III show that the preoperative clinical-radiographic diagnosis was in error in 50% of the cases. Thus, the results of biopsy led to significant changes in therapy postoperatively. Both metastatic carcinoma and nonneoplastic conditions were underdiagnosed preoperatively. Patients in whom tumor was suspected but not confirmed at biopsy have not deteriorated postoperatively in such a way as to suggest a missed diagnosis. Solitary metastatic nodules in the brainstem were found in 4 patients, only 1 of whom had a known primary tumor. He, and 1 of the 3 patients with an occult systemic malignancy, are alive and well at follow-up 1 and 1½ years respectively after external beam radiotherapy.

The 1 patient in whom lymphoma was diagnosed was receiving immunosuppressive therapy for leukemia and thought to have a brainstem abscess. Antibiotic therapy was stopped and radiation therapy initiated after the biopsy showed primary CNS lymphoma.

Discussion

Although many authors agree in principle to the surgery of brainstem lesions for diagnostic and therapeutic purposes, the choice of surgical approach and the extent of resection remain controversial [1, 4–7]. Stereotactic biopsy and aspiration techniques with CT guidance and multiplanar image reformation now permit the safe, accurate, and reliable diagnosis of intra-axial brainstem lesions with acceptable operative and anesthetic risk [2, 3]. Serial biopsy specimens along a single probe trajectory are obtained, minimizing the incidence of nondiagnostic exploration. In selected cases, the aspiration of cystic lesions, monitored by intraoperative CT, allows the reduction of local mass effect as well as the restoration of CSF pathways.

The transfrontal probe trajectory to the midbrain with the patient under local anesthesia has a long record of safety in stereotactic operations for movement disorder and pain. The transcerebellar approach to targets in the ventral or lateral pons at the level of the middle cerebellar peduncle represents the safest, shortest and most direct route to that region. The trajectory avoids all major extra-axial vascular and cranial nerve structures while eliminating the need to traverse the incisura or puncture the tentorium. Anesthetic times have been short with the patient in the prone position, and no complications have occurred.

This series of patients demonstrates that CT-guided stereotactic exploration of mass lesions in the brainstem is both productive and safe. The empiric treatment of patients harboring such lesions based on the reluctance to expose them to the risks of prolonged anesthesia and open operation is no longer necessary.

References

1 Baghai, P.; Vries, J.K.; Bechtel, P.C.: Retromastoid approach for biopsy of brainstem tumors. Neurosurgery *10:* 574–579 (1982).

2 Beatty, R.M.; Zervas, N.T.: Stereotactic aspiration of a brainstem hematoma. Neurosurgery *13:* 204–207 (1983).

3 Bosch, D.A.; Beute, G.N.: Successful stereotaxic evacuation of an acute pontomedullary hematoma. J. Neurosurg. *62:* 153–156 (1985).

4 Hacker, R.J.; Fox, J.L.: Surgical treatment of brainstem carcinoma: case report. Neurosurgery *6:* 430–432 (1980).

5 Lassiter, K.R.L.; Alexander, E.; Davis, C.H.; Kelly, D.L.: Surgical treatment of brainstem gliomas. J. Neurosurg. *34:* 719–725 (1971).

6 O'Laoire, S.A.; Crock, H.A.; Thomas, D.G.T.; Gordon, D.S.: Brainstem hematoma: a report of six surgically treated cases. J. Neurosurg. *56:* 222–227 (1982).

7 Villani, R.; Gaini, S.M.; Tomei, G.: Follow-up study of brainstem tumors in children. Child's Brain *1:* 126–135 (1975).

Dr. R.J. Coffey, MD, Department of Neurological Surgery, Box J-265, JHM Health Center, Gainesville, FL 32610 (USA)

Proc. 9th Meeting World Soc. Stereotactic and Functional
Neurosurgery, Toronto 1985
Appl. Neurophysiol. *48:* 472–476 (1985)

Cell Kinetics of Neuroepithelial Tumors in Serial Stereotactic Biopsies. A New Combined Approach[1]

G. Broggi[a], *A. Franzini*[a], *A. Costa*[b], *A. Melcarne*[a], *A. Allegranza*[a]

[a] Department of Neurosurgery, Service of Functional Neurosurgery, Istituto Neurologico 'C. Besta', and [b] Istituto Nazionale per lo Studio e la Cura dei Tumori, Milan, Italy

Key Words. Cell kinetics · Stereotactic biopsies · Glial tumors · Stereotactic surgery

Abstract. 33 consecutive patients with brain glial tumors underwent serial stereotactic biopsies and (^{3}H)-thymidine in vitro investigation. The labeling index has been determined in each case and matched with the WHO histological classification. The feasibility and the accuracy of cell kinetics study applied to stereotactic biopsies are discussed in view of future application for prognostic purposes. Particular attention is given to the description of the method.

Introduction

Prognosis and therapeutic possibilities in patients with deep-seated glial tumors, investigated by serial stereotactic biopsies, are usually established according to the histological diagnosis and neuropathological grading as proposed by the WHO Committee [8]. Nevertheless, the expected survival may vary widely despite homogeneous histological classification of tumors. For instance, statistical investigations performed in a histologically ascertained low-grade astrocytoma series show survival periods ranging between a few years and more than 10 years [3–5]. To obtain more reliable prognostic data in glial tumors, their proliferative activity has been investigated by *Hoshino* et al.

[1] Supported by grant No. 84.00474.44 from the Consiglio Nazionale delle Ricerche, Rome, Italy.

[3, 4]. These authors proposed the intravenous administration of (^{3}H)-thymidine in patients undergoing surgical removal of the lesion, followed by an autoradiographic study on the resected neoplastic tissue. This method detects the amount of cells in the S phase of the proliferating cycle, which are labeled by (^{3}H)-thymidine. The ratio between the number of cells in S phase and the number of viable cells represent the labeling index (LI) that is related to the prognosis and survival. In different tumors other than gliomas, the LI has been determined by an in vitro procedure, the prognostic value of which has been confirmed [6, 7]. This procedure has been applied to stereotactic biopsies of deep unresectable tumors in which only conservative treatment can be performed. The advantages of this combined methodology are discussed in a mature astrocytoma series, an anaplastic astrocytoma series and in glioblastoma.

Materials and Methods

33 patients, 24 males and 9 females, aged between 6 and 60 years (average 37 years), were included in this study. The lesions were located within the brainstem in 2 cases, the basal ganglia in 12 and within the white hemispheric matter in 19 cases. Histologic diagnosis and tumor grading were obtained from multiple tissue samples taken during CT stereotactic biopsy including intraoperatively guided transtumoral impedance monitoring. Depth EEG recording from the neoplasm and surrounding tissues was also performed in 10 patients affected by associated symptomatic epilepsy [1, 2].

The definitive histologic diagnosis demonstrated low-grade astrocytoma in 14 patients, anaplastic astrocytoma in 7 patients and glioblastomas in 12 patients.

The cell kinetic study was performed on fragments obtained from each biopsy sample. In 11 patients, four different targets within the neoplastic mass were sampled, three targets in 17 patients and only two targets in 5 patients.

After sampling, the fragment of tissue was immediately placed in a nutrient medium (RPMI 1640; Gibco, Grand Island, N.Y.) supplemented with 20% fetal calf serum plus antibiotics (Gibco) and incubated in nutrient medium containing (^{3}H)-thymidine (6 μCi/ml; spec. act. 5 Ci/mmol; Radiochemical Centre, Amersham, UK) for 1 h at 37 °C in a Dubnoff shaker (Valentini, Milan, Italy). After the incubation, the (^{3}H)-thymidine was removed and the specimen rinsed once in Hank's BSS (Gibco), fixed in Bouin's solution for 1 h, dehydrated, embedded in paraffin and cut into sections 4 μm thick. Autoradiography was performed on deparaffinized slides according to the stripping film technique (Kodak AR10; Kodak, UK). After 10 days of exposure, the autoradiographs were developed in Kodak D 19b for 5 min at 18 °C and fixed in Kodak F5. The slices were finally stained with hematoxylin and eosin at 4 °C. The LI was determined by counting la-

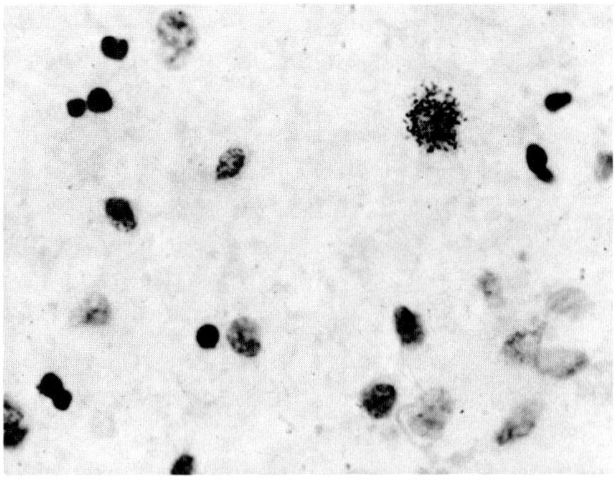

Fig. 1. Histological finding in anaplastic astrocytoma specimen treated by (^{3}H)-thymidine in vitro processing and HE stain (× 500). One labeled nucleus is clearly shown with multiple black grains; pyknotic cells and viable glial cells are present.

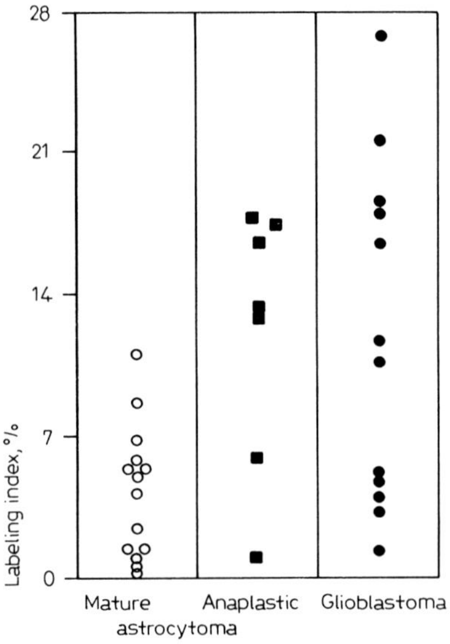

Fig. 2. Scattergrams of LI ranges in mature astrocytoma (14 cases); anaplastic astrocytoma (7 cases) and glioblastoma (12 cases).

belled nuclei per total viable glial cells through the entire sections; 1,000–10,000 total cells per tissue sample were evaluated. The total number of grains per nucleus in labeled cells was always more than 10. The final appearance of labelled cells and viable cells is shown in figure 1.

Results

The average of LI the values determined in the different areas of each single tumor has been considered representative of the potential proliferative activity. The final value of LI was matched with the definitive histological diagnosis. In low-grade astrocytomas, the LI ranged between 0.2 and 11%, in anaplastic astrocytoma between 2.7 and 17.7% and in glioblastoma between 1.4 and 26.8%. The distribution of LI values in these three histological classes shows that higher LI values are present in malignant gliomas (fig. 2). Nevertheless, certain anaplastic astrocytomas and glioblastomas are characterized by low LI values, and this suggests the possible existence of different kinds of tumors within the same morphologically identified class.

Further analysis and long-term follow-up studies are necessary to understand the prognostic value of these preliminary findings. The feasibility of the described combined approach is demonstrated and the field of kinetics and growth studies can be explored further by stereotactic techniques.

References

1 Broggi, G.; Franzini, A.: Value of serial stereotactic biopsies and impedance monitoring in the treatment of deep brain tumors. J. Neurol. Neurosurg. Psychiat. *44:* 397–401 (1981).
2 Broggi, G.; Franzini, A.; Giorgi, C.; Spreafico, R.; Avanzini, G.: Depth recording and neuropathological aspects in symptomatic tumoral and nontumoral epilepsy. Acta neurochir. *33:* suppl., pp. 97–103 (1984).
3 Hoshino, T.: A commentary on the biology and growth kinetics of low-grade and high-grade gliomas. J. Neurosurg. *61:* 895–900 (1984).
4 Hoshino, T.; Barker, M.; Wilson, C.B.; Boldrey, E.B.; Fewer, D.: Cell kinetics of human gliomas. J. Neurosurg. *37:* 15–26 (1972).
5 Laws, E.R.; Taylor, W.F.; Clifton, M.B.; Okazaki, H.: Neurosurgical management of low-grade astrocytoma of the cerebral hemispheres. J. Neurosurg. *61:* 665–673 (1984).

6 Livingston, R.B.; Ambus, U.; George, S.L.; Freireich, E.J.; Hart, J.S.: In vitro determination of thymidine ^{3}H-labeling index in human solid tumors. Cancer Res. *34:* 1376–1380 (1974).
7 Silvestrini, R.; Daidone, M.G.; Costa, A.; Sanfilippo, O.: Cell kinetics and in vitro chemosensitivity as a tool for improved management of patients. Eur. J. Cancer clin. Oncol. *21:* 371–378 (1985).
8 WHO: Histological classification of tumors of the nervous system (WHO, Geneva 1979).

Prof. G. Broggi, Istituto Neurologica 'C. Besta', Via Celoria 11,
I-20133 Milano (Italy)

Proc. 9th Meeting World Soc. Stereotactic and Functional
Neurosurgery, Toronto 1985
Appl. Neurophysiol. *48:* 477–480 (1985)

Survey of CT-Guided Stereotactic Surgery

Philip L. Gildenberg, Patricia Franklin

Recognizing that the marriage of computerized tomographic scanning with stereotactic techniques (CT-SET) has created a resurgence in stereotactic surgery with new applications in many clinical conditions, an informal survey was recently conducted to determine the use of CT-SET techniques.

A questionnaire was prepared and distributed to the members of the World Society for Stereotactic and Functional Neurosurgery and, through the courtesy of several manufacturers [Radionics, Inc., Burlington, Mass., and PMT Corp., Minneapolis, Minn.], to neurosurgeons who had recently purchased stereotactic equipment or instruments. The questionnaire was designed to collect information from surgeons currently performing CT-SET, as well as those who anticipate beginning such procedures within the year.

The information requested included: (1) type of stereotactic apparatus; (2) type of CT scanner; (3) where the procedures were performed (OR, CT suite, etc.); (4) approximate numbers of cases performed for various indications, and (5) an estimated number of procedures anticipated for the next year.

Completed questionnaires were received from 67 neurosurgeons who actually perform CT-SET (58 WSSFN members and 9 nonmembers) and 25 who anticipate beginning in 1986. While the informal nature of the survey precludes statistical analysis of the information, the survey results (fig. 1–4) and comments from the respondents confirm that: (1) CT stereotaxis will have an increasing role in neurosurgical management; (2) CT biopsy will become the procedure of choice for deep-seated brain tumors; (3) several applications will become much more widely employed in the future: (a) interstitial irradiation; (b) stereotactic insertion of chemotherapeutic agents; (c) CT functional procedures; (4) MRI stereotaxis and PETT stereotaxis will become available in the near future.

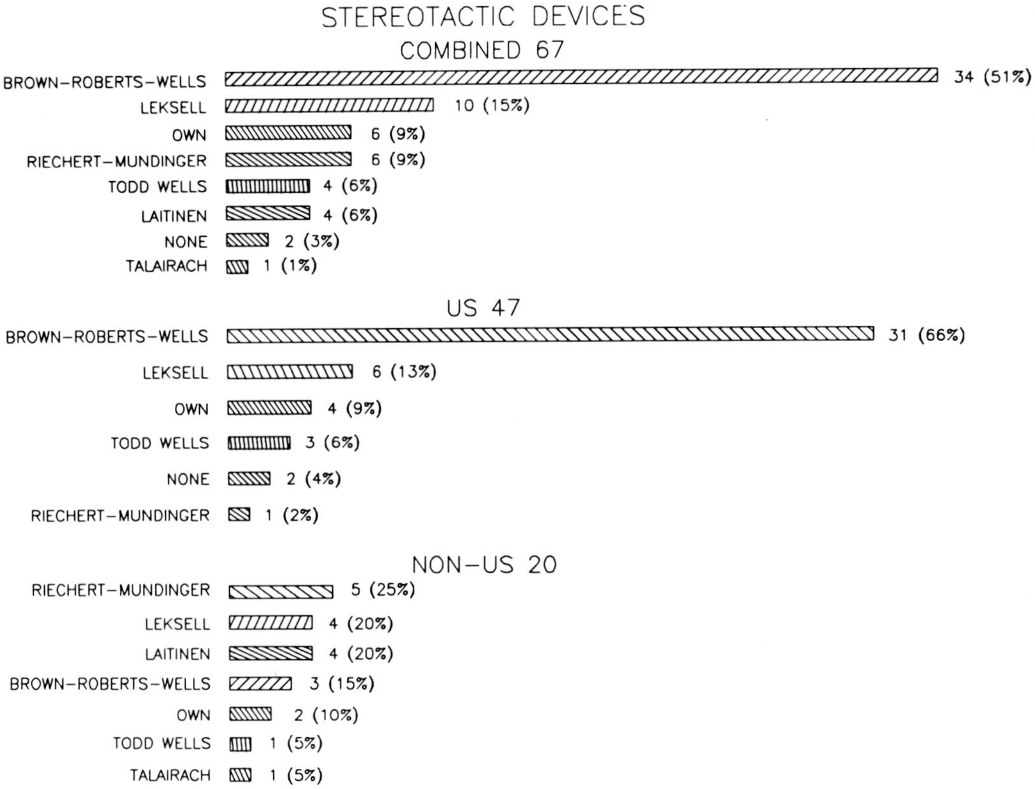
STEREOTACTIC DEVICES
COMBINED 67
BROWN-ROBERTS-WELLS 34 (51%)
LEKSELL 10 (15%)
OWN 6 (9%)
RIECHERT-MUNDINGER 6 (9%)
TODD WELLS 4 (6%)
LAITINEN 4 (6%)
NONE 2 (3%)
TALAIRACH 1 (1%)
US 47
BROWN-ROBERTS-WELLS 31 (66%)
LEKSELL 6 (13%)
OWN 4 (9%)
TODD WELLS 3 (6%)
NONE 2 (4%)
RIECHERT-MUNDINGER 1 (2%)
NON-US 20
RIECHERT-MUNDINGER 5 (25%)
LEKSELL 4 (20%)
LAITINEN 4 (20%)
BROWN-ROBERTS-WELLS 3 (15%)
OWN 2 (10%)
TODD WELLS 1 (5%)
TALAIRACH 1 (5%)

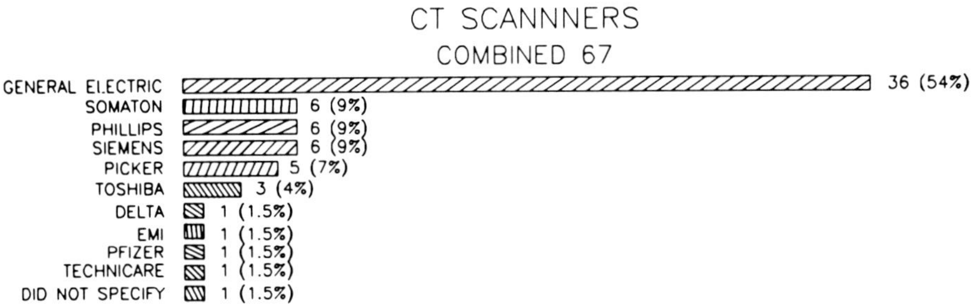
CT SCANNNERS
COMBINED 67
GENERAL ELECTRIC 36 (54%)
SOMATON 6 (9%)
PHILLIPS 6 (9%)
SIEMENS 6 (9%)
PICKER 5 (7%)
TOSHIBA 3 (4%)
DELTA 1 (1.5%)
EMI 1 (1.5%)
PFIZER 1 (1.5%)
TECHNICARE 1 (1.5%)
DID NOT SPECIFY 1 (1.5%)

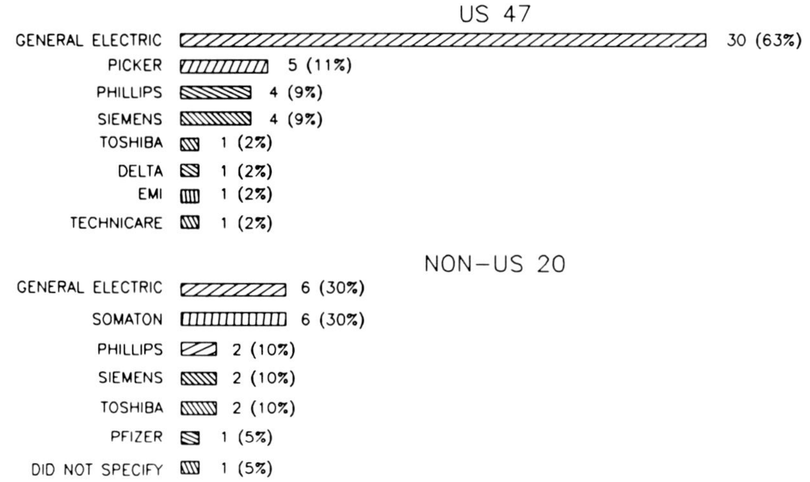
US 47
GENERAL ELECTRIC 30 (63%)
PICKER 5 (11%)
PHILLIPS 4 (9%)
SIEMENS 4 (9%)
TOSHIBA 1 (2%)
DELTA 1 (2%)
EMI 1 (2%)
TECHNICARE 1 (2%)
NON-US 20
GENERAL ELECTRIC 6 (30%)
SOMATON 6 (30%)
PHILLIPS 2 (10%)
SIEMENS 2 (10%)
TOSHIBA 2 (10%)
PFIZER 1 (5%)
DID NOT SPECIFY 1 (5%)

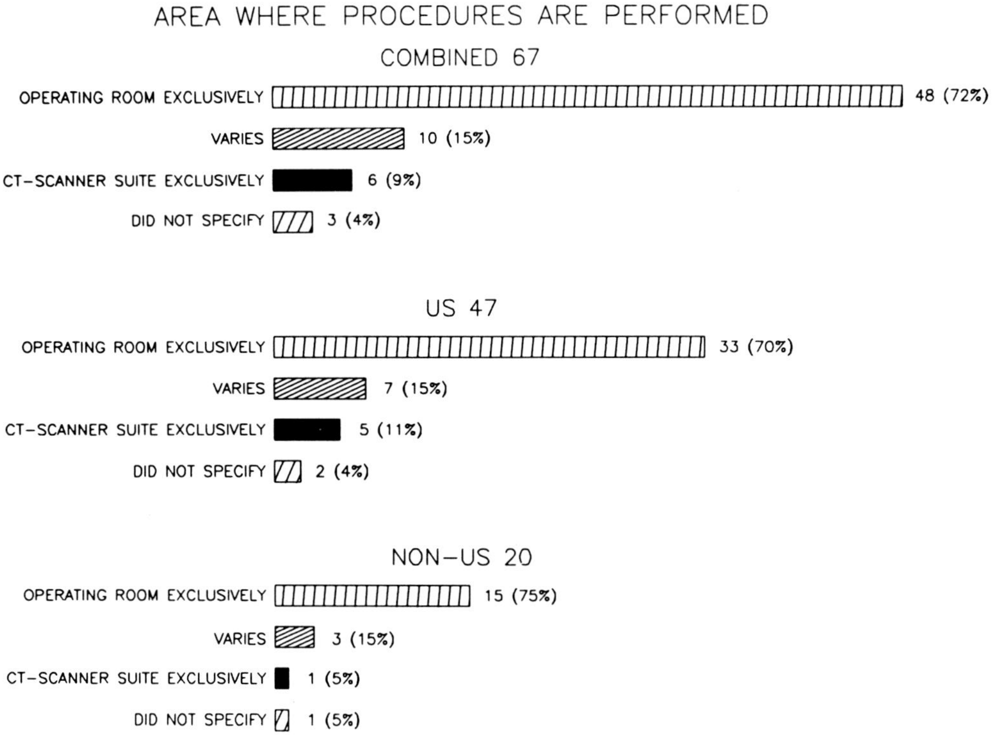
AREA WHERE PROCEDURES ARE PERFORMED
COMBINED 67
OPERATING ROOM EXCLUSIVELY 48 (72%)
VARIES 10 (15%)
CT-SCANNER SUITE EXCLUSIVELY 6 (9%)
DID NOT SPECIFY 3 (4%)
US 47
OPERATING ROOM EXCLUSIVELY 33 (70%)
VARIES 7 (15%)
CT-SCANNER SUITE EXCLUSIVELY 5 (11%)
DID NOT SPECIFY 2 (4%)
NON-US 20
OPERATING ROOM EXCLUSIVELY 15 (75%)
VARIES 3 (15%)
CT-SCANNER SUITE EXCLUSIVELY 1 (5%)
DID NOT SPECIFY 1 (5%)

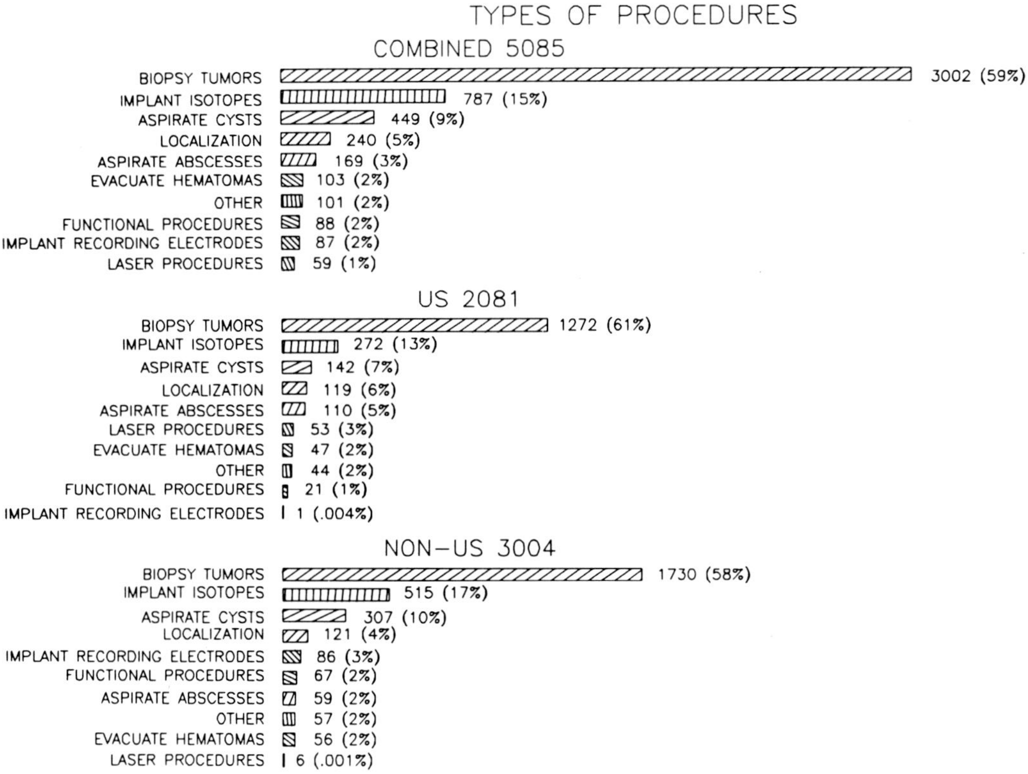

P.L. Gildenberg, PhD, 6560 Fannin, No. 1530, Houston, TX 77030 (USA)

Proc. 9th Meeting World Soc. Stereotactic and Functional
Neurosurgery, Toronto 1985
Appl. Neurophysiol. *48:* 481 (1985)

A Stereotactic Guide for Approach Through the Foramen ovale and Foramen jugulare

Lauri V. Laitinen

Department of Neurosurgery, University Hospital, Umeå, Sweden

A new, fully stereotactic instrument, called a 'Trigeminus Stereoguide', has been used for 2 years in the percutaneous treatment of trigeminal and glossopharyngeal neuralgia [1]. The instrument is based on the Cartesian rectilinear principle. The target, a selected part of the foramen ovale or pars nervosa of the foramen jugulare, is visualized in axial and lateral radiography and defined with x, y and z coordinates. A spherical system consisting of a cylinder and a 90° arc with an electrode carrier is so positioned at the lateral surface of the frame that the mid-point of the spherical system coincides with the target which can be reached accurately from a suitable bone-free direction.

One hundred and seven patients with trigeminal and 2 with glossopharyngeal neuralgia were treated with the new instrument. A graded electrocoagulation was produced with a Radionics Lesion Generator Model RFG-3B. In the last 75 patients the desired part of the foramen was reached accurately without correction of the direction of the electrode. The average time of surgery was 30 min instead of 90 min with the previous free-hand technique. The Trigeminus Stereoguide has opened a new era in the percutaneous treatment of tic douloureux.

Reference

1 Laitinen, L.V.: Trigeminus stereoguide: an instrument for stereotactic approach through the foramen ovale and foramen jugulare. Surg. Neurol. *22:* 519–523 (1984).

L.V. Laitinen, Department of Neurosurgery, University Hospital,
S-90185 Umeå (Sweden)

Proc. 9th Meeting World Soc. Stereotactic and Functional
Neurosurgery, Toronto 1985
Appl. Neurophysiol. *48:* 482–487 (1985)

Intracranial Tumor Biopsy – CT-Guided Stereotactic Surgery

M. Poza[a], *M.A. Perez-Espejo*[a], *J.F. Martinez-Lage*[a],
J.A. Esteban[a], *V. Climent*[b], *J. Sola*[c]

[a] Regional Neurosurgical Centre, [b] Neuroradiological Unit, and
[b] Pathology Department, El Palmar, Murcia, Spain

Key Words. Brain biopsy · Brain tumor · CT stereotaxis · Stereotactic surgery

Abstract. A modification of Gildenberg's technique for brain tumor biopsy is described. Marking the light beam of the gantry on the scalp with a pencil, when the lesion appears on the screen, no ScoutView is necessary. With radiopaque marks on the drawn lines, the levels of the slice are transferred to a lateral conventional X-ray, for calculation of the 'Z' coordinate. 'X' and 'Y' coordinates are determined on the CT scanner.

Introduction

During the last decade, the combination of CT and stereotactic surgery has been used for brain tumor biopsy, mainly in cases of deep lesions. *Gildenberg* [4] has done a complete review of different methods. Most of the techniques employed up to now have needed a special frame to determine the coordinates of the lesion. However, in the past 5 years, a few works have been published that deem the use of the said frame unnecessary [3, 5, 6]. We carry on this system, with some modifications of the technique, as described by *Gildenberg* [3].

Materials and Methods

Thirty-three patients have been operated on with this technique. One patient required a second operation, the first one was unsuccessful.

With the suspicion of a space-occupying lesion, a CT scan is done, beginning at the basal plane (Somaton D2). When the lesion first appears, the light beam in the gantry is switched on, which traces a line around the scalp (fig. 1). With a dermographic pencil or

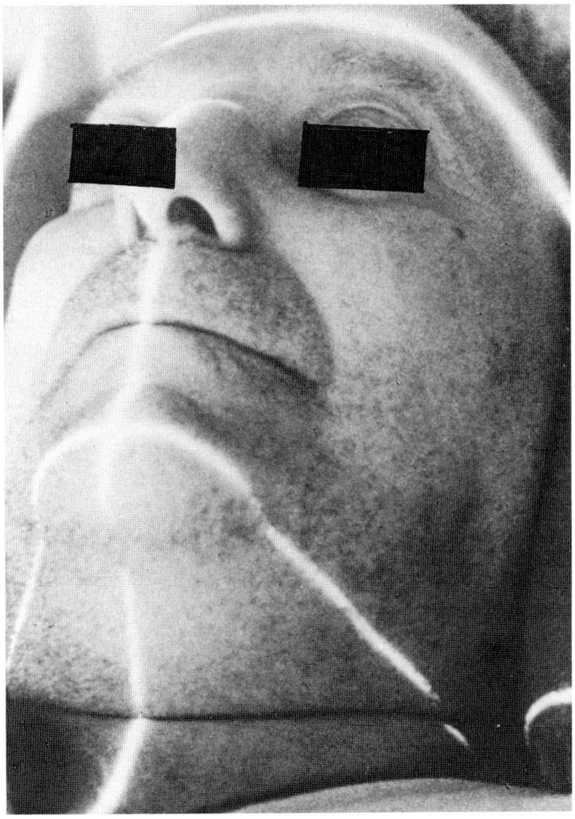

Fig. 1. Light beam marking a plane.

a pin, several dots or scratches are marked on the skin, following the aforementioned line. We continue ascending in cuts of 4 or 8 mm, according to the size of the tumor, until the lesion disappears from the screen.

The examination is repeated in the suspicious planes, after injection of contrast material. Again, only the ideal planes are marked on the skin. The head must be shaved before this second CT scanning, particularly in cases of small size lesions.

The computer defines the coordinates 'Y' and 'X' of the target lesions, taking as references the outer table of the frontal or occipital bone at the sagittal plane, and the midline of the skull for the coronal plane.

The patient may then be transferred to his room and operation scheduled for a convenient day. The lines on the skin must be kept indelible until surgery is performed.

Once in the theater, the patient is operated on with local anesthesia, except in children. The stereotactic guide is placed on the head, after making the burr hole, with the

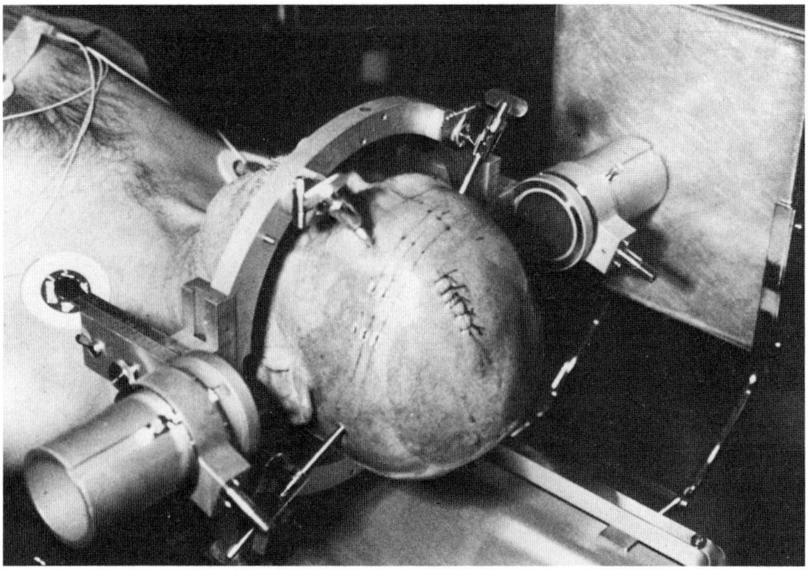

Fig. 2. Lines indicating slices of interest. Small radiopaque cottonoids are seen at intervals along the lines.

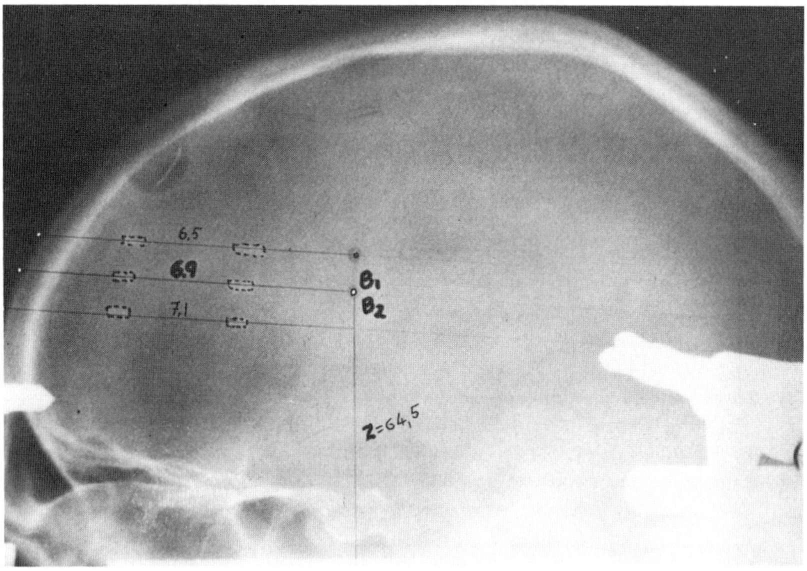

Fig. 3. Lateral film showing three 'Y' coordinates and 'Z' coordinate.

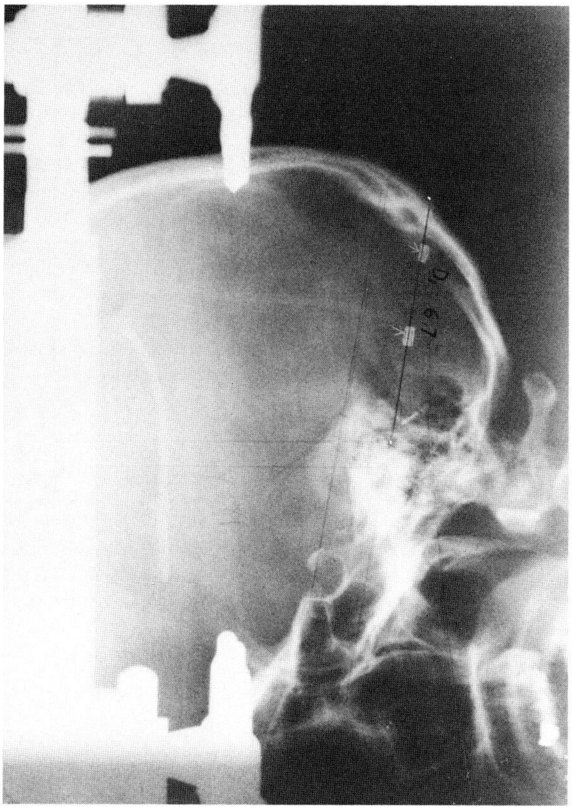

Fig. 4. Lateral film illustrating the coordinates of a pontine tumor.

plane of the frame parallel to the dermographic lines. A lead filament or moistened cottonoids with a radiopaque strip are placed on the dotted lines on the skin at each selected plane (fig. 2). A lateral film is taken from an X-ray source 4 m from the patient, or nearer if a corrective rule is used for magnification. The last coordinate, 'Z', is calculated from the 'zero' point of the guide to the plane selected for biopsy (fig. 3). The microforceps (1.8 mm in diameter) is inserted, and new X-ray films are taken in conventional biplane radiography to verify the position. The neuropathologist crushes and stains the fresh tissue. Two or three biopsies are taken from different parts of the tumor or its surroundings. The reliability of the crushing technique had been tested many times with samples of tumors removed in open craniotomy.

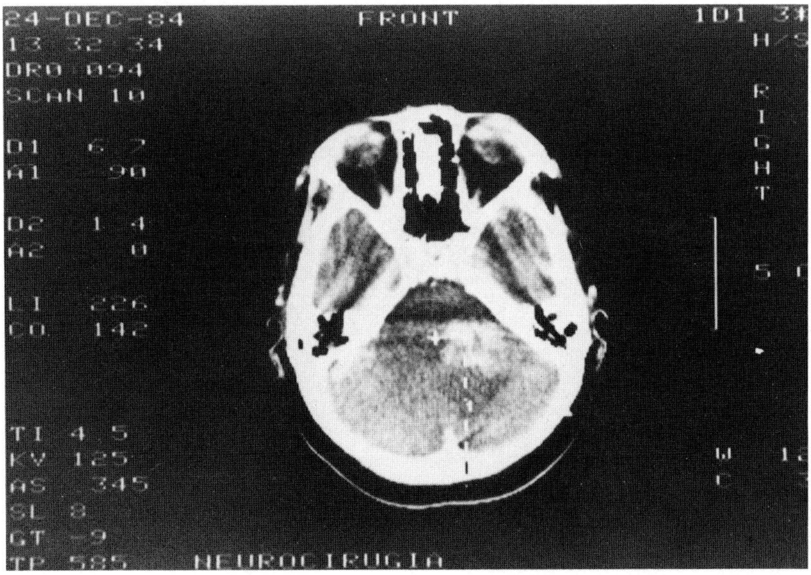

Fig. 5. Pontine tumor. The coordinates 'X' and 'Y' are graphically shown and numbers are seen on the left (D1, D2).

Results

Thirty-four operations were performed on 33 patients, aged 2–80 years. Thirty-two patients had deep-seated lesions in the cerebral hemispheres and 1 patient had a pontine tumor (fig. 4, 5). Four cysts were aspirated through a cannula after biopsy of the wall. There were 15 malignant gliomas (8 glioblastomas), 7 astrocytomas, 2 oligodendrogliomas, 1 ependymoma, 1 pineocytoma, 1 tuberculoma, 1 infarct, 4 metastatic carcinomas and 1 unspecific inflammatory process. Two patients died during the stay in hospital, 1 of the deaths related to the procedure.

Discussion

Candidates were selected for stereotactic surgery in preference to open craniotomy for deep intracerebral lesions suspicious of being tumors. The technique must be simple, reliable and with no additional frames [4]. One must not use CT scanner time unnecessarily.

No significant difference of accuracy has been found with the use of the CT-guided stereotactic frame and the method proposed by *Gildenberg* [3]. With *Gildenberg*'s technique, the patient's head must be fixed, without any movement between the first and the last plane of the CT scanning. This modified method eliminates the need of the Scout-View and reduces the risk of error by head movements, because attention is centered on the slices where the lesion appears. Only very small tumors require slices of 4 mm thickness. The presence of an neuropathologist in a room close to the theater permits one to get several biopsies in different parts of the tumor and infiltrated areas, so that it is possible to get more information about the hypercellular zone and the infiltrating areas of malignant gliomas [2].

References

1 Bullard, D.E.; Nashold, B.S.; Osborne, D., et al.: Experience using two CT-guided stereotactic biopsy methods. Appl. Neurophysiol. *46:* 188–192 (1983).
2 Burger, P.C.: Pathologic anatomy and CT correlations in the glioblastoma multiforme. Appl. Neurophysiol. *46:* 180–187 (1983).
3 Gildenberg, P.L.: Calculation of stereotactic coordinates from computed tomography scan. Neurosurgery *10:* 580–586 (1982).
4 Gildenberg, P.L.: Stereotactic neurosurgery and computerized tomographic scanning. Appl. Neurophysiol. *46:* 170–179 (1983).
5 Lee, S.H.; Vilafana, T.; Lapayoker, M.: CT intracranial localization with a new marker system. Neuroradiology *16:* 570–571 (1978).
6 Piskun, W.S.; Stevens, E.A.; Lamorgese, J.R., et al.: A simplified method of CT-assisted localization and biopsy of intracranial lesions. Surg. Neurol. *11:* 413–416 (1979).

M. Poza, Regional Neurosurgical Centre, El Palmar, Murcia (Spain)

Proc. 9th Meeting World Soc. Stereotactic and Functional
Neurosurgery, Toronto 1985
Appl. Neurophysiol. *48:* 488 (1985)

CT-Guided Stereotactic Biopsy of Lower Brain Stem Lesions

K.S. Sahni, N.R. Ghatak, Harold F. Young

Medical College of Virginia Hospital, Richmond, Va., USA

CT-guided stereotactic biopsies for deep-seated brain stem lesions, as reported in the literature, have been performed either via the transtentorial approach or the posterior fossa approach. We have used a different technique of approaching these deep brain stem lesions. The idea was obtained from the mesencephalotomies performed by stereotactic surgeons in the past. We approached these lesions through a twist drill, slightly anterior to the coronal sutures in a transincisural fashion thus not penetrating the tentorium. We used the Brown-Robert-Wells stereotactic system.

Four patients with brain stem lesions were biopsied with this technique. Appropriate tissue diagnosis was made in 3 out of 4 patients. The only patient in which an accurate diagnosis could not be achieved was a patient who had been previously treated by radiation and chemotherapy without any tissue diagnosis. In this particular patient the only diagnosis that could be established was that of 'necrosis'.

Diagnosis of brain stem lesions has always been a matter of controversy for neurosurgeons. We believe, with the availability of this relatively simple technique, all brain stem lesions should be biopsied to obtain a precise tissue diagnosis prior to commencing any treatment. The only complication involved with this technique was diplopia in 3 out of 4 patients. In 1 of the patients this disappeared spontaneously, and in the other 2 it persisted. Other than this oculomotor dysfunction, no other complications were noted in any of the cases. We also believe that the potential for future use of this technique may also include aspiration of cysts, abscesses and also implantation of isotopes for brain stem gliomas.

K.S. Sahni, MD, Medical College of Virginia Hospital,
Richmond, VA 23298 (USA)

Proc. 9th Meeting World Soc. Stereotactic and Functional
Neurosurgery, Toronto 1985
Appl. Neurophysiol. *48:* 489–490 (1985)

Lettre de M. le Professeur *J. Talairach* à la «World Society for Stereotactic and Functional Neurosurgery»

Je suis particulièrement sensible à l'honneur que me fait la Société Mondiale de Neurochirurgie Fonctionnelle. Mais je pense que cette distinction a surtout le mérite de rappeler aux plus jeunes non pas l'«évidente» vertu des plus anciens (ils sont toujours vertueux... à cet âge...) mais une autre notion qui les dépasse de loin pour nous englober tous. Car, en face d'une spécialité aussi récente que la nôtre, qui essaye, avec courage et difficulté, de comprendre le dysfonctionnement cérébral et d'y remédier, vous devrez affronter, vous aussi, avec votre propre originalité, des problèmes théoriques et techniques aussi difficiles et contraignants que les nôtres avant de devenir, à votre tour, les plus anciens... donc les plus méritants.

La recherche de résultats thérapeutiques dans des domaines jusqu'alors inaccessibles est, vous le savez, souvent décevante. Mais, lorsqu'elle est couronnée de succès, elle fait partie des grandes joies de la vie. Une intervention nouvelle, en particulier de type stéréotaxique, ne va pas sans poser des problèmes théoriques et pratiques de tous ordres, et, peut-être plus qu'ailleurs, d'ordre éthique. Vous avez déjà appris que cette recherche, perdue dans un monde de connaissances encore bien incertaines, n'est pas toujours entourée de beaucoup de sollicitude et que l'on se trouve souvent bien seul avec ses doutes.

Rappelez-vous alors que si nous étions tous passionnés et pleins d'espoirs, la majorité de nos collègues restait naturellement assez indifférente, parfois méprisante sinon hostile, à l'égard de cette nouvelle voie neurochirurgicale.

On a de la peine à se souvenir, à l'aube de ce Congrès Mondial, que notre spécialité fut considérée en ses débuts comme: «anti-chirurgicale et aveugle» par ses nouvelles techniques peu sanglantes, à voies d'abord réduites et multiples; «retardataire» et «sans avenir», en raison de certaines de ses conceptions sans doute parfois trop réductionnistes mais opposées à un globalisme stérile; «inutilement compliquée» et «obsessionnelle» dans ses efforts à mettre en valeur les rapports des structures cérébrales avec leurs anomalies, dans un espace tridimensionnel exact et à situation spatiale connue par rapport au chirurgien; «immorale», enfin, par ses techniques en partie dérivées de l'expérimentation animale.

On sait aujourd'hui, malgré ces appréciations caricaturales, ce que cette méthodologie a apporté à la neurophysiopathologie humaine, aux thérapies ionisantes, à la neurochirurgie classique, mais également à la neuroradiologie. En effet, celle-ci va se trouver dans l'obligation d'adopter, dans un avenir proche, la précision stéréotaxique pour exprimer le volume. Elle devra mettre en valeur, pour chacune de ses explorations, les trois dimensions de l'espace à partir d'un système de référence commun et exactement situé dans l'espace... et faire ainsi (sans doute avec l'aide de l'ordinateur) de la stéréotaxie... sans le savoir!

Il m'est très agréable de constater que notre spécialité est particulièrement riche en ouvertures nouvelles, grâce à vous, mais aussi, il faut le rappeler, grâce à ceux qui comme notre élève et ami *G. Szikla,* nous ont quittés trop tôt après avoir tant œuvré.

Ces nouvelles recherches ne manqueront pas d'être exposées dans votre Congrès auquel je souhaite, sous la présidence de notre ami *J. Siegfried,* beaucoup de succès et auquel je regrette de ne pouvoir assister.

J. Talairach

Proc. 9th Meeting World Soc. Stereotactic and Functional Neurosurgery, Toronto 1985
Appl. Neurophysiol. *48:* 491 (1985)

Summary of the Letter of Prof. J. Talairach Read by Dr. Munari to the World Congress of the World Society for Stereotactic and Functional Neurosurgery

I am particularly flattered by the honour given me by the World Society for Stereotactic and Functional Neurosurgery. But I think that this distinction has above all the merit of reminding the younger among you not of the 'obvious' virtue of older colleagues (they are always virtuous at that age...), but of a notion which is far beyond them and includes all of us. Because, confronted with a new difficult speciality like ours, which tries courageously to understand and remedy cerebral dysfunction, you will have, in your turn and in your own way, to tackle the same compelling theoretical and technical problems prior to becoming the elder, that is the most deserving.

You know how disappointing results may be, but successes may be a source of great joy. A new type of intervention, especially stereotactic interventions always entail various kinds of problems: theoretical, practical and above all ethical.

It is difficult to remember today that our speciality was first considered antisurgical and blind, backward and without future, unnecessarily complicated and obsessive, and immoral, since it was directly derived from animal experiments.

However, in spite of such a caricatural picture, this approach provided important contributions to neurophysiopathology, radiotherapy and classical neurosurgery. As a matter of fact, neuroradiology is and will be more and more obliged to use a spatial reference system for exploring the three-dimensional cerebral space – in other words, neuroradiology is becoming 'stereotactic' without knowing it.

Finally, I have enjoyed the quality of the new perspectives in our speciality, and remember the important contributions of those like my pupil and friend, Gabor Szikla who left us too early. I am convinced that this congress, presided by J. Siegfried, to which I regret not to be able to participate, will be a success. *J. Talairach*

Author Index

Subject Index